The Great Nation in Decline

T0230592

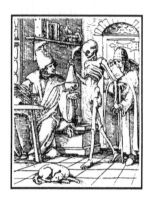

The History of Medicine in Context

Series Editors: Andrew Cunningham and Ole Peter Grell

Department of History and Philosophy of Science
University of Cambridge

Department of History
The Open University

Titles in this series include:

Hospital Politics in Seventeenth-Century France
The Crown, Urban Elites and the Poor
Tim McHugh

Melancholy and the Care of the Soul
Religion, Moral Philosophy and Madness in Early Modern England
Jeremy Schmidt

A Cultural History of Medical Vitalism in Enlightenment Montpellier
Elizabeth A. Williams

The Great Nation in Decline
Sex, Modernity and Health Crises in Revolutionary France *c.*1750–1850

SEAN M. QUINLAN

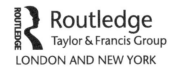

Routledge
Taylor & Francis Group
LONDON AND NEW YORK

First published 2007 by Ashgate Publishing

2 Park Square, Milton Park, Abingdon, Oxon OX14 4RN
711 Third Avenue, New York, NY 10017, USA

Routledge is an imprint of the Taylor & Francis Group, an informa business

First issued in paperback 2016

British Library Cataloguing in Publication Data
Quinlan, Sean M.
   The great nation in decline: sex, modernity and health crises in revolutionary France
   c.1750–1850. – (The history of medicine in context)
1. Public health – France – History – 18th century 2. Public health – France – History – 19th century
3. France – Social conditions – 18th century 4. France – Social conditions – 19th century
   I. Title
   362.1'0944'09033

Library of Congress Cataloging-in-Publication Data
Quinlan, Sean M.
   The great nation in decline: sex, modernity, and health crises in revolutionary France
   c.1750–1850 / Sean M. Quinlan.
     p.; cm. – (History of medicine in context)
   Includes bibliographical references.
ISBN 978-0-7546-6098-9 (hardback: alk. paper) 1. Public health– France– History–18th century. 2. Public health–France–History–19th century. 3. Hygiene, Sexual–France–History–18th century. 4. Hygiene, Sexual–France–History–19th century. 5. Social medicine–France–History–18th century. 6. Social medicine–France–History– 19th century. 7. Degeneration–France–History–18th century. 8. Degeneration–France–History–19th century. I. Title. II. Series.
[DNLM: 1. Hygiene–history–France. 2. History, 18th Century–France. 3. History, 19th Century–France. 4. Morals–France. 5. Physician's Role–history–France. 6. Social Conditions–history–France. QT 11 GF7 Q7g 2007]
   RA499.G73 2007
   362.1094409033–dc22

                                                                        2007007386

ISBN 978-0-7546-6098-9 (hbk)
ISBN 978-1-138-26548-6 (pbk)

For Julien and Adrien

Contents

Acknowledgements

This book would never have been finished without much personal and financial support, and I am very pleased to acknowledge these debts here. My deepest thanks goes to the late William B. Cohen, who supervised the thesis upon which this book is based. His vast understanding and love of French history – as well as his boundless willingness to engage, nurture and indulge each one of his students – has never failed to amaze and overwhelm. My life is incomparably richer for having had him as a teacher.

A number of other teachers, colleagues and friends have left their mark on this project. As members of my thesis committee, John M. Efron, James C. Riley and Dror Wahrman made detailed comments on the original draft and helped me rethink the material. In 1998–2000, at the *American Historical Review*, Michael Grossberg and Jeffrey Wasserstrom broadened my horizons and opened intellectual doors. In 2000–01, at the Humanities Consortium at the University of California, Los Angeles, directors Peter Reill, Vincent Pecora and Henry Ansgar Kelly made me feel welcome and provided a rigorous but friendly intellectual environment; and my 'fellow fellows' – Daniel Brownstein, Andreas Killen, Jennifer Mason, Abigail Firey and Scott Sprenger – challenged my thinking on every level. Beginning in 2001, at the University of Idaho, my colleagues Katherine Aiken, Iván Casteñeda, Dale Graden, Ellen Kittel, Richard Spence and Adam Sowards helped me establish my research programme and encouraged me every step of the way. William L. Ramsey, especially, changed how I write and taught me about the historian's responsibility in the public realm – and in wildly unpredictable ways.

Institutional funding gave me extended time to work in specialized archives: in 1996–97, a Fulbright IIE grant at the École des Hautes Études in Paris; in 1997, an Ezra Friedlander fellowship from Indiana University; in 2000–01, an Andrew Mellon postdoctoral fellowship at the Humanities Consortium at the University of California, Los Angeles; in 2002 and 2004, faculty seed grants from the University of Idaho Graduate School; and in 2004, summer stipend fellowship from the National Endowment for the Humanities. I should like to thank the archivists and librarians at the Bibliothèque Interuniversitaire de Médecine (BIUM), the Académie Nationale de Médecine, Archives de l'Assistance Publique, Archives Nationales, Bibliothèque Nationale de France and the National Library of Medicine, who helped me track down manuscripts and obscure printed sources.

Earlier parts of this work were given as presentations at the Humanities Consortium at UCLA (2001), the Northeastern American Society of Eighteenth-Century Studies (2002), the annual meeting of History of Science Society (2002), the International Society for Eighteenth-Century Studies (2003), and annual meetings of the American Association for the History of Medicine (2004 and 2005). I should like to thank all the commentators and attendees for their feedback, but I particularly need to signal out Clifford Conor, Helen Deutsch, Pascale Gramain, James R. Jacob, Margaret C. Jacob, Robert A. Nye, Dorothy Porter, Matthew Ramsey, Dorothée Sturkenboom, Jason Szabo, Randolph Trumbach, Anne Verjus, Anne C. Vila and Elizabeth A. Williams.

Earlier drafts or parts of chapters were originally published as 'Colonial Bodies, Hygiene and Abolitionist Politics in Eighteenth-Century France', *History Workshop Journal*, no. 42 (1996); 'Physical and Moral Regeneration after the Terror: Medical Culture, Sensibility and Family Politics in France, 1794–1804', *Social History* 29 (2004); and 'Inheriting Vice, Acquiring Virtue: Hereditary Disease in French Enlightenment Medicine', *Bulletin of the History of Medicine* 80 (2006). I thank the editors and publishers for allowing me to reproduce that material here.

Further acknowledgements are in order. Ever since our first trans-Atlantic phone conversation, when I was a naive undergraduate hoping to study French history, Rachel G. Fuchs has taken enormous interest in my career and intellectual development. From her, above all, I have learned the historian's craft. She has left an ineffaceable imprint on my work and remains a model of academic excellence, engagement and wit. I owe her more than words can say. My dear friend and colleague Stephen Toth has provided staunch support and intellectual camaraderie. He has listened – with a patience befitting Job – to my most inchoate thoughts and waded through numerous drafts of this book. In him, I have found a true friend, and we've endured more together than I could have possibly imagined. Mary Terrall has become a wonderful mentor and friend, and her good sense has greatly shaped this project. She has provided real inspiration and confidence.

I owe the most to my beloved partner, Sandra Reineke. She has constantly encouraged my work and allowed me to persevere in the face of my gravest doubts. Her laughter has kept my own 'physical and moral faculties' from becoming too disorganized. From her own intellectual interests, I have learned and continue to learn much; and she has shaped the content of my work. Her love fills my every day with infinite joy and turns the smallest details into the greatest pleasures.

I dedicate this book to our two young boys, Julien and Adrien. In the last days of preparing the typescript, Julien kept me company by sitting by my desk and writing a book about dinosaurs.

List of Abbreviations

AAFM	Anciennes Archives de la Faculté de Médecine de Paris
AM	Archives de l'Académie Nationale de Médecine (Académie Royale de Médecine)
AN	Archives Nationales, Paris
ANM	Bibliothèque de la l'Académie Nationale de Médecine
AP	Assistance Publique
ARS	Archives de l'Académie des Sciences
BN	Bibliothèque Nationale de France, Paris
FMP	Bibliothèque de la Faculté de Médecine
SEM	Archives de la Société de l'École de Médecine
SME	Archives de la Société d'Émulation Médicale
SRM	Archives de la Société Royale de Médecine

Introduction:
Degeneration, Regeneration and Health Panics in Modern France

A half century ago, historians had an easy way to explain the development of public health. For them, it was the story of the triumph of humanitarianism and scientific progress. At the dawn of the modern age, they said, well-meaning doctors advanced how they understood sickness and health and learned to prevent disease on the collective level. Although hygiene was as old as Western medicine itself, this new form of public health – what they called social medicine – was novel because it self-consciously treated the health of populations, not individuals. Social medicine was born in the Enlightenment, came of age with Victorian social reforms and fully matured when governments implemented their social security systems in the mid-twentieth century. This history was written by a generation of doctor–historians such as George Rosen and Henry Sigerist, scholars who in many ways embodied the ideas of 1950s progressive humanism and believed that health was a right and a responsibility for every government to provide.[1] Looking at the broad-scale social reforms implemented after World War II, they reasonably concluded that, in the near future, every person across the globe would be able to avoid deadly pathogens, as governments would build the infrastructure needed to contain infectious diseases and give their citizens access to reliable medical care. As Félix Marí-Ibáñez confidently declared in his preface to Rosen's *History of Public Health* (1958), 'Medicine has evolved into the Preventive Medicine – ultimate goal of Public Health – of today, which anticipates the Medicine of Tomorrow'.[2]

Beginning in the 1960s, this historiographical narrative came under critical scrutiny. In the decades following Sigerist and Rosen's pathbreaking studies, a new generation of historians wrote a different history of public health. These scholars came from a different methodological and political context: they were trained in the methods and theories of social history, not medical science, and wanted to write history 'from below', from the perspective of ordinary people of the past. On the one hand, left-leaning historians were likely inspired by the idealism and populism of the 1960s and were suspicious of professional and bureaucratic authority; on the other hand, more conservative historians rejected social engineering and criticized government power and the social security system. Despite their ideological differences, both groups of scholars believed that government experts and professional authorities – the 'best and the brightest' – used science and technology,

---

1   See, for example, Henry Sigerist, *Medicine and Human Welfare* (New Haven, 1941); and George Rosen, *A History of Public Health* (New York, 1958).
2   Félix Martí-Ibáñez, 'Foreword', in Rosen, *History*, p. 14.

not for good, but to control or repress their fellow citizens. In many ways, they were responding to the recent horrors of eugenics, concentration camps, colonial wars, and Soviet gulags and asylums, and were critiquing the 'warfare-welfare' state of 'administered living'.[3] For them, Rosen's 'Medicine of Tomorrow' was in fact a 'Medical Nemesis' (as Ivan Illich put it), a medicine more at home in Aldous Huxley's *Brave New World* than in L.-S. Mercier's *The Year 2440: A Dream If Ever There Was One*.[4] Health was not a right, a responsibility, or even something a person might actually want to enjoy. Quite the contrary, as some sociologists claimed, health was an 'imperative', a coercive force imposed by public authorities and scientific experts to maintain productivity and conformity.[5] Social control masqueraded under the guise of rationality and progress.

The most important thinker in this regard was philosopher Michel Foucault. In his highly influential studies, which appeared in the 1960s and 1970s, Foucault argued that social medicine was part of a new model of 'biopower' that has tried to control all elements of modern human life, a practice he called 'governmentality'.[6] He thus identified an ideological or 'discursive' partnership between the state, professions and social elites – a kind of disciplinary nexus that worked together to exercise power upon a given polity or population.[7]

With this shift in historical thinking, scholarship reached a certain impasse, each side with its own myths and merits, and even detailed and scrupulous archival studies have produced fascinating but widely divergent results.[8] Earlier historians correctly emphasized medical innovations and how doctors expanded modern health services and brought care to larger segments of the general population. At the same time, however, they overlooked that power and prejudice sometimes inspired health policies – most notoriously with the cases of eugenics and labelling and controlling the 'deviant'. By contrast, social and cultural historians have explored how ordinary people experienced health and sickness and how they interacted with medical authorities and tried to make sense of their own bodily experiences. As

---

3   Herbert Marcuse, *One-Dimensional Man: Studies in the Ideology of Advanced Industrial Society*, 2d edn (Boston, 1991), pp. 48–55.

4   Ivan Illich, *Medical Nemesis: The Expropriation of Health* (New York, 1982).

5   For typical examples, see Peter Conrad and Joseph W. Schneider, *Deviance and Medicalization: From Badness to Sickness*, 2d edn (Philadelphia, 1992); Deborah Lupton, *The Imperative of Health: Public Health and the Regulated Body* (London, 1995); and Alan Peterson and Deborah Lupton, *The New Public Health: Health and Self in the Age of Risk* (London, 1996).

6   Michel Foucault, *The History of Sexuality: An Introduction*, trans. Robert Hurley (New York, 1990 [1978]), pp. 138–9. For a similar take on the biopower theory, see Giorgio Agamben, *Homo Sacer: Sovereign Power and Bare Life*, trans. Daniel Heller-Roazen (Stanford, 1998).

7   Michel Foucault, 'Governmentality' and 'The Political Technology of Individuals', in *Power*, vol. 3, *The Essential Works of Foucault 1954–1984*, ed. James D. Faubion (New York, 2000), pp. 201–22, 403–17, at p. 219.

8   On this point, see Lindsay Wilson, *Women and Medicine in the French Enlightenment: The Debate over 'Maladies des femmes'* (Baltimore, 1993), pp. 1–2. For a superb overview of the recent historiography of public health, see Dorothy Porter, *Health, Civilization, and the State: A History of Public Health from Ancient to Modern Times* (London, 1999).

these historians have powerfully reminded, medical practitioners were potentially motivated by issues of power and interest and their altruistic claims should not be taken at face value, arguing that we should study the experience of sickness and treatment from the perspective of the ordinary patient.[9]

Nevertheless, the biopower model has a number of weaknesses. Most obviously, there was no biopower lobby, movement, group, party, platform or spokespersons; nor does it seem likely that political elites in a variety of national contexts could uniformly agree upon such a far-reaching policy. Consequently, social control theorists often appeal to vast, unconscious forces at work in society – usually global capitalism – and thus turn history into a story of impersonal processes that lack historical agents and conscious acts. Though historical forces sometimes obey their own inner logic, it is important to remember that people make their own history just as that history shapes their own actions and perceptions of social reality. Public health is no exception. Many observers across the political spectrum wanted to promote health policies for their nation, but they were motivated by radically different reasons: some altruistic, some controlling, some plain expedient. In this sense, the most important factors often depended upon conflict and contingency.

More significantly, perhaps, it is possible to overlook an important point: that health activism – whatever the ostensible motivation – can make a significant difference in people's lives. When social critics attack medical authority and big government – and sometimes do so with good reason – they can potentially forget that doctors do in fact save lives and that public health services can vastly increase the quality and quantity of human life across the globe. In the starkest possible terms, medical activism can save and improve individual life through public services, hospital care, urban planning and social welfare, though sometimes individuals have to give up elements of personal autonomy in order to reap the benefits of medical care.[10] In some ways, medical critics have perhaps drunk too deeply at the well of negative liberty, inadvertently suggesting that people cannot afford – or should not even want – a great society.

In the following pages, I tell a different story about the birth of modern health care, but that is because I approach the matter differently from both the progressive and neo-Foucauldian historians. This book examines how doctors contributed to a much broader public discussion about physical degeneracy and depopulation in France between roughly 1750 and 1850, a period in which leading intellectuals and public officials believed that the 'great nation' was menaced by decadence and decline. It uncovers a rich and far-ranging medical debate in which four generations of

---

9   For a good summary, see Olivier Faure, 'La médicalisation vue par les historiens', in Pierre Aïach and Daniel Delanoë (eds), *L'ère de la médicalisation: Ecce homo sanitas* (Paris, 1999), pp. 53–68.

10   On this point, see the impassioned work by Paul Farmer, *Pathologies of Power: Health, Human Rights, and the New War on the Poor* (Berkeley, 2003); and Richard Hofrichter, 'The Politics of Health Inequities: Contested Terrain', in Hofrichter (ed.), *Health and Social Justice: Politics, Ideology, and Inequity in the Distribution of Disease* (San Francisco, 2003), pp. 1–56.

health activists hoped to use biomedical science to transform the self, sexuality and community in order to regenerate a sick and decaying nation. Doctors called this programme 'physical and moral hygiene'. By promoting this programme, these doctors redefined their public personas, casting themselves as moral crusaders and health activists, and thereby invented a new field of social medicine – a medicine concerned with health of large-scale populations. At the same time, doctors imparted biomedical ideas and language that allowed lay people to make sense of bewildering sociopolitical changes, thereby giving them a sense of agency and control over these revolutionary events. Medicine thus became a primary ideological force in shaping the social and political configurations of old regime, revolutionary and post-revolutionary France. In this manner, this book highlights the complex and contradictory ideological forces that have motivated doctors and public authorities to reform health conditions and why they came to believe these reforms were so pressing and important.

In terms of modern public health, this chronological period and this national setting are crucial for two reasons. First, the years between 1750 and 1850 formed a key period in the making of modern health care. During this period, doctors first articulated that health was a universal right and a desired goal for all enlightened societies. In their efforts to extend health-care services and institutions, these activists built the foundations for public authorities to implement the later bacteriological breakthroughs pioneered by Louis Pasteur and Robert Koch in the 1880s. At the same time, they also established important precedents for early social reform, which helped policy-makers to create the welfare state and extend public services in the late nineteenth century.[11] Second, the national setting is important because modern medicine was arguably born in revolutionary France. During the 1790s, doctors and legislators overhauled medical schools and hospitals, and created a staggering number of medical specializations: clinical teaching, the modern hospital ward, morbid anatomy, experimental physiology, forensic medicine, psychiatry and physical anthropology. Following these reforms, France became the acknowledged world leader in medical teaching and research, and Paris schools and hospitals attracted a cadre of students and admirers from all over Europe and the Americas.[12]

---

11   On this early history of public health in France, see the excellent surveys by Bernard P. Lécuyer, 'L'hygiène en France avant Pasteur', in Claire Bayet-Salomon (ed.), *Pasteur et la Révolution Pastorienne* (Paris, 1986), pp. 65–139; and Matthew Ramsey, 'Public Health in France', in Dorothy Porter (ed.), *The History of Public Health and the Modern State* (Amsterdam, 1994).

12   On the rich historiography on French medicine in this period, see especially Jacques Léonard, *Les médecins de l'ouest au XIXe siècle* (3 vols, Lille, 1978); François Lebrun, *Se soigner autrefois: médecins, saints et sorciers aux XVIIe et XVIIIe siècles* (Paris, 1983); Matthew Ramsey, *Professional and Popular Medicine in France: The Social World of Medical Practice* (Cambridge, 1987); Toby Gelfand, *Professionalizing Modern Medicine: Paris Surgeons and Medical Science and Institutions in the Eighteenth Century* (Westport, 1980); Jan Goldstein, *Console and Classify: The French Psychiatric Profession in the Nineteenth Century* (Cambridge, 1987); Elizabeth A. Williams, *The Physical and the Moral: Anthropology, Physiology, and Philosophic Medicine in France, 1750–1850* (Cambridge, 1994), and *A Cultural History of Medical Vitalism in Enlightenment Montpellier* (Aldershot,

In this setting, medical luminaries forged a new science of public health, one that would inspire unprecedented health activism.

During this period, as this study shows, doctors were not simply concerned with the expansion of biomedical knowledge in its own right. Rather, they wanted to apply their specialized knowledge to improve the health of the social body in the broadest possible terms. In this endeavour, doctors moved from specific concerns over patient care and public health to think about how they could build a more perfect polity. These concerns radiated across several interconnected levels. Applied medical knowledge, doctors argued, could improve the citizenry and make a more harmonious social order. Medical science allowed policy-makers to reform social elements that threatened the health of the polity, elements that ranged from fashionable elites to the urban working classes. It promised to transform domestic relations by identifying the natural parameters between men and women, and by emphasizing women's roles as wives and mothers within the domestic sphere. Finally, through pronatalist policies and sexual hygiene, doctors could help the government regulate demographic behaviour within the metropole and overseas colonies.

To regenerate the nation, doctors created one key idea: physical and moral hygiene. This idea differs essentially from the public health policies usually associated with infectious disease, hospital care, welfare services, sanitation and vaccination. As doctors saw it, physical and moral hygiene could potentially transform mind and body and alter man's total relation with nature and society. As such, doctors approached mind, body and society in largely holistic terms, seeing these three domains as fundamentally interconnected and interdependent. To study these relations, doctors borrowed key ideas from physiology, physical anthropology and demographic science, hoping to discover what kinds of morals and manners best promoted human health and happiness. By engaging in these modes of inquiry, they hoped to create a blueprint for a better society – or, at the very least, to create a society that could better alleviate dire health conditions.

Consequently, health activists dealt less with real-world health problems than ideal forms of personal conduct and behaviour: the ways things ought to be and how to make them so. Medical practitioners thus explored problems that we do not always associate with public health: ideal health and beauty; how men and women should behave and what roles they should play in public and private life; how parents should raise and teach their children; and how to improve sexual hygiene and fertility. At times, physicians focused upon real or imagined behaviour in particular groups of people, and they changed their objects of study and approbation as the political and social context changed over the age of revolution.

Medical practitioners put ideas about moral and physical hygiene in the service of political and social agendas. Often, they wavered between utopian and pragmatic

---

2003); and Roselyne Rey, *Naissance et développement du vitalisme en France de la deuxième moitié du 18e siècle à la fin du Premier Empire* (Oxford, 2000). On hospital and charity reform, see Colin Jones, *The Charitable Imperative: Hospitals and Nursing in Ancien Régime and Revolutionary France* (London, 1990); and Dora B. Weiner, *The Citizen-Patient in Revolutionary and Imperial Paris* (Baltimore, 1993). The best overview remains Lawrence Brockliss and Colin Jones, *The Medical World of Early Modern France* (Oxford, 1997).

policies: they hoped to diagnose social problems and cure or prevent them, but usually within the limits set by nature and social realities. In so doing, doctors put all of society on the sick bed and examined it with the tools of biomedical science; they hovered around the bedside and diagnosed and predicted, arguing what caused social diseases and how they could best cure or prevent them. They were drawn to this bedside for a variety of reasons – some moral, some humanitarian, some professional, some ideological – and they came from diverse backgrounds – some therapeutic, political, socioeconomic and regional. But whatever the apparent differences, doctors shared two crucial beliefs: they believed that an ounce of prevention was worth a pound of cure, and that doctors had important insights about society and thus lay people should treat them as moral and social authorities. Here, doctors saw themselves as the true defenders of moral values and patriotism, earnest professionals who knew what was best for the present and future health of the nation.

What drove this health activism was a series of health panics about physical degeneracy and demographic decline. These panics touched social elites deeply, raising troubling questions about the family, sexuality and national power and prestige. At times, they seemed to shake the social order itself and challenge what it meant to be French. With the term *health panic*, I am taking a key idea in sociological literature called moral panics, following what historian Nancy Tomes has done with her pioneering work on American 'germ panics'.[13] In moral panics – whether fears about epidemics, pederasty, youth gangs or homosexuality – people react strongly to something, whether real or imagined, that seems to threaten the community, undermining the social order or 'some idealized part of it'.[14] Consequently, the community reacts in disproportionate ways to the perceived threat, often scapegoating particular groups of people and sometimes becoming violent against them. In this context, a number of figures become self-conscious crusaders and public spokespersons by not only diagnosing the problem and offering cures, but by inspiring sympathetic observers to organize and act as well. In some cases, social change and stress can instigate moral panics, but these are not absolute preconditions. Indeed, moral panics are so interesting because they often have a random dimension to them and lack identifiable causes. Though they obviously crystallize community malaise or uncertainty, it is difficult to identify what concrete interests and agendas motivate the panics or the crusaders who lead them – whether personal gain, political expediency, class consciousness, professional jealousies or moral values and so on.[15] In the case of the health panics in France, health crusaders were not motivated by straightforward epistemological, professional or ideological factors (indeed, these doctors came from a variety of social, therapeutic, and political persuasions); rather, I argue, they felt so compelled to speak about the social order because they were such an intrinsic part of it and gave so much to defining its boundaries and self-identity.

---

13 Nancy Tomes, 'The Making of A Germ Panic, Now and Then', *American Journal of Public Health* 90 (2000): 191–98.

14 Kenneth Thompson, *Moral Panics* (London, 1998).

15 See Erich Goode and Nachman Ben-Yehuda, *Moral Panics: The Social Construction of Deviance* (Oxford, 1994).

In these health panics, health crusaders entered a broad public debate about the health and fertility of the French nation. As the crucial work by Robert A. Nye, Karen Offen and Rachel G. Fuchs (amongst others) has shown, this debate continues to this day, and is absolutely central to understanding politics and public policy in modern France. From the 1700s onwards, public authorities and intellectuals believed that demographic growth absolutely determined socioeconomic health and great power status. Consequently, population became France's most pressing national security issue, as the government obsessively focused upon demographic trends and the policy initiatives – both public and private – that could influence sexual behaviour and fertility within certain groups of people. Authorities were particularly anxious about anything that could subvert idealized sexual relations and negatively affect fertility.[16] Whereas recent scholarship has focused upon fears about degeneracy and depopulation during the fin-de-siècle period, this study locates the origins of this discourse in an earlier historical context – during the protracted cultural crisis of old regime France.

In this discourse, medical practitioners believed their profession could advise the government on family and other demographic policies because they best understood, with their specialist knowledge, the biological realm of human experience. As they told receptive audiences, chronic sociopolitical crises – associated with war, revolution, urban change and industrialization – had made people sick in body and mind and caused the population to degenerate and decline. Between 1750 and 1850, doctors variously blamed key groups for France's moral and physical degeneracy – fashionable elites, intellectuals, women, sickly children, the urban poor, urban tradesmen, industrial workers and even radical Jacobins and sansculottes – and they targeted them for programmes of health rehabilitation. These groups could be regenerated by adapting medical ideas about domestic hygiene, sexual behaviour, public assistance, occupational health, urban planning and rural improvement.

Physicians drew their ideas about physical and moral hygiene from important developments in the fields of physiology and demography, which gave them a conceptual language to discuss these problems and make a coherent plan for intervention. The most important influence was what Elizabeth A. Williams has recently called 'physiological' or 'anthropological' medicine.[17] Between the eighteenth and early nineteenth century, a number of self-styled 'enlightened physicians' [médecins-philosophes] pioneered a new physiological study of human nature, a study they linked to the so-called 'science of man'. This problematic was distinct from the disciplines that we now know as anthropology, ethnography, psychology and sociology (though the historical antecedents are clear).[18] Following

---

16 On this point, see Rachel G. Fuchs, 'France in Comparative Perspective', in Elinor Accampo, Rachel Fuchs and Mary Lynn Stewart (eds), *Gender and the Politics of Social Reform in France, 1870–1914* (Baltimore, 1995), pp. 157–83; and Robert A. Nye, 'Biology, Sexuality, and Morality in Eighteenth-Century France', *Eighteeth-Century Studies* 35 (2002): 235–38, at p. 236.

17 Williams, *Physical and the Moral*.

18 On the science of man, see especially Domenico Bosco, *La decifrazione dell'ordine: morale e antropologia in Francia nella prima età moderna* (2 vols, Milan, 1988); Sergio Moravia, *La scienza dell'uomo nel settecento* (Bari, 1978); Martin S. Staum, *Cabanis:*

the Cartesian divide between the formal spheres of mind and body, the science of man involved a holistic meditation upon the psycho-physiological sources of the human self, as well as the political and social practices to be derived from this knowledge. Consequently, as a number of prominent philosophers made clear – from Blaise Pascale to Nicolas Malebranche, David Hume, Voltaire, G.-L. Leclerc de Buffon and J.-J. Rousseau – the science of man was the first of all sciences, since it boasted the greatest import for human affairs.[19]

In the science of man, the fundamental concern was a relation called '*le physique et le moral*'. This expression sheltered a vast repository of cultural and ideological associations, long since buried and forgotten, that are difficult to exhume, dissect and display. As Clifford Geertz and Robert Darnton have argued, however, it is precisely when scholars have encountered such recurring linguistic figures that they know they have dug up an important relic of past cultural experience.[20] To continue with this archaeological metaphor, when excavating these meanings, we find that this discourse on the physical and moral was not solely embedded in the biomedical domain; quite the contrary, it was disseminated through a dazzling array of texts and contexts, zigzagging through numerous traditions, genres and modes of inquiry. On one level, contemporaries used the term as a kind of shorthand to describe qualities of mind and body and, in particular, the variable and unpredictable interactions between the two substances. In this sense, the physical and the moral raised powerful associations – often with explicit metaphysical connotations – about the flesh, the soul, will, reason and desire. Quite simply, then, contemporaries believed that the physical and the moral formed the basis for understanding the totality of human experience, starting with the abstract quality of the 'self'.

On another level, however, I should emphasize that contemporaries used the 'physical and the moral' to discuss what we might call the sociocultural *products* of mind–body interaction. By this I mean that thinkers not only believed that physical and moral relations determined basic mental faculties – instinct, sense, memory, reason, judgment, foresight and industry – but they also influenced social phenomena writ large in terms of manners, morality, letters, the arts and science, wealth and industry. In the broadest sense, society itself – including all the pressing issues associated with tradition and authority – could be traced back to the mind–body problematic. As such, the physical and the moral harboured a powerful ideological dimension. Not only did its practitioners describe *how* mind–body interaction occurred, but they also explained how it *ought* to work and, in the cases of deviation, how reformers might go about rectifying these dysfunctions. In this sense, contemporaries conflated the 'moral' world of the mind or soul with explicit issues about politics and personal

---

Enlightenment and Medical Philosophy in the French Revolution (Princeton, 1980); Goldstein, *Console and Classify*, pp. 49–55. See also the fundamental surveys by Georges Gusdorf: *La révolution galiléenne* (2 vols, Paris, 1969), vol. 2, pp. 178–290, *L'avènement des sciences humaines au siècle des Lumières* (Paris, 1972), and, more generally, *Dieu, la nature, l'homme au siècle des Lumières* (Paris, 1972).

19   François Azouvi, *Maine de Biran: la science de l'homme* (Paris, 1995).

20   See Clifford Geertz, *The Interpretation of Cultures: Selected Essays* (New York, 1973); and Robert Darnton, *The Great Cat Massacre and Other Episodes in French Cultural History* (New York, 1984).

morality – especially in periods of profound social upheaval. In the words of Dr Louis de Lacaze:

> By this, we can easily understand the first physical reason behind our mores [*moeurs*] and talents; it even demonstrates how the faculties can be perfected, destroyed, or even transformed according to the manner in which they are cultivated and how they are habitually practiced … . [Hence] we can easily see at what point it is necessary to cultivate the talents that one wants to maintain and how we can determine at the same time the limits that we should prescribe.[21]

For their part, medical practitioners had an important stake in this abstract philosophical debate because they saw mind and body as an integrated whole, and wanted to discover a unifying physical principle that could explain all facets of life, health and pathology. For them, the science of man could create a more exact therapeutic approach and help formulate health reforms, thereby allowing medical practitioners to participate in broader political and philosophic debates.

From the closing decades of the old regime to the early years of the July monarchy, the medical community approached the mind–body problematic through a concept they called sensibility – that is, the organism's unique capability to receive and to respond to external and internal sensation. Medical practitioners here engaged themselves in a wide cultural dialogue about the meanings of 'sensibility', a term famously associated with the sentimental or 'pre-Romantic' literature of Samuel Richardson, J.-J. Rousseau and Johann Wolfgang Goethe. In rough terms, intellectuals believed that sensibility allowed people to feel and experience life; it described how people responded – in moral, intellectual and emotional terms – to experience and sensation.[22] As the pathbreaking work by G. S. Rousseau, Christopher Lawrence and John Mullan has demonstrated, sensibility had a significant biomedical dimension, because it raised powerful ideas about the relation between corporeal factors and individual feeling, sentiment and consciousness itself. For prominent doctors and naturalists, this sensible faculty depended upon the brain and nervous system, which allowed the individual to experience the inner and outer world and act upon these sensations.[23] Sensibility thus became the vital force that animated all living beings and gave them the power to feel and to be sociable; it was a dynamic faculty

---

21 Louis de Lacaze, *Idée de l'homme physique et moral* (Paris, 1755), pp. 399–401.

22 On the literary and philosophic dimensions of sensibility, see Northrop Frye, 'Towards Defining an Age of Sensibility', *English Literary History* 23 (1956): 144–52; Janet Todd, *Sensibility: An Introduction* (London, 1986); G. J. Barker-Benfield, *The Culture of Sensibility: Sex and Society in Eighteenth-Century Britain* (Chicago, 1992); Frank Baasner, *Der Begriff 'sensibilité' im 18. Jahrhundert: Aufstieg und Niedergang eines Ideals* (Heidelberg, 1988); and John C. O'Neal, *The Authority of Experience: Sensationist Theory in the French Enlightenment* (University Park, 1996).

23 G. S. Rousseau, 'Nerves, Spirits, and Fibres: Towards Defining the Origins of Sensibility', in R. F. Brissendon and J. C. Eade (eds), *Studies in the Eighteenth Century*, vol. 3 (Canberra, 1976), pp. 137–57; Christopher Lawrence, 'The Nervous System and Society in the Scottish Enlightenment', in Barry Barnes and Steven Shapin (eds), *Natural Order: Historical Studies of Scientific Culture* (Beverly Hills, 1979), pp. 19–40; and John Mullan, *Sentiment and Sociability: The Language of Feeling in the Eighteenth Century* (Oxford,

that provoked sympathy and benevolence, two moral impulses that every human community needed in order to live together and survive.

In France, as the important studies by Elizabeth A. Williams and Anne C. Vila have shown, sensibility became a kind of 'bridging concept' that moved between scientific, literary and philosophic domains of thought, spilling into all levels of learned discourse.[24] In the eighteenth and early nineteenth centuries, the discourse on sensibility owed much to vitalist theories pioneered by doctors of the Montpellier medical school, notably François Boissier de Sauvages, Théophile de Bordeu and P.-J. Barthez, and the later doctors associated with the Paris health schools, such as Pierre Cabanis, Philippe Pinel, Xavier Bichat and B.-A. Richerand. These doctors rejected the reductive aspects of mechanistic philosophy (associated with the Cartesians and Newtonians) and instead pioneered physiological models to express the dynamic qualities in living beings. As they saw it, sensibility regulated a variety of complex physiological functions – ranging from sense, volition, reflex, development and reproduction – and allowed the body to react to internal and external stimuli.[25] Sensibility became the key vital principle, if not the defining feature of life.

By emphasizing experience and sensation, medical practitioners turned the nervous system into the central part of the human self. For doctors, the nerves mediated mind–body relations and linked the unitary organism to its physical and social environment. From here, it was a small leap for them to say that that nerves determined all forms of health, pathology and human nature itself.[26] Following this insight, doctors began the ambitious task of charting nervous sensibility across all levels of human experience, as it related to sex, age, temperament, occupation and geography. This point is of capital importance. As I show in the following analysis, medical crusaders used these categories to explain variations in individual sensibility to diagnose the health conditions of specific groups and improve their physical and moral health: sensibility gave them the conceptual language to understand health panics, while simultaneously imparting therapeutic and preventive responses for perceived 'high-risk groups'.

In all this, it should be emphasized, doctors imparted a complex and ambivalent view of the human body and mind. Though medical practitioners came from a variety of religious, ideological and philosophic backgrounds, they often believed that material or physical factors influenced, in various degrees, the moral dimensions

---

1990). On this historiography, see my 'Sensibility and Human Science in the Enlightenment', *Eighteenth-Century Studies* 37 (2003–04): 296–301.

24   Williams, *Physical and the Moral*, and *Cultural History of Medical Vitalism*; and Anne C. Vila, *Enlightenment and Pathology: Sensibility in the Literature and Medicine of Eighteenth-Century France* (Baltimore, 1998).

25   Roselyn Rey, *Naissance et développement du vitalisme*; Georges Canguilhem, *La connaissance de la vie*, 2d edn (Paris, 1969), pp. 83–100; and Jacques Roger, *Les sciences de la vie dans la pensée française au XVIIIe siècle: la génération des animaux de Descartes à l'Encyclopédie*, 3d edn (Paris, 1993), pp. 614–53.

26   Mario Galzinga, 'L'organismo vivente e il suo ambiente: nascita di un rapporto', *Rivista critica di storia della filosofia* 34 (1979): 134–61.

of human experience.[27] In this attitude, doctors paradoxically undermined both sacred and more secular ideas about mind–body dualism: for traditionalists, doctors challenged metaphysical ideas about the soul, life and death itself by emphasizing that material factors determined moral qualities; for secularists, doctors challenged cherished ideas about rationality and self-control because problems such as muscle reflex and irritability overturned the idea of a specific *locus* of sensation and will (whether in the brain or nerves).[28] Consequently, doctors literally 'decentralized' the body and promoted a vision of human nature that was incredibly dynamic but potentially unstable. As a sensible being, the human organism experienced all sorts of irrational forces that shaped mind and body, for better or for worse, and made humans who they were as individuals. These complex physical impulses suggested that people were never quite in control of their minds and bodies; at the point of excess, sensibility could command mind and body relations and manifest itself in pathological display. Consequently, doctors urged their compatriots to discipline themselves, demanding, in the words of Anne C. Vila, 'not just elucidation but control'.[29] As we shall see, this problem was particularly pressing during the period of revolutionary upheaval, as medical practitioners claimed that sociopolitical changes battered individual sensibility, thereby causing nervous degeneracy and infertility.

Beyond these ideas about sensibility, doctors also borrowed key concepts from demography and the human sciences: in fact, the two proved complementary. When doctors studied sensibility, they often approached health and sickness in terms of collective behaviour and thus emphasized group profiles and 'risks' in making health policy. As they concluded, physical and moral degeneracy affected specific groups or *populations* of people. Therefore, health crusaders should approach physical and moral hygiene on the macro-level of population, and they looked for new ways to study demographic phenomena to transform the fundamental causes of natural discord in society.[30] In this context, health activists feared that excessive sensibility and nervous degeneracy were causing the population to decline, and they turned to demographic inquiry to help formulate public policy responses.

As with concerns over sensibility, hygienists contributed to a broader scientific and philosophic debate. During this period, intellectuals first used 'population' as a discreet category of social analysis.[31] Public authorities and intellectuals believed that population was the absolute measure of national power, productivity and overall

---

27 Sergio Moravia, 'Philosophie et médecine en France à la fin du XVIIIe siècle', *Studies on Voltaire and the Eighteenth Century* 89 (1972): 1089–151, and 'Dall' "homme machine" all' "homme sensible": meccanicismo, animismo e vitalismo nel secolo XVIII', *Balfagor* 29 (1974): 633–48.

28 On how vitalist physiology challenged Enlightenment beliefs, see Williams, *Cultural History of Medical Vitalism*.

29 Vila, *Enlightenment and Pathology*, p. 6.

30 James C. Riley, *Population Thought in the Age of Demographic Revolution* (Durham, NC, 1985), p. 37.

31 Foucault, *History of Sexuality*, pp. 25–6; Keith Tribe, *Governing Economy: The Reformation of German Economic Discourse, 1750–1840* (Cambridge, 1988), p. 29; and Joseph J. Spengler, *French Predecessors to Malthus: A Study in Eighteenth-Century Wage and Population Theory* (Durham, NC 1942), pp. 22–26.

health, and so they concluded that social inquiry should begin with demographic analysis.[32] In Michel Foucault's celebrated formulation, 'Governments perceived that they were not dealing simply with subjects, or even with a "people", but with a "population", with its specific phenomena and its peculiar variables.'[33] To understand demography and all its possible 'variables', then, social observers needed to study all physical and moral influences that acted upon the individual, just like physiologists studied mind and body from a holistic perspective to make sense of health, life and pathology.

To provide one example: the most sophisticated demographic approach was pioneered by Jean-Baptiste Moheau, in his *Recherches et considérations sur la population de la France* (1778). In this book, Moheau argued that social observers should evaluate all the environmental, social and biological influences that affected population patterns. He had a profoundly political and utilitarian agenda. As he saw it, public authorities and policy-makers must use the empirical methods of the Scientific Revolution and apply them to society. As he put it, the government should follow scientific emphasis on experimentation, research and calculation and then use these ideas to rationalize public policy. Moheau sought to situate demographic phenomena within the totality of human experience, using enlightened policy to improve the general population's health.[34]

Demographers like Moheau influenced health crusaders in two ways. First, physicians used demographic categories to study diseases within particular groups, distinguishing carefully between fashionable elites, fellow intellectuals, women, children, the poor, the working classes and African slaves. Second, they connected these categories with prevailing theories about disease categories and causation. In the early modern period, medical practitioners created broad taxonomies of human illnesses through case histories and clinical observation, taxonomies they called 'nosologies'. Drawing upon naturalist classification systems, above all those of Carl Linnæus, these nosologies tried to reduce diseases 'to definite and certain *species* … with the same care we see exhibited by botanists in their phytologies'.[35] In these systems, physicians transcribed every possible disease symptom, as though this linguistic sifting of signs could actually materialize the sickness and allow them to treat it.[36] Drawing upon this approach, medical crusaders juxtaposed nosological and demographic categories, hoping to classify the gamut of social diseases by isolating

---

32   See Joachim Faiguet de Villeneuve, *Discours d'un bon citoyen sur les moyens de multiplier les forces de l'État et d'augmenter la population* (Brussels, 1760), pp. 146–47; P.-H. Thiry d'Holbach, *Système social ou principes de la morale de la politique, avec un examen de l'influence du gouvernement sur les moeurs* (3 vols, London, 1773), vol. 3, p. 34.

33   Foucault, *History of Sexuality*, p. 25.

34   Jean-Baptiste Moheau, *Recherches et considérations sur la population de la France* (1778; Paris, 1994), pp. 53, 307–08.

35   Thomas Sydenham, *The Works of Thomas Sydenham*, trans. R. G. Latham (London, 1848), vol. 1, p. 13, quoted in Lester S. King, 'Boissier de Sauvages and Eighteenth-Century Nosology', *Bulletin of the History of Medicine* 40 (1966), p. 43.

36   Jean-Pierre Peter, 'Le corps du délit', *Nouvelle revue de psychanalyse*, no. 3 (1971), p. 90, and 'Les mots et les objets de la maladie: remarques sur les épidémies et la médecine dans la société française de la fin du XVIIIe siècle', *Revue historique*, no. 246 (1971), pp. 16, 19.

risk factors such as age, sex, occupation, lifestyle and social environment.[37] In the words of one physician, 'a common predisposing cause exists anytime a disease genus is shared among a considerable number of individuals, and one must search for it in the habits of those who are subordinate to the action of that cause'.[38] In this manner, medical practitioners combined physiological and demographic ideas to study particular 'high-risk groups' in aggregate terms and then craft health policies to regenerate a sick and decaying society.

Structurally, the book combines a chronological and thematic approach. The six chapters trace how medical practitioners began their health crusading during the mid-Enlightenment; how this activism flowered during the French Revolution; and how doctors revised their views during the period of post-revolutionary reaction. In Chapter 1, the analysis shows how medicine entered political life in France between 1750 and 1770. In this period, doctors involved themselves in a broader public debate about morality, social class and the family, and the health means to reform upper-class mores. Social critics believed that libertinism, luxury and changing gender roles had corrupted traditional elite values and threatened the health of the French nation. Elites thus needed a new lifestyle and new values to combat physical degeneracy, and physicians saw themselves as the vanguard of this search. As they said, a flamboyant and effeminate lifestyle among elites had caused nervous disease and sexual degeneracy, and the most likely victims were women and children.

In response, doctors looked to new models of human nature and universal laws that promoted physical and moral health, and drew upon recent physiological work to understand proper health regimen. In turn, they eagerly applied these insights to high-risk groups such as fashionable elites, intellectuals, women and children, thereby endorsing a lifestyle of sobriety, domesticity and useful works. Accordingly, women had to rehabilitate their compromised sensibility through domestic care and maternal breast-feeding (as notoriously promoted by J.-J. Rousseau). In order to diminish child morbidity and mortality, doctors further promoted programmes of physical education that involved wet-nursing controls, improved diet, dress reform and maternal devotion. Finally, ambitious doctors outlined sexual hygiene and human breeding projects to combat degeneracy and depopulation. Appealing to virtue and patriotism, these practitioners provided a sustained critique of urbane society and countered with new moral values sanctified under the halo of medical authority. Like Caron de Beaumarchais's character Figaro, though, they were willing to accept the status quo so long as elites mended their ways and conformed to middle-class standards of behaviour.

In the last two decades of the old regime, as Chapter 2 shows, medical practitioners turned from luxury and libertinism and instead focused upon the health

---

37   SRM 168, d. 3, Marre, report of 6 Sept. 1787; SRM 168, d. 3, Trinque, 'Mémoire sur une maladie épidémique qui règne à Balagué', 18 Aug. 1786; Dr Raymond, 'Mémoire sur les épidémies', *Histoire de la Société royale de médecine* (10 vols, Paris, 1779–98), vol. 4, pt 2, pp. 2, 37, 78.

38   SRM 196, d. 10, Molin, 'Essai sur quelques parties de la gymnastique appliqués aux hôpitaux' (n.d.).

of French society in general. For the first time, doctors and administrators thought systemically about the health and hygiene of all people in the rural and urban environment. To improve health and fertility, they said, every person – regardless of social status – should learn basic hygiene. What drove this new medical activism was a deepening panic about the quantity and quality of the French population, a perceived demographic crisis that motivated administrative inquiries by prestigious bodies like the Royal Academy of Sciences. These observers concluded, contrary to current historical understanding, the French population was declining. In part, these fears and anxieties responded to the military struggles of the War of Austrian Succession (1740–48) and the Seven Years War (1756–63). At this time, social critics argued that luxury, libertinism and rural backwardness had weakened the human constitution and caused the population to decline – thereby threatening the international status of the great nation.

To respond to this perceived demographic crisis, reform-minded doctors wanted a national health agency to overhaul health care and public welfare. As a result, Louis XVI created the Royal Society of Medicine in 1776–78 to coordinate medical correspondence and advise on public health reform. In turn, country doctors elaborated detailed reform projects to improve local health and combat folk medicine. Above all, the Royal Society wanted to create a national medical topography. In this massive inquiry, which was never completed, doctors planned to map all the environmental factors that caused disease so public officials could plan large-scale sanitary reform. In so doing, doctors highlighted, perhaps unintentionally, poverty and work hazards in the towns and countryside. What emerged was not a Rousseauvian, idyllic vision of the country, but rather a disturbing portrait of squalor, ignorance and deadly disease.

To a greater degree, medical topographies shaped health policies in the towns. Both the Royal Society and the Academy of Sciences interested themselves in working-class disease and urban sanitation. By the late 1780s, the Royal Society pushed a major programme of urban renewal, hoping to close cesspools and cemeteries in metropolitan sites throughout France. It achieved a major victory in 1786–88, when it relocated the venerable cemetery of Saint-Innocents in Paris. In these efforts, however, doctors emphasized sanitary measures over social reform, thereby avoiding explicit discussion about the relations between class and disease.

Chapter 3 shows that physical and moral hygiene extended to colonial possessions in the New World. In the waning years of the Old Regime, doctors engaged themselves in bitter public exchanges over slavery and health in France's overseas territories – especially that economic gem of the Americas, Saint Domingue (present-day Haiti). Following the humiliating territorial losses after the Seven Years War, social observers hoped to modernize the plantation system and improve productivity. Again, demographic concerns proved crucial. Commentators decried the high rates of morbidity and mortality within the slave community and believed this depopulation caused a corresponding increase in the slave trade. In particular, colonial doctors believed that tropical disease threatened productivity and hoped to improve the health of white settlers and black slaves. But in voicing these concerns, doctors raised explosive questions as they suggested that sicknesses were racially specific and contingent upon free or slave status.

As doctors saw it, whites and blacks faced different health problems. For them, white settlers must adapt their tender bodies to the pathological climate by learning health control. Medical and lay commentators, such as M.-L.-E Moreau de Saint-Méry and J.-F. Lafosse, stressed how the body reacted to the tropical environment, saying that only self-control and propriety protected the colonist from acclimatization and physical degeneration. By contrast, doctors argued that blacks were biologically different from whites, predisposing them to chattel slavery and various diseases as well. At the same time, degrading conditions also caused slave morbidity and mortality. To harness this racially adapted workforce, doctors wanted to lower abuses and asked public authorities to improve slave treatment (although they never challenged the peculiar institution directly).

On the eve of the French Revolution, antislavery activists such as Daniel Lescallier and Lecointe-Marsillac followed medical critiques and claimed that slavery and the slave trade caused black health problems, and that abolition would restore physical and moral health to Africans. These writers believed that physical and moral hygiene could help assimilate the liberated slave and, in some cases, it should precede slave emancipation. In so doing, abolitionists transposed racist ideas about degeneracy that were often advanced by proslavery apologists, and thus undermined the moral arguments against slavery and colonial exploitation. Antislavery writers abandoned full support for emancipation, a radical move only taken in 1794 to respond to the slave revolution in Saint Domingue.

Though medicine had entered the political theatre during the old regime, the French Revolution truly put it on centre stage. Chapter 4 explores how medicine became central to political projects for the 'physical and moral regeneration' of French society. Indeed, regeneration was one of the great aspirations of the French Revolution. In making the new nation, French people received a new identity – that of the citizen – and this event promised to transform their lives completely. revolutionaries thus invented new cultural practices to emphasize rebirth and freedom from a sick and degenerate regime. For them, the revolution offered not just liberty but also the chance for better health and beauty. Crucially, doctors contributed to this culture of social rebirth, but over the course of the revolution their views became more conservative and they insisted that regeneration should be mediated by domestic restraint.

In 1789, regeneration denoted three agendas. It could mean the reform of laws and institutions (especially fiscal policy); the rehabilitation of specific social groups (libertines, slaves, Jews, women and so on); or to change the whole social body (the nation-state and all its people). In the radical phases of the revolution, health activists, such as F.-X. Lanthenas and J.-M. Audin-Rouvière, imagined a sanitary utopia to improve the health of the labouring classes. But the Reign of Terror changed everything. Contemporaries rejected radical health agendas and instead hoped that hygiene could regenerate traditional law and custom, especially in terms of family law. Following radical changes in medical science and institutions, doctors brought new clinical and physiological insights upon health projects, arguing that physical passions and gender confusion had enervated French society and caused anarchy and terror. They hoped to contain Jacobin excess and popular agitation by using hygiene and public instruction.

This debate took a number of forms. As doctors such as Pierre Cabanis and Xavier Bichat argued, recent clinical discoveries showed that human nature was less malleable than earlier revolutionaries had thought. Therefore, emotional and physical self-control, taught by doctors and internalized within the family, could heal civil society and improve society. This medical programme had three levels: first, a health regimen aimed at controlling limited amounts of vital energy in the human body; second, a physical and moral rehabilitation of women – as suggested by J.-L. Moreau de la Sarthe and others – to anchor females in the domestic sphere; and, finally, reproductive strategies, proposed by L.-J.-M. Robert and J.-A. Millot, to breed a new generation of healthy citizens. In their efforts to combine moderate republicanism with traditional law and custom, doctors turned away from radical politics and contributed to the patriarchal family law of the 1804 Civil Code, which denied women active citizenship and made the family into the basic legal unit.

Chapter 5 shows that the conservative backlash continued to change physical and moral hygiene. During the Napoleonic Empire and the Restoration of the monarchy (1804–30), doctors further revised their ideas about self and society, diverging in their attitudes towards health activism in degree, form and function. At the same time, they pushed government and scientific support for greater medical intervention in society. Generally, medical historians have studied this new health movement in terms of the aetiological debate over contagion vs. infection: conservatives supported quarantine policies, while liberals believed in atmospheric infection and rejected government regulations, preferring instead environmental sanitation. By contrast, this chapter examines health activism in terms of the long-term medical discussion about human nature and society. Post-revolutionary doctors explored what an ideal healthy community should look like, how medicine could help make it, and whether government should finance and implement these programmes. In a major revision of Old Regime and revolutionary attitudes, doctors now focused upon the limits of human change and whether people had a born identity, one they could not change; whether sociological factors influenced health and morality; and whether or not unchecked demographic growth was beneficial to the polity. Increasingly, doctors raised moral questions about the labouring classes in health thought and framed them in socio-statistical terms.

As a result, three major approaches to social medicine emerged following the Napoleon regime: that of the pragmatic hygienists and forensic specialists such as Paul Mahon and F.-E. Fodéré, who wanted to create a so-called *médecine politique* that reflected the legal, administrative and political realities of the Napoleonic and Restoration states; that of the idealistic and religious reformists associated with the former Idéologues, Eclectics and social Christians, such as J.-J. Virey and P.-J.-B. Buchez; and that of the sanitarians who led the new public health movement of the 1820s, such as L.-R. Villermé and Alexandre Parent-Duchâtelet, who focused upon Malthusian policies, socio-statistical methods and the moral condition of the labouring classes. By the July Revolution of 1830, the liberal sanitarian approach triumphed in public health circles, and expressed an increasing pessimism about progressive change and the social conditions of early industrial France.

Finally, Chapter 6 shows medical attitudes about human nature, sexuality and society changed in dramatic ways under the July Monarchy (1830–48). New forms of class conflict drove health activism. In the wake of urban migration, industrialization and pauperization, health activists advanced radically different ideas about social hygiene and poverty. These doctors saw human nature and social change in dim terms, and they believed that dirt and immorality caused disease and disorder. They rejected government interference in private life, and looked to paternalist manufacturers to regulate the health and welfare of the labouring poor.

In this context, the 1832 cholera epidemic moved these beliefs to the forefront of health activism. L.-F. Benoiston de Châteauneuf's cholera inquest of 1834 – a landmark in the history of public health – telescoped unprecedented attention upon what practitioners called the 'conditions of existence' in the towns and manufacturing centres – especially Paris. Given degenerative conditions, doctors concluded that the labouring classes were maladapted to their living environment and were losing a biological struggle for existence. Prominent doctors such as B.-A. Richerand rejected earlier pronatalist policies and instead argued that disease eliminated a superfluous (and seditious) element of the population. In the 1840s, doctors and social economists, including L.-R. Villermé and H.-A. Frégier, espoused similar beliefs, concluding that working-class sloth and immorality caused poverty, disease and unrest.

These beliefs only deepened following the 1848 revolutions, as doctors argued that a hereditary predisposition caused disease, deviance and dearth. For instance, in their influential studies on hereditary disease, Prosper Lucas and B.-A. Morel claimed that social dislocation stemmed from a sexually contagious, ever-expanding degeneration, and they sought for new forms of social hygiene to control working-class sexuality. Thus, doctors suggested that descent and heritage limited social change and rejected the revolutionary heritage of the French middle classes. In this sense, the liberal crisis that followed the 1848 revolutions first emerged within early nineteenth-century medical circles, transforming how doctors thought about social change and melioration.

CHAPTER ONE

A Medical Diagnosis of Social Crisis, *c.* 1750–1776

In 1783, Delaporte, a Paris doctor, forwarded the following memoir to the prestigious Société Royale de Médecine, the institutional body that coordinated health policy for king Louis XVI. In the opening paragraphs, Delaporte warned:

> Cries about the degeneration of the human species are heard everywhere … . A flagging, weak and less vivacious generation has replaced, without succeeding, that brilliant [Frankish] race, those men of combat and hunting, whose bodies were more robust, cleaner and of greater height than those of today's civilized peoples. All these blights, without doubt, have been produced by laxity and abuse of physical education.
>
> It is undeniable that this alienation, this general corruption, prepares insensibly, over the course of centuries, the decadence of empires, and that it is quietly digging a grave for the human species. Already, innumerable diseases, unknown in those primitive times when exercise and frugality used to form the inviolable morals of citizens, afflict in every sense those beings who know neither pain nor death; and, considering the fact that more ghastly and destructive disease modifications are multiplying every day, these illnesses will have an increasingly fatal influence on the progress of enervation and physical and moral impotence.[1]

In warning against racial miscegenation and national decline, Delaporte seems out of place in the Age of Reason. His words evoke, rather, the fin-de-siècle fears about degeneracy and depopulation usually associated with Gustave Le Bon and Émile Zola, fears that appeared after the Franco-Prussian War and Paris Commune of 1870–71.[2] But Delaporte was neither crank nor quack. Indeed, many eighteenth-century thinkers were obsessed about degeneracy and decline and, as this chapter will show, a number of doctors – both prominent and provincial – shared these beliefs as well. In Grenoble, Dr P.-J. Nicolas wrote, 'We often complain that the human species is degenerating and weakening every day, and that the number of individuals is considerably diminished'.[3] In Paris, Dr Landais observed, 'Everyone complains constantly about the degeneration of the human species. We are weaker and less

1   SRM 120, d. 2, Delaporte, 'Mémoire sur l'éducation physique des enfans' (1783).

2   Robert A. Nye, *Crime, Madness, and Politics in Modern France: The Medical Concept of National Decline* (Princeton, 1984); Daniel Pick, *Faces of Degeneration: A European Disorder, c. 1848–c. 1918* (Cambridge, 1989); and Sander Gilman and J. Edwards Chamberlin (eds), *Degeneration: The Dark Side of Progress* (New York, 1985).

3   P.-F. Nicolas, *Le cri de la nature en faveur des enfans nouveaux-nés* (Grenoble, 1775), pp. 111–12.

robust than our fathers; we cannot conceal this truth from ourselves'.[4] According to Pierre Amoreux, a prominent doctor at the Montpellier medical school, a weak and effeminate education had caused the 'very manifest and proven abbreviation of life, depopulation and the degeneration of the human species'.[5] Nicolas, Landais and Amoreux were clear. French society was sick. Their compatriots had abandoned civic virtue, patriotism and family values. They blamed an unhealthy lifestyle, and they said their profession should not stand idle.

This alarmist language, which saturates the medical literature of the Enlightenment, marks a new development in French cultural history. In the 1750s, doctors abruptly entered the political culture of pre-revolutionary France, and began commenting upon a wide array of concerns not usually associated with public health: ideal health and beauty, upper-class morals and manners, the place of women in society, child education and sexual hygiene. Political timeliness, not scientific breakthroughs, drove this new assertiveness. At this point, socially engaged doctors injected themselves into a public debate about morality and social class in Enlightenment France, a debate in which contemporaries discussed how they could reform what were perceived to be debauched upper-class mores. Moral crusaders claimed that high society had been corrupted by luxury, libertinism and disorderly women – and urban elites needed moral hygiene to halt this decadence and decline.

As this chapter shows, ambitious physicians joined this crusade. These doctors tried to distinguish themselves from other moral pundits, saying that they could better diagnose the physical causes of these social pathologies, the people or groups at highest risk, and the proper therapeutic or preventative responses. They hoped to use new scientific insights about mind and body to improve society, claiming that a depraved lifestyle had caused the population to degenerate and decline.[6] As an antidote, they projected an ideal world that promoted health and moral values – a world characterized by self-restraint, paternal authority, happy motherhood and sexual control. In this discourse, medical practitioners argued that the family could best regenerate morals and manners because it was a healthy or natural institution that could best nurture the individual. This new domesticity encouraged physical and moral health and could build a more perfect polity. Playing to virtuous and patriotic sentiments, medical crusaders attacked urbane society, countering with a new lifestyle of self-restraint, family values and useful works – all sanctified under the halo of medical authority. In this process, they identified four high-risk groups: fashionable elites, intellectuals, women and children. All four groups, medical crusaders stressed, needed health discipline in order to regenerate French society.

---

4   Landais, *Dissertation sur les avantages de l'allaitement des enfans par leurs mères* (Geneva and Paris, 1781), pp. 42–45.

5   SRM 120, dos. 3, Amoreux, 'Des maladies héréditaires, pour servir de réponse à la question proposée à leur sujet par la Société royale de médecine', 2 Apr. 1790.

6   On eighteenth-century libertinism, see Robert Darnton, *The Forbidden Best-Sellers of Pre-Revolutionary France* (New York, 1996), p. 90; and J.-M. Goulemot, 'Toward a Definition of Libertine Fiction and Pornographic Novels', trans. A. Greenspan, *Yale French Studies*, no. 94 (1998): 133–45.

Diagnosing degeneracy in the 1750s: Le Camus, Brouzet de Béziers and Vandermonde

At first glance, it seems astonishing that eighteenth-century thinkers were so obsessed about degeneracy and decline. This was, after all, the Age of Enlightenment, an era in which leading *philosophes* claimed that reason would free people from ignorance and squalor and make society a better place to live. Their chosen word was *perfectibility*. By this, the *philosophes* meant that people had an innate faculty to perfect or improve themselves in body and spirit. The word was first used in the 1750s by the reformer A.-R. Turgot, and *philosophes* such as C.-A. Helvétius, P.-H. Thiry d'Holbach and A.-N. Condorcet soon picked it up and made it into their credo.[7] As several historians have shown, however, not all intellectuals shared this exaggerated optimism, and medical thinkers, especially those associated with the Montpellier medical school, formed an important critical voice.[8] The *philosophe* Denis Diderot, for example, said that physical qualities constrained the mind and that only an elect few could perfect themselves.[9] The best-known critic, of course, was J.-J. Rousseau, who claimed that modern letters and science had destroyed moral values. Though many intellectuals rejected Rousseau's primitivism and political radicalism, they did agree that morality was declining and feared that decadent behaviour threatened France's great power status. In their eyes, people had lost moral and physical self-restraint and this loss had torn apart the moral fabric of French civilization. This moral panic inspired health reform movements in the old regime.

Many factors contributed to this intellectual ferment, which exploded in an unprecedented cultural crisis in the early 1750s. Although France experienced a prolonged economic boom during the 1740s and 1750s – historian Alfred Cobban has even called these two decades the golden age of eighteenth-century France – a number of disasters, including failed harvests, famine, population movements and lost wars, created a profound sense of malaise amongst the upper classes.[10] As a consequence, a diverse groups of intellectuals, ranging from C.-P. Duclos to the Physiocrat economists, took this malaise and framed it in moral terms, denouncing

---

7   R. Wokler, 'Rousseau's Perfectibilian Liberalism', in A. Ryan (ed.), *The Idea of Freedom* (New York, 1979), pp. 233–52; and John Passmore, *The Perfectibility of Man* (New York, 1970), pp. 149–211.

8   On general anxieties about progress and decline, see Harry G. Payne, *The Philosophes and the People* (New Haven, 1976); and Harvey Chisick, *The Limits of Reform in the Enlightenment: Attitudes Toward the Education of the Lower Classes in Eighteenth-Century France* (Princeton, 1981). On medical concerns, see Elizabeth A. Williams, *A Cultural History of Medical Vitalism in Enlightenment Montpellier* (Aldershot, 2003).

9   Andrew Curran, 'Monsters and the Self in the *Rêve de d'Alembert*', *Eighteenth-Century Life* 21 (1997): 48–69.

10   Alfred Cobban, *A History of Modern France* (London, 1963–65), vol. 1. On old regime socioeconomic change, see Colin Jones, 'Bourgeois Revolution Revivified: 1789 and Social Change', in Colin Lucas (ed.), *Rewriting the French Revolution* (Oxford, 1991), pp. 69–118, and 'The Great Chain of Buying: Medical Advertisement, the Bourgeois Public Sphere, and the Origins of the French Revolution', *American Historical Review* 101 (1996): 13–40.

what seemed to be the 'excessive depravation', 'disorder' and 'moral degradation' of their times.[11] As they saw it, their compatriots had lost the moral virtue and patriotic sentiments needed to keep the nation strong and healthy, and they blamed luxury and libertinism amongst elites.[12] To regenerate society, fashionable elites needed new morals and manners to help mend their debauched ways. In the 1740s and 1750s, prominent writers and artists picked up this crusade. This didacticism framed the sentimental literature of the eighteenth century, which sought both to criticize fashionable elites and exhort them to moral reform. The best-known examples are the influential novels by Samuel Richardson and J.-J. Rousseau or the morally edifying images by J.-B. Greuze and J.-L. David.[13] Underneath these criticisms lurked a fierce class consciousness. For social critics, personal character, not privilege and property, determined social status, and the surest markers of it were individual morality, work ethic, patriotism and, above all, propriety.

Ambitious doctors joined this crusade. Like other intellectuals, they wanted to regenerate moral values. They too saw decay and rot in French society. Following other crusaders, physicians linked social status and character, but they portrayed sickness as a consequence of immoral behaviour. For them, physical and moral degeneracy was not just figurative hyperbole. High society was truly sick. Their dealings with patients had convinced them of this fact. Luxury and libertinism had corrupted a prophylactic instinct needed to keep society virtuous and healthy. Quite simply, the upper classes had lost control of their bodies to modern life: 'The dikes have burst, the earth has been flooded with the waves of need and the races have degenerated'.[14] The wound was self-inflicted, and in their correspondence with central authorities and other medical institutions, medical crusaders documented the symptoms of moral rot: gout, stones, obstructions, intestinal disorders, cold sores, ulcers, inflammations, suppurations, headaches, migraines, sensitive eyes, insomnia, somnolence, lethargy, dropsy, consumption, tumors, birth defects, scirrhus, apoplexy,

---

11   C. P. Duclos, *Considérations sur les moeurs de ce siècle* (Amsterdam and Paris, 1751), p. 107, quoted in Jacques Rustin, *La vice à la mode: étude sur le roman français du XVIIIe siècle de Manon Lescaut à l'apparition de la Nouvelle Héloïse (1731–1761)* (Paris, 1979), pp. 42–43.

12   See Roger Chartier, *The Cultural Origins of the French Revolution*, trans. Lydia G. Cochrane (Durham, NC, 1991), pp. 92–135; Sarah Maza, 'Luxury, Morality, and Social Change: Why There Was No Middle-Class Consciousness in Prerevolutionary France', *Journal of Modern History* 69 (1997): 199–229; Sarah Maza, 'The Diamond Necklace Affair Revisited (1785–1786): The Case of the Missing Queen', in Lynn Hunt (ed.), *Eroticism and the Body Politic* (Baltimore, 1991), pp. 63–89. See also Antoine de Baecque, *The Body Politic: Corporeal Metaphor in Revolutionary France, 1770–1800*, trans. Charlotte Mandell (Stanford, 1993), pp. 29–75.

13   See Warren Roberts, *Morality and Social Class in Eighteenth-Century French Literature and Painting* (Toronto, 1974); and Joan Landes, *Women and the Public Sphere in the Age of the French Revolution* (Ithaca, 1988), pp. 17–65.

14   Alphonse Leroy, *Recherches sur les habillemens des femmes et des enfans* (Paris, 1772), pp. 2–3.

enervation, convulsions and delirium. These diseases fell under one master pathology: nervous disease.[15]

By emphasizing nervous disease, medical crusaders took new ideas about sensibility that were developed by prominent medical theorists such as Albrecht von Haller, Charles Bonnet and Théophile de Bordeu and used them to diagnose a felt social crisis. As they saw it, luxury and libertinism had exasperated the body's sensibility and caused a plague of nervous disease.[16] In St Étienne, Dr Noudeau complained that nervous diseases have 'become so frequent every day'.[17] In Grasse, Dr Rossignolly warned that decadence had 'thickened the sum of human deformities and filled our cities with hysterics and hypochondriacs'.[18] In Lausanne, the famed medical writer Samuel Tissot insisted that nervous diseases 'have become more common, in a more considerable proportion than others, and I am not afraid to say that if they used to be more infrequent, then today they are more frequent, especially in the cities'.[19] For these doctors, this plague signified everything that was wrong with contemporary morals and manners; and to cure it, the upper classes needed a health programme to restore their physical and moral health. Their lifestyle had undermined the moral claims that justified their social and economic authority. The health and security of the body politic demanded it. In this case, 'nervous disease' should be viewed in a much broader framework than described by Michel Foucault as a 'great fear of madness', one centred on disciplinary definitions of madness and the central role of institutions like the asylum.[20] Rather, alarmed practitioners claimed nervous disease was consuming the whole of the body politic in an alarming and ever-shifting flood of illnesses.

Members of the medical establishment responded to this felt crisis. Between 1753 and 1756, three physicians published books on moral degeneracy and outlined ways to prevent or cure these pathologies. These path-breaking works included Antoine Le Camus's *Médecine de l'esprit* (1753), N. Brouzet de Bézier's *Essai sur l'éducation médicinale des enfans* (1754) and C.-A. Vandermonde's *Essai sur la manière de perfectionner l'espèce humaine* (1756), works which were written in general terms for colleagues, educators, public authorities and other concerned readers. Hoping to form healthy and moral individuals, these authors framed moral malaise in medical terms; in turn, their ideas about moral hygiene began to shape public discourse in new and unexpected ways.

The first doctor to pick up these themes was Antoine Le Camus in his *La Médecine de l'esprit* (1753). Le Camus was a prominent figure at the Paris medical school

---

15   S.-A. Tissot, *De la santé des gens de lettres* (Lausanne, 1768), pp. 182–86 n. l; and Jacques Ballexserd, *Dissertation sur l'éducation physique des enfans* (Paris, 1762), pp. 23–29.

16   SRM 116, d. 2, L'Enuë de la Vallée, 'Mémoire au concours sur les affections de l'âme, les maladies nerveuses, l'hystéricisme, l'hypchondriacisme, la mélancholie', 7 Mar. 1786.

17   SRM 185, d. 3, Noudeau, 'Réflexions sur l'utilité des frictions sêches dans les maladies nerveuses, avec observation', 12 May 1787.

18   SRM 200, d. 1, Rossignolly, 'Mémoire sur les maladies nerveuses proprement dittes [sic]', 7 Mar. 1786.

19   S.-A. Tissot, *Traité des nerfs et leurs maladies* (5 vols, Paris and Lausanne, 1778), vol. 1, pp. iii–iv.

20   Michel Foucault, *Histoire de la folie à l'âge classique* (Paris, 1972), pp. 382–83.

and was extensively engaged in mid-century medical and philosophic concerns. His book belonged to a new medical literature, appearing in the 1740s and 1750s, in which self-proclaimed 'enlightened physicians' [*médecins-philosophes*] claimed that biomedical science could explain the mind–body problematic and thus contribute to metaphysical debate. These studies included C.-N. Le Cat's *Traité des sens* (1742), Julien Offray de La Mettrie's *L'histoire naturelle de l'âme* (1745) and *L'Homme-machine* (1748), Louis de Lacaze's *L'idée de l'homme physique et moral* (1755) and Antoine Louis's *Essai sur la nature de l'âme* (1757). Though medical practitioners usually affirmed a conventional Cartesian dualism – the materialist La Mettrie was a notorious exception – they did insist that many so-called afflictions of the soul had a physical basis and that only a well-trained doctor could treat them.[21] They thus put the soul on the doorstep of medical practice and made medicine into an arbiter in theological and metaphysical debate.

This philosophic and health-based engagement had an underlying professional agenda. Books like Le Camus's must be seen within the context of a shifting medical epistemology, internecine corporate politics and broader critiques levelled at the social and political institutions of the old regime. Between roughly 1750 and 1776, a broad constellation of events – including the rise of the surgeons at St Côme, passionate disputes over physicians' and surgeons' corporate privileges, the decline of religious sentiments surrounding medical practice, the growth of unlicensed medical personnel, and the criticisms levelled at hospital care and poor relief – undermined the traditional medical authority found in universities and guilds.[22] According to the cantankerous medical critic J.-E. Gilibert, for example, a state of 'medical anarchy' reigned in the French kingdom,[23] and numerous doctors wanted to radically reform existing medical institutions and regulations. As one physician complained:

> Without doubt, there are abuses to correct in the exercise of medicine, abuses that are dangerous to the health, even the life, of man, abuses that infinitely impede the art of healing, which debase, in some ways, the doctor's reputation by prohibiting him from any emulation, by ruining the success of his practice and by preventing [patients] from having recourse to his knowledge at the beginning of an illness, that is to say, at those moments when the doctor's insight is most necessary.[24]

---

21   See Ann Thomson, *Materialism and Societey in the Mid-Eighteenth-Century: La Mettrie's Discourse préliminaire* (Geneva, 1981); and Kathleen Wellman, *La Mettrie: Medicine, Philosophy, and Enlightenment* (Durham, NC, 1992).

22   See especially Matthew Ramsey, *Professional and Popular Medicine in France: The Social World of Medical Practice* (Cambridge, 1987), pp. 17–70; Toby Gelfand, *Professionalizing Modern Medicine: Paris Surgeons and Medicial Science and Institutions in the Eighteenth Century* (Westport, 1980), pp. 67–79; and Jan Goldstein, *Console and Classify: The French Psychiatric Profession in the Nineteenth Century* (Cambridge, 1987), pp. 15–40.

23   J.-E. Gilibert, *L'anarchie médicale, ou la médecine considérée comme nuisible à la société* (3 vols, Neuchâtel, 1772).

24   SRM 132, d. 52, Duverin, 'Essai sur les abus à corriger dans l'exercise de la médecine', 8 Mar. 1777. See also FMP, ms. 2006, fol. XXXVII, 'Motifs qui doivent déterminer l'arrest du conseil provisionnel et lettres patentes' (n.d.); and SRM 131, d. 36, 'Mémoire présenté à la Société ou Correspondance royale de médecine établie à Paris par arrêt de conseil du 29 avril 1776'.

These demands converged with mounting criticism of medical epistemology. Internal detractors, notably the famed comparative anatomist Félix Vicq d'Azyr, charged that medicine had failed to keep abreast of scientific and philosophic advances, and they pressed for their colleagues to perfect medical knowledge, skills and institutions.[25] Apparently, leading doctors had digested the criticisms by Étienne de Condillac (amongst others), who claimed that medicine remained one of practical sciences still bound to formal rationalism and 'abstract hypotheses'.[26]

According to Sergio Moravia, reform projects involved three main points: medicine had to claim its proper autonomy and resist being subjugated by the physical and chemical sciences; doctors should perfect their instruments and methods to respond to medical sceptics and 'empiricists'; and, finally, the discipline must reach a level of epistemological sophistication, not simply in therapeutic practice, but rather in 'nosological' or 'bioanthropological' systems. Medicine must become a true 'science of man', that is, a discipline that contemplated the human self in all its physical and moral dimensions.[27] Although this 'medical anthropology' promised to improve the doctor's skill and prestige, it also envisioned a social mission for medical personnel, who could use this knowledge to alleviate the human condition. As one doctor wrote, 'The science of man has always appeared the most sublime and most necessary', yet for others it was 'the most cultivated but least advanced' of all.[28]

Though Le Camus's book constitutes part of this medical literature, he significantly moved beyond his colleagues. By studying the mind–body problem, he said, doctors could to cure, 'by mechanical means', physical and moral vice and thus improve the human spirit: in his mind, he wanted to create a true 'man of spirit', a person who 'does not search for his ideas with difficulty, who reasons readily and judges exactly'.[29] Abstract medical knowledge thus bore upon practical (if not more humanistic) questions about self-formation and self-mastery, thereby moving from theory to practice. And, despite his anti-materialist sentiments, he situated himself squarely in Enlightenment epistemology, both in terms of method and approach.

Throughout, Le Camus used the empirical psychology of John Locke and Étienne de Condillac as a practical medical guide, and he echoed their belief that sensory experience formed human identity. In contrast to traditional Lockean psychology, however, Le Camus emphasized the ways in which corporeal factors shaped the individual self. According to him, the individual was comprised of two substances:

---

25   AN F^{17}1246, no. 292, *Arrest du Conseil d'État du Roi, qui établit une Commission de Médecins à Paris, pour tenir une correspondance avec les médecins de provinces* (Paris, 1776).

26   Étienne de Condillac, *Oeuvres complètes* (32 vols, Geneva, 1970), vol. 2, pp. 262–64.

27   Sergio Moravia, 'Philosophie et médecine en France à la fin du XVIIIe siècle', *Studies on Voltaire and the Eighteenth Century* 89 (1972): 1089–151, and 'Dall' "homme machine" all' "homme sensible": meccanicismo, animismo e vitalismo nel secolo XVIII', *Balfagor* 29 (1974): 633–48.

28   SRM 138, d. 14, Estienne, médecin à Auriol, letter of 29 Apr. 1786; P.-J. Barthez, *Nouveaux élémens de la science de l'homme*, 2d edn (2 vols, Paris, 1806), vol. 1, pp. 1–2; J.-P. Marat, *De l'homme* (3 vols, Amsterdam and Paris, 1775–76), vol. 1, pp. i, xvii–xix.

29   Antoine Le Camus, *Médecine de l'esprit* (2 vols, Paris, 1753), vol. 2, p. 51.

one material and corruptible (the body) and the other pure and immaterial (the soul). Because the soul came from God, it was perfect; therefore, its impurities developed only after it was united with the flesh. But this carnal weakness offered an opportunity. Doctors simply needed to discover the physical mechanism that governed understanding; afterwards, they could fine-tune the body to make the soul work at the highest possible level.[30]

In searching out this mechanism, Le Camus entered an acrimonious medical debate about the physiological basis of feeling and sensation, a European-wide debate that had split between various factions of mechanists such as Hermann Boerhaave and Freidrich Hofffmann, on the one hand, and vitalists such as François Boissier de Sauvages and Robert Whytt, on the other. For his part, Le Camus followed neo-mechanistic physiologists such as Albrecht von Haller and C.-N. Le Cat, who said that the nerves contained a subtle fluid called the 'animal spirits' in an effort to maintain the formal Cartesian division between mind and body. According to these thinkers, this spirituous fluid was filtered in the brain and communicated the soul's will though the nerves and muscles and then carried feelings back to the soul. For these reasons, the immaterial soul could not function in a body with impaired nervous properties.[31]

To maintain the nervous system, Le Camus said that the doctor must help the patient mould what was called 'temperament'. Temperament was an ancient idea that dated back to ancient Greco-Roman medicine, and signified a person's total physical disposition. It was formed by a unique balance of humoral fluids – blood, phlegm, black and yellow bile – as well as other contingent factors, including climate, geography, age, sex, occupation and diet. These combined qualities shaped an individual's constitution and personal type (whether sanguinary, bilious, phlegmatic or melancholic), and explained possible disease susceptibility, treatment and prevention for each person.[32]

Le Camus amplified these ideas about personal temperament and predisposition, putting this medical knowledge in the service of a moral agenda. By changing temperament, he promised, the doctor could improve and perfect the spirit, thereby sculpting a more harmonious whole. The key was child education, because an infant's first experiences – from the moment it left the womb – formed its entire life. For this reason, the doctor must recognize two kinds of education: a spiritual education that shaped the child's morality and common sense; and a corporal education that shaped the body in which the soul would reside and act.[33] But on this important topic of corporeal education, which seemed so important for his programme of regeneration, Le Camus offered little practical advice other than breast-feeding, arguing that hired wet-nurses potentially communicated moral and physical vices to infants.[34]

---

30   Ibid., vol. 1, p. xviii.

31   Ibid., vol. 1, pp. 58–59.

32   Ibid., vol. 2, p. 308.

33   Ibid., vol. 1, pp. 260, 271.

34   Ibid., vol. 1, pp. 276, 278–79. On wet-nursing, see George Sussman, *Selling Mother's Milk: The Wet-Nursing Business in France, 1715–1914* (Urbana, 1982); and Nancy Senior, 'Aspects of Infant Feeding in Eighteenth-Century France', *Eighteenth-Century Studies* 16 (1983): 367–88.

Though Le Camus broached the problem of corporeal education as but one part of his larger work, his words hit a nerve, because the subject was taken up the following year by Dr N. Brouzet de Béziers, in his book *Essai sur l'éducation médecinale des enfans* (1754). Brouzet is a relatively obscure figure in eighteenth-century medicine – indeed, this book seems to have been his only publication – but his book put child hygiene at the front of public discussions about moral degeneracy and decline. Throughout, he stressed repeatedly to his readers that child illnesses were often fatal, and that the physician should never let nature take its own course: he needed to act and act quickly.[35] Brouzet's book proved so pathbreaking that it inspired an entirely new medical genre about child hygiene and even sparked a passionate crusade on behalf of child health by doctors such as J. C. Desessartz, Joseph Raulin, Jacques Ballexserd and P.-J. Nicolas, long before J.-J. Rousseau had picked up these anxieties in his *Émile*. Soon prominent medical and literary societies were fervently debating the causes of child mortality.[36]

There were grim reasons for this medical activism. In the old regime, a third of all newborns died before their first birthday, and roughly half of all children lived to age ten. In urban areas, parents often abandoned their children and the death rates in foundling homes and orphanages approached a staggering 90 percent.[37] In the mid-century, moral critics and doctors denounced this state of affairs and demanded that concerned parents and public authorities do something about it.[38] Two things apparently changed attitudes. The first was a new sensibility about childhood. In writings and images, as Philippe Ariès and Anne Higonnet have shown, contemporaries created a new image of family life by celebrating childhood and parental love; they emphasized that children had an autonomous identity and that childhood itself was a significant stage in human growth.[39] Because contemporaries believed childhood

---

35   N. Brouzet de Béziers, *Essai sur l'éducation médicinale des enfans et sur leurs maladies* (2 vols, Paris, 1754), vol. 1, pp. xix–xx.

36   M.-F. Morel, 'Ville et compagne dans le discours médicale sur la petite enfance au XVIIIe siècle', *Annales: E.S.C.* 32 (1977): 1007–24; Jacques Donzelot, *The Policing of Families*, trans. Robert Hurley (New York, 1979); and Gilbert Py, *Rousseau et les éducateurs: étude sur la fortune des idées pédagogiques de Jean-Jacques Rousseau en France et en Europe au XVIIIe siècle* (Oxford, 1997), pp. 253–314.

37   Alain Bideau, Jacques Dupâquier and Hector Gutierrez, 'La mort quantifiée', in Dupâquier (ed.), *Histoire de la population française*, vol. 2, *De la Renaissance à 1789* (Paris, 1988), pp. 222–43. On child abandonment, see Claude Delasselle, 'Les enfants abondonnés à Paris au XVIIIe siècle', *Annales: E.S.C.* 30 (1975): 187–218; and Dora B. Weiner, *The Citizen-Patient in Revolutionary and Imperial Paris* (Baltimore, 1993), pp. 45–76, 191–222.

38   For example, see SRM 141, d. 6, J.-L. Fourcroy de Guillerville to Clermont Beauvoisis, 22 Apr. 1777. Like Fourcroy, a number of physicians used hospital and parish records to detail child morbidity and mortality. See also: SRM 136, d. 17, Delaporte and Carrère, 'Rapport du mémoire de M. Bret, intitulé *Essai sur l'éducation physique des enfans et sur la conduite que les femmes doivent tenir après leur accouchement*' (1783); SRM 134, d. 34, Munnicks, 'Mémoire sur la mortalité infantile', 31 Aug. 1784; and SRM 134, d. 32, Marignes, 'Mémoire sur cette question: Quelle est la cause de la disposition au calcul et autres affections analogues auxquels les enfans sont sujets?' 7 Mar. 1786.

39   The classic analyses are Philippe Ariès, *Centuries of Childhood: A Social History of Family Life*, trans. Robert Baldick (New York, 1962); D. G. Charlton, *New Images of the*

shaped the adult self, and that children themselves deserved sentimental love and affection, they empathized more strongly with children, especially the spectacle of child suffering, and they also began to identify with parents who had lost their young. The second reason was more ideological. After Le Camus and Brouzet, medical crusaders saw child mortality as a symptom of degeneracy and decline, and they used this issue as a vehicle to attack upper-class morals and manners. As these writers saw it, urban elites preferred to live a corrupt life of luxury and libertinism, so they left their children with wet-nurses and domestic servants and thereby caused child sickness and death.[40] Those children who did survive lacked the physical and moral fortitude needed to become virtuous, patriotic citizens. By keeping children healthy and clean, parents could substantiate their love of family and country – but if they failed to do so, doctors and public authorities should intervene and regulate their children's health.[41]

Brouzet divided his book into two parts. The first traced child development from conception to puberty and stressed proper hygiene and moral precautions; the second part identified specific child diseases and tried to classify them in nosological terms, specifying whether they were acute, external, internal or chronic. In all this, he insisted that child disease was a continuum that stretched across physical and moral development. Drawing upon naturalist G.-L. de Buffon's anthropological study of the human life cycle, he divided childhood into eight distinct stages, moving from conception to adolescence, and then tried to identify the diseases and health risks that characterized each. To do so, Brouzet looked to new physiological models that came from the Montpellier medical school: in particular, he was impressed by Théophile de Bordeu's pioneering studies on endocrinology, which had argued that a physical sensibility regulated vital functions and caused physical crises that culminated in fevers and discharges. As such, Brouzet saw childhood as inherently pathological: it was a disease that started at birth and continued until it resolved itself in the crisis of puberty. Just like a fever that built to a heightened pitch and suddenly broke, childhood had its own symptoms and dramatic resolutions. In this sense, the child's sensibility made it live and grow, giving it the energy needed to become an adult, but it could also consume the body and make it sick. For this reason, children easily became hypersensible and died from nervous convulsions.[42]

Brouzet believed that a number of factors threatened the child's delicate sensibility. Children might languish under a bad diet and breathe bad air; they potentially suffered from hereditary diseases; and they might also be afflicted with irresponsible wet-nurses and abusive governesses. In this litany of failures, he often blamed parents for neglecting proper domestic hygiene and inadvertently causing child illness and

Natural in France: A Study in European Cultural History (Cambridge and New York, 1984), 135–77; and Anne Higonnet, *Pictures of Innocence: The History and Crisis of Ideal Childhood* (London, 1998).

40 L. J. Jordanova, 'Naturalizing the Family: Literature and the Bio-Medical Sciences in the Late Eighteenth Century', in Jordanova (ed.), *Languages of Nature: Critical Essays on Science and Literature* (London, 1986), pp. 86–116.

41 SRM 120, d. 2, Delaporte, report to the Société Royale de Médecine (n.d.).

42 Brouzet, *L'éducation médicinale des enfans*, vol. 2, pp. 1–2, 3.

death. To fix this sorry state of affairs, Brouzet believed that children needed a new form of education and he even gave it a name: *medicinal education*.[43] This 'physical education', as later medical practitioners called it, helped form healthy and vigorous children, and cared for them from the womb to puberty – and some medical writers stated their express hope that it could inculcate civic virtue and patriotism.[44] In the words of one physician:

> The present question must have the greatest influence on our century and for the times to come. It is to take the human species in its infancy, it is to renew, so to speak, the source; it is to meliorate the race; it is to prepare for the nation subjects who are most dignified to serve it and are in better condition to support force and splendour.[45]

Like Le Camus, Brouzet focused upon breast-feeding. In the 1750s, some doctors called upon mothers to nurse their newborn children, claiming it was healthy for mother and child; others said that it gave the mother sensual pleasures that compensated for conjugal abstinence after birth (medical and moral writers often believed that sex while breast-feeding corrupted a mother's milk). J.-J. Rousseau, of course, famously made maternal breast-feeding the centrepiece of his moral campaign. But not all doctors supported breast-feeding, and many roundly attacked Rousseau for his health advice. For example, J.B. Van Helmont and Philippe Hecquet found a mother's milk so revolting that they urged mothers to only feed their children cereal porridges.[46] Brouzet agreed, though he stressed other reasons. On one level, he feared that upper-class mothers had simply become too sickly and degenerate to nurse their children, and he cautioned that mother's milk might be transmitting hereditary diseases. On another level, he hoped that non-nursing mothers might resume conjugal duties and thus help the population grow.[47] Following Brouzet's ideas, sympathetic doctors qualified their attitudes towards breast-feeding and urged women to consult their doctors making any firm decisions about infant nursing. One manuscript at the Paris medical faculty gave detailed advice on how to make this difficult decision. The author explained to his fellow doctors that they should look at the woman's birth history, the size and shape of her breasts, her temperament, diet and personal hygiene. If parents hired an outside nurse, they should vigilantly observe her actions and keep her from having sex with the other domestic help.[48] The message, though, was clear: urban women were probably too degenerate to nurse

---

43   Ibid., vol. 1, pp. i–ii.

44   SRM 197, d. 4, Daube, 'De l'éducation physique des enfans' (1784); see also ANM, ms. 10, Procès-verbaux de la SRM, 6 Apr. 1784.

45   SRM 120, d. 2, Amoreux, 'Les abus à réformer dans l'éducation physique'.

46   For an overview of these theories, see ANM, ms. 1025, fol. 179, Coutouly, 'Maladies des enfans du premier âge' (n.d.); Hermann Boerhaave, *Traité des maladies des enfans*, trans. M. Paul, rev. by Gerard van Swieten (Avignon and Paris, 1759), pp. 5–6, 28, 30–31; and Nicolas Chambon de Montaux, *Des maladies des enfans*, 2 vols. (Paris, Year VII), vol. 1, pp. 325–30.

47   Brouzet, *L'éducation médicinale des enfans*, vol. 1, 148, 151–52, 164, 181–82; Joseph Raulin, *De la conservation des enfans* (2 vols, Paris, 1768), vol. 2, pp. 169, 173–75, 198–99.

48   FMP, ms. 2082, 'Traité du régime et des maladies les plus fréquentes des enfans' [mid-1700s].

their own children, and doctors needed to regenerate the family by other means. Maybe contemporaries needed a broader programme of family hygiene.

In this anxious cultural setting, Charles-Auguste Vandermonde, one of Le Camus's colleagues at the Paris medical faculty, published his *Essai sur la manière de perfectionner l'espèce humaine* in 1756, right at the onset of the traumatic Seven Years War. With this important book, he helped define medical consensus about moral decline and degeneracy, and he decisively linked inheritance and moral hygiene.[49] Three years earlier, he had penned a lengthy dictionary on personal hygiene, specifically addressed to lay readers, but his *Essai* was far more ambitious and sophisticated in its scope and content. This text followed Le Camus and Brouzet de Béziers, but now framed social criticisms in terms of sex and heredity. Moving beyond moral hygiene and physical education, Vandermonde promised his readers that sexual hygiene could improve humanity. As he declared, 'If chance can degenerate the human species, medicine [*l'art*] can also perfect it'.[50] With this text, Vandermonde broke with a whole range of erotic books such as Nicolas Venette's *Conjugal Love or the Pleasures of the Marriage Bed* (1685) and Claude Quillet's *Callipaedia* (1655), books that often taught readers how to control sex and fertility.[51] Unlike these eighteenth-century sex writers, Vandermonde wrote specifically for those doctors and bureaucrats who worried about fertility, the primary agent of state power. For him, the French population urgently needed sexual hygiene, because luxury and libertinism had disrupted natural bonds and caused the species to degenerate.[52] In his words:

> Man is the only being who has risen from his initial condition by weakening his natural conformation and by altering every aspect of his original imprint ... . Our body languishes, weakens and loses the beautiful proportions that it had received from nature. Our reason is obscured, our spirit is enervated and we no longer find in man the *chef-d'oeuvre* of the Creator.[53]

When Vandermonde spoke of perfecting the race, he meant that people should regain the primordial, virtuous body that modern man had lost when he abandoned

---

49   Vandermonde's text has but recently attracted historical and critical interest: see Anne C. Vila, *Enlightenment and Pathology: Sensibility in the Literature and Medicine of Eighteenth-Century France* (Baltimore, 1998), pp. 88–91; K. A. Wellman, 'Physicians and Philosophes: Physiology and Sexual Morality in the French Enlightenment', *Eighteenth-Century Studies* 35 (2002): 267–77. See also Georges Vigarello, *Le sain et le malsain: santé et mieux-être depuis le Moyen Âge* (Paris, 1993), pp. 156–64.

50   C.-A. Vandermonde, *Essai sur la manière de perfectionner l'espèce humaine* (2 vols, Paris, 1756), vol. 1, pp. 91–92.

51   Roy Porter, '"The Secrets of Generation Display'd": *Aristotle's Master-piece* in Eighteenth-Century England', in Robert Purkis MacCubin (ed.), *'Tis Nature's Fault: Unauthorized Sexuality During the Enlightenment* (New York, 1987); and, most recently, Mary E. Fissell, 'Making a Masterpiece: The Aristotle Texts in Vernacular Medical Culture', in Charles E. Rosenberg (ed.), *Right Living: An Anglo-American Tradition of Self-Help Medicine and Hygiene* (Baltimore, 2003), pp. 59–87.

52   Vandermonde, *Essai*, vol. 2, pp. 31–32, 106–07.

53   Ibid., vol. 1, pp. iv–v.

the state of nature – not the decadent world of novels and salons, but the *belle nature* that still lived on in humanity. In some ways, Vandermonde grappled with the same question that had haunted J.-J. Rousseau: both writers wondered how contemporaries could reconcile natural qualities of mind and body with the pressures of modern life. Unlike Rousseau – who, while advocating personal hygiene, had notoriously criticized medical expertise – Vandermonde instead promised that medicine and science could lend a helping hand to create a more 'natural' and virtuous kind of man. As he informed his readers, health and beauty were objective categories and could be studied (and improved) with all the tools available to modern science. For example, doctors and aesthetes had shown that they could quantify form and symmetry in Greco-Roman sculpture – what they saw was the pinnacle of artistic accomplishment – and could thus properly measure individual beauty (these beliefs were later developed by physiognomists such as Peter Camper and Johann Lavater).[54] Consequently, Vandermonde urged doctors to gaze carefully into the human face and study its appearance and proportion. Skin colour provided another sign of beauty; few doctors and naturalists believed, Vandermonde said, that black Africans were more beautiful than white Europeans. Above all, the beautiful body was a healthy body and it thus needed good bones, muscles and nerves. He concluded:

> It is therefore [the body itself] that we must perfect. We must renew the corrupted source of our humors and spirits. We must repair our organs and change, fortify, and meliorate all the forces of our machine. It is by taking this route that we can break the chain of most rebellious diseases and the most tumultuous passions, and that, by perpetuating in the human species our beauty, force, and health, we can sow the germ of virtue and push the spirit to its highest force.[55]

In his breeding programme, Vandermonde drew upon the new theories of sexual reproduction pioneered by naturalists such as Pierre Maupertuis and G.-L. de Buffon. These naturalists revived the Aristotelian model of epigenesis and incorporated new microscopic and experimental work on generation. Often, epigenesists claimed that the embryo developed sequentially from a mass of organic molecules, believing that chemical attraction or an interior mould determined form and embryonic growth. In this manner, epigenesists emphasized that both mothers and fathers contributed material qualities to their offspring, and thus explained a wide range of issues about development and anomalies, including hereditary disease.[56]

Though indebted to these epigenetic thinkers, Vandermonde offered his own original take on generation, arguing that the reproductive organs filtered a humour

---

54 L. J. Jordanova, 'The Art and Science of Seeing: Physiognomy, 1780–1830', in W. F. Bynum and Roy Porter (eds), *Medicine and the Five Senses* (Cambridge, 1993), pp. 122–33.

55 Vandermonde, *Essai*, vol. 1, p. vii.

56 See Jacques Roger, *Les sciences de la vie dans la pensée française au XVIIIe siècle: la génération des animaux de Descartes à l'Encyclopédie*, 3d edn (Paris, 1993); Elizabeth B. Gasking, *Investigations Into Generation, 1651–1828* (Baltimore, 1967); Pierre Darmon, *Le mythe de la procréation à l'âge baroque* (Paris, 1981); and especially Mary Terrall, *The Man Who Flattened the Earth: Maupertuis and the Sciences in the Enlightenment* (Chicago, 2002), pp. 218–21.

that contained 'an infinity of parts proper to form a like individual'.[57] When the male and female reproductive fluids combined, the organic particles – which resembled encased spirals that spun in perpetual motion – organized themselves according to their intrinsic levels of oscillation; in this process, parental characteristics blended together and formed a new individual – except when determining biological sex (if the more active particles dominated, a male resulted).[58] This model allowed Vandermonde to explain inherited and acquired vices. Ideally, when the reproductive matter fused together, the molecular spirals joined in tightly linked bonds (rather like the wedges of a puzzle); but if this did not happen, an asymmetrical union caused erratic development and an imperfectly formed embryo. In the case of disease, the vitiated molecules failed to bind properly with the partner's reproductive molecules and thus caused a permanent hereditary stain. According to Vandermonde, these contaminated particles preserved their ancestral memories, causing hereditary traits to revert or to jump across generations.

Because parents could pass along acquired diseases and anomalies – both moral and physical – Vandermonde believed that people needed a combination of sexual hygiene and physical education in order to regenerate themselves. This physical rebirth needed a form of racial intermixing: '[it is necessary] to renew the races, by mixing them every generation; this is the best means of perfecting the works of nature'.[59] He was impressed by recent experiments with hybridization and acclimatization conducted at the Jardin du Roi and the Académie des Sciences, which suggested that human agents could transform the natural qualities of living things.[60] Drawing upon botanical analogies, Vandermonde argued that when the same seeds were planted in the same soil, they inevitably degenerated; therefore, one must sow them in virgin lands, transporting the pollen from the city to the countryside, or vice versa. For him, racial intermixture caused greater vitality and beauty for upper-class and royal lineage. In his argument he used anthropological and travel literature to illuminate sexual and child-raising habits across the globe – showing what Mary Louise Pratt has called the planetary consciousness of Enlightenment thought – and he praised the racial miscegenation that had occurred since the discovery of the New World.[61]

In all this, Vandermonde underscored how heredity could transmit particular diseases from parents to children. He claimed that blind parents spawned deaf, dumb, or blind progeny; and he believed that syphilis, scrofula, scurvy and cancer were also hereditary. For these reasons, individuals should choose their partners with an eye for height, weight, size and temperament, and people with similar physical deformities should avoid marrying under any circumstances. After a couple had consummated

---

57   Vandermonde, *Essai*, vol. 1, p. 145.

58   Ibid., vol. 1, p. 159.

59   Ibid., vol. 1, p. 103. See also FMP, ms. 5116, 'Recueil d'observations tant de médecine que de chirurgie, avec un traité de la génération de l'homme et la manière de perfectionner l'espèce humaine et un recueil de plantes propres à chaque maladie', Oct. 1756.

60   Emma C. Spary, *Utopia's Garden: French Natural History from Old Regime to Revolution* (Chicago, 2000), pp. 112–14.

61   Mary Louise Pratt, *Imperial Eyes: Travel Writing and Transculturation* (London, 1992).

their union, they must stay monogamous, lest they exhaust their sexual energy and debase their offspring. In particular, Vandermonde cautioned against precocious and aged unions, and he noted that European Jews demonstrated the dangers of consanguinity, a custom that 'had degenerated that people'.[62] Following doctors like Brouzet, he also believed that urban women were too degenerate to nurse their children and he therefore encouraged doctors to find other ways to keep children well-fed and healthy.[63]

Le Camus, Brouzet and Vandermonde defined how medical and lay readers thought about moral degeneracy and decline. Their works inspired an entire medical writing on moral vices, as health crusaders explored the physical causes of degeneracy and depopulation. Many of these books – like abbé Lignac's *De l'homme et de la femme* (1772) and Gabriel Venel's *Essai sur la santé* (1776) – claimed that luxury and libertinism infected the family and was causing the French population to degenerate. Slowly but surely, they warned, degeneracy undermined European vitality.[64] Other physicians even doubted whether the present and future generation could assume the duties of an enlightened society. Dr Joseph Raulin asked, 'Feeble fathers, debilitated or valetudinarian mothers, given over or subject to such abuses, could they fertilize embryos, engender foetuses and form children who would not participate in their disorders or their effects and who were not their pathetic victims?'[65] Consequently, some medical crusaders argued that they must spread the gospel of moral hygiene by putting it in the hands of ordinary readers.

Self-help for sick elites: the example of Samuel Tissot

While the works of Le Camus, Brouzet and Vandermonde shaped public debate about physical and moral degeneracy, some medical crusaders apparently felt that their works were too abstract and erudite for a general readership. If high society were to reform itself, patriotic doctors should put this knowledge into a more accessible framework, so readers could grasp the magnitude of the problem and to learn how to regenerate themselves. J.-J. Rousseau's physician, Achille Le Bègue de Presle, conceived of such a project when he himself was recovering from a deadly illness. 'How many times', he wrote, 'has one risked his health and even his life, often for reasons that he would blush to admit, and for pleasures of which the intensity,

---

62   Vandermonde, *Essai*, vol. 1, pp. 112–13. Abbé Henri Grégoire approvingly incorporated Vandermonde's remarks about the physical degradation of European Jews into his pro-emancipationist tract, *Essai sur la régénération physique, morale et politique des juifs* (Metzt, 1788).

63   Vandermonde, *Essai*, vol. 2, pp. 51–54.

64   Jacques Ballexserd, *Dissertation sur cette question: quelles sont les causes principles de la mort d'un grand nombre d'enfans* (Geneva, 1775), pp. 1–2; Abbé de Lignac, *De l'homme et de la femme considérés physiquement dans l'état du mariage* (2 vols, Paris, 1772), vol. 1, p. 4–6.

65   Raulin, *De la conservation*, vol. 1, pp. xii–xiv.

grandeur or length are not worth the smallest price of evil with which they were purchased?'[66]

By posting such questions, doctors like Le Bègue were exploited a general interest in personal health. In the wake of secularism and rising bourgeois norms, 'health' became an ideal to be pursued for its own intrinsic value – to live, not for the next life, but instead for personal well-being in this one. During the Enlightenment, there appeared a large number of books that told aristocratic and bourgeois readers how to prevent disease and to live a long and healthy life. These books included Levache de Préville's *Méthode aisée pour conserver sa santé* (1752), C.-A. Vandermonde's *Dictionnaire portatif de santé* (1753), Duhamel de Monceau's *Moyens de conserver la santé* (1755) and James Mackenzie's *Histoire de la santé* (French edn, 1761).[67] In these books, hygienists identified with an upper-class clientele and gave their readers advice that substantially differed from what they prescribed for the poor and labouring classes. To remain healthy, they said, the reader must learn the 'six things non-natural', a key idea inherited from Galenic and Arabic medical corpus. Though traditional humoral medicine was declining, the doctrine of the non-naturals suited both the social realities and ideological outlook of the mid-eighteenth century.[68] Quite simply, the non-naturals were the external factors that caused disease. The 'six articles necessary for life' included the air, meat and drink, sleep and watching, exercise and rest, evacuations and obstructions, and the passions of the mind. These forces acted upon the individual's 'naturals' – the humours, the temperaments and faculties – while disregard caused the so-called 'contra-naturals' – diseases, their causes and their symptoms.[69] By learning the non-naturals, and the corollaries of hygiene and regimen, individuals could control their own bodies, especially in terms of diet, exercise and personal cleanliness.[70] Hygienists thus encouraged middle-class readers to look beyond present experiences and calculate future health and vitality. According to Dorinda Outram, these writers separated the exogenous (exterior) and endogenous (interior) sources of disease, and thereby 'abstracted' the body from its environment and isolated one person's bodily experience from another.[71] Only personal initiative determined health. Nothing else mattered.

Starting in the 1750s, medical reformers took this health interest and put it in the service of a more concrete social agenda, arguing that the leisured classes needed new health rules to cure immorality and physical degeneracy. In this discussion,

---

66 Achille Le Bègue de Presle, *Le conservateur de la santé* (Paris, 1763), p. ix.

67 Georges Vigarello, *Le propre et le sale: l'hygiène du corps depuis le moyen âge* (Paris, 1985), pp. 107–24.

68 William Coleman, 'Health and Hygiene in the *Encyclopédie*: A Medical Doctrine for the Bourgeoisie', *Journal of the History of Medicine and Allied Sciences* 29 (1974): 399–421.

69 ANM, ms. 1023, 'Cours d'hygiène, commencé le 18 aoust 1774'; and FMP, ms. 5067, Dr Dubernard, 'Cours des élémens d'hygiène', Toulouse, Year V [1797]. See Oswei Temkin, *Galenism: Rise and Decline of a Medical Philosophy* (Ithaca, 1973), pp. 103–08; and Peter H. Niebyl, 'The Non-Naturals', *Bulletin of the History of Medicine* 45 (1971): 486–92, at p. 491.

70 *Encyclopédie, ou dictionnaire raisonné des sciences, des arts et des métiers*, eds Denis Diderot et al. (36 vols. Geneva, 1777–79), s.v. 'Régime'.

71 Dorinda Outram, *The Body and the French Revolution: Sex, Class, and Political Culture* (New Haven, 1989), p. 47.

reformers walked a fine line as they simultaneously criticized and placated aristocrats and fashionable elites. After all, these two groups remained highly lucrative (and powerful) patients and patrons, and reformers knew their professional status and success needed their favour and grace. So enterprising health crusaders approached moral reform in an unusual but enterprising way, by drawing upon a literary device: the sentimental novel. As is well known, the modern novel emerged during the mid-1700s, as writers used new narrative techniques to give their books greater psychological depth and realism (what contemporaries called verisimilitude). In many ways, sentimental fiction dramatized conflicts within elite society, focusing upon lachrymose scenarios involving parental brutality, infidelity, incest, lust, greed, luxury and libertine violence.[72] These books allowed readers to explore values in conflict and to work through the consequences of individual choice and agency. In this literature, sentimental writers often used the body to incarnate qualities of vice and virtue. A famous example appears in P.-A.-F. Choderlos Laclos's *Les liaisons dangereuses* (1782), in which the villainous Marquise de Merteuil was disfigured by smallpox.[73] Medical reformers used similar tactics. Taking cues from novelists, they tried to show that personal hygiene promoted sentimental virtue while moral vice caused disease and death. They dramatized the struggle between virtue and vice as a struggle between health and sickness, while teaching how the iniquitous could find the path towards healthy righteousness. With good reason, some reviewers called these books a kind of 'medicinal novel', the doctor's version of sentimental fiction.[74]

Of this medical literature, Samuel Tissot offered the most scathing critique of French society. Tissot was a well-known figure in French science and letters who has attracted much recent scholarship. A tireless medical crusader who came from a Swiss Calvinist background, Tissot wrote a series of wildly popular books on personal health and hygiene, which he directed towards educated lay readers and provincial elites: *L'Onanisme* (1760), *Avis au peuple sur sa santé* (1761), *De la santé des gens de lettres* (1768) and *Essai sur les maladies des gens du monde* (1770). These themes converged in his magnum opus, a five-volume study of nervous disease that he published in 1778. In these books, Tissot pioneered a decidedly sentimental and novelistic style when discussing health issues, and his work had a wide resonance. In the course of his medical activism, Tissot befriended major medical reformers and met with prominent *philosophes* such as J.-J. Rousseau, who admired his dire warnings against masturbation. Like Rousseau, Tissot saw himself as an active 'friend of the people' and campaigned vigorously for health reform. As recent historiography has shown, he corresponded widely with patients and admirers from across Europe, and

---

72   Rustin, *La vice à la mode*, p. 36; and Lynn Hunt, *The Family Romance of the French Revolution* (Berkeley, 1992), pp. 17–52.

73   P.-A.-F. Choderlos de Laclos, *Les liaisons dangereuses*, ed. René Pomeau (Paris, 1996), pp. 511–12.

74   See Francis Bacon Lee's translation of S.-A. Tissot, *An Essay on the Disorders of People of Fashion* (London, 1771), p. vi.

advised his devotees on everything from the common cold to sick barnyard animals. Even queen Marie Antoinette owned copies of his books.[75]

Tissot took careful aim at the intelligentsia and fashionable elites. There was good reason to target these two groups: after all, intellectuals and patrician elites were the two groups that made up the Enlightenment 'republic of letters'. But this very novelty made moral critics suspicious of this alliance, and they concluded that it lacked cultural legitimacy. In response, intellectuals tried to justify themselves by showing that they did useful and important things, diligently exercising their minds for the benefit of humanity.[76] But doctors like Tissot doubted their claims, countering that Rococo high society had made people sick and infertile because of a flaccid and sensible lifestyle.[77] Whereas the poor died from dearth and hard work, fashion and manners killed the rich. As a consequence, Tissot wanted to unify 'the science of manners and that of health', giving his readers health advice so they could live more moral, healthy and productive lives.[78] Like sentimental novelists, then, Tissot exploited literary conventions to press a social agenda about class and sexual behaviour.

For Tissot, intellectuals suffered unique health problems. 'Quite some time ago', he said, 'it was remarked that the study of science was unfavourable to the health of the body. Men of letters consecrate their life to studies that are often useless, while they neglect the art of health'. Scholars suffered from two delirious habits, 'the assiduous travails of the spirit, and the continual inactivity of the body'. Using new models of the sensible body (also used by Brouzet and Vandermonde), Tissot argued that intellectual labour overwhelmed the brain, degenerated the medulla and exacerbated the body's sensibility. At first, the man of letters experienced anxiety and melancholia; soon the stomach and bowels became irritable and hypersensible. Hypochondria followed. He wrote, 'With my own eyes, I have seen those sick people who have been punished by this literary intemperance ... by spasms, convulsions and, finally, by the deprivation of all their senses'.[79]

But more was at stake than 'literary intemperance'. In short, he said, men of letters lived a totally unhealthy lifestyle. At their desks, they sat in ways that ruined good posture and digestion. Their studies were dark and damp. They burned the midnight oil and inhaled noxious fumes from their candles and fireplaces. They neglected personal hygiene and diet; they had bad teeth and gums; and they were always constipated and irritable. Ultimately, they turned into misanthropes because their intellectual pursuits consumed their minds and frazzled their nerves. In this polemic, Tissot excepted priests and doctors. These two occupations, he said, studied the most important things of all – the body and the soul – but they didn't learn about

---

75   On Tissot, see Antoinette Emch-Dériaz, *Tissot: Physician of the Enlightenment* (New York, 1992).

76   Daniel Roche, *Les républicains des lettres: gens de culture et Lumières au XVIIIe siècle* (Paris, 1988), pp. 219, 225–26, 229–32; Dena Goodman, *The Republic of Letters: A Cultural History of the French Enlightenment* (Ithaca, 1994), pp. 90–135.

77   S.-A. Tissot, *Essai sur les maladies des gens du monde*, 2d edn (Lausanne, 1770), pp. 2, 133.

78   Tissot, *De la santé*, p. 7.

79   Ibid., pp. 14–15, 28–29.

them in the abstract. Rather, they applied their learning in the real world by tending to the moral and physical needs of their respective flocks. Men of letters couldn't claim to do such useful and virtuous work: they even refused human company.

When Tissot attacked intellectual misanthropy, he was underscoring what was, for him, an even deeper problem. For him, the arts and sciences had alienated modern man; the republic of letters had turned from the human community and made itself sick and depraved. People should always cultivate civil life before they cultivated the arts and sciences; otherwise, one engendered the 'decadence of letters'.[80] He railed against intellectuals who became obsessed by their studies; a fixed object of desire, he maintained, made people mentally and physically unstable. But men of letters were blind to all this. As Tissot thought, they refused to admit that they had a dangerous occupation and that they needed to change their lives.

Here, Tissot drew an analogy between the man of letters and the republic of letters. To be healthy, people needed three things: good circulation, strong fibres and taut nerves. But scholarly life ruined all three: the nerves were frazzled, the blood didn't circulate and the muscles atrophied. The body weakened so much it couldn't discharge its accumulated waste. Imprisoned by his studies, the retentive scholar was literally overcome by his own excrement, much as the republic of letters was overcome by the worthless knowledge that spewed from Europe's printing presses. When discussing Leydian historian Juste-Lipse, a constipated hypochondriac, Tissot connected learning and excrement:

> He was only healed after he had defecated a mass shaped in the figure and colour of his intestines. *It was a gluey and viscous pituit, the fruit of his sedentary life and his studies,* which had little by little filled the intestinal canal; this pituit, having degenerated into rot, had attacked the entire animal economy; but the source having been destroyed, the patient quickly recovered his health. (my emphasis)[81]

For Tissot, the health of men of letters showed that not everyone could lead an enlightened life. He evoked Rousseau's words in the *Discourse on Sciences and Arts*: 'Let us not chase after a reputation which would escape us, and in the present state of things would never be worth what it cost'.[82] But Tissot amplified Rousseau's criticisms. In his eyes, some men were born geniuses, but not all men could become great thinkers. When second-rate people went beyond their native intelligence, they strained their minds and bodies, making themselves sick and socially worthless. By abandoning their natural place, men of letters caused themselves to degenerate.

Although Tissot believed that an unnatural lifestyle had made men of letters sick, he felt this was doubly true for the upper crust of French society. He explored this theme in his *Essai sur les maladies des gens du monde* (1770), in which he moved from the world of letters to the world of wealth and privilege. He targeted people of rank and fashion, what contemporaries called *les grands* or *le monde*. The shift is crucial. In *De la santé des gens de lettres*, Tissot had berated people of his

---

80 Ibid., p. 57.

81 Ibid., pp. 65–66.

82 J.-J. Rousseau, *The First and Second Discourses*, trans. Judith R. Masters (New York, 1964), p. 64.

own class and educational background; but in the *Essai*, he flatly told the privileged and wealthy that they were morally and physically depraved and that they were no longer respected by their social inferiors.[83] As he stated, he was forced to write this book because of what he had observed, from a distance, in high society. Fashionable elites had totally 'shattered' their health: they suffered irregularity, depression and 'continual anguish'. Therefore, he set out to tell his upper-class readers about their dangerous 'manner of living' and 'recall them to one less detrimental'. Tissot combined both scare tactics and moral exhortation, as he gave readers 'a general table of the *Errors of regimen*, and their evil consequences'. 'I repeat', he stressed, '*This subject was not my choice.*'[84]

To convince readers, Tissot gave his book a decided literary quality by comparing and contrasting, on every health issue, the imagined lifestyle of the decadent rich with that of rustic farmers, focusing upon diet, exercise, housing, air quality and so on. As Tissot saw it, people of fashion lived a dissolute life filled with 'luxury and dissipation' and, as a consequence, their health and sanity had declined precipitously. Tissot diagnosed the causes: a 'love of rank', cupidity, ambition, vanity, avarice, luxury, sensualism. Fashionable elites had 'disordered' their nerves because of passion, pleasure and peer pressure. Their bodies became sensible and weak and could not endure the most 'tender impressions'. They could neither understand nor control what they felt and experienced; everything excited them, everything consumed them. Like men of letters, people of fashion lost touch with their own bodies, becoming hypochondriacs and hysterics. As a consequence, they 'are often out of order without being able to assign the cause', and thus found 'in their nerves an insurmountable obstacle to happiness'.[85]

If misanthropy killed men of letters, socializing did in the upper crust. As Tissot saw it, urban elites were trapped in a vacuous world of appearance and style. Because they were so 'disagreeably inactive', people of fashion tried to 'kill time' with dissolute pleasures and 'factitious subterfuges'. The rich soon filled up their meaningless existence with socializing and consumer goods. As he noted, 'Unhappily, this false taste is contagious, for from those who invented it through necessity, it hath past as a fashion to such as it detriments very much. It is generally among the well-educated, who seem to propose it as the principle object of their pursuit.' By degrading taste, luxury degraded morality. In the end, the upper crust could only amuse themselves when they overturned 'the order of nature' and violated all the things that made normal people healthy and happy.[86]

In this sad state of affairs, the doctor could only try to diagnose and cure. But once the disease set in, it sapped energy and strength, weakening people in body and mind. Reason itself became useless as the nerves 'murder[ed] the mental faculties'. But since all of high society behaved in a depraved and decadent way, their compatriots accepted these habits as normal and desirable and even imitated them. And when the trendsetters become sick and degenerate, the sycophants imitated them again. As

---

83   On this point, see Vila, *Enlightenment and Pathology*, 188–96.
84   Tissot, *Essay*, pp. xii, 3, 163.
85   Ibid., pp. xiv, 3, 29–30, 35–36, 48, 62.
86   Ibid., pp. 11–12.

Tissot saw it, health and morality had simply become *unfashionable* in high society. 'What fashion', he exclaimed, 'is it but a fashion which renders it impossible to be happy and to discharge our duty properly?'[87]

To cure this insanity, urban elites must reject 'the pleasures of fashion' and recognize 'those pleasures that are real'. In short, real pleasure meant hard work, rustic simplicity and family love. But Tissot didn't want the upper crust to work, eat and dress like labourers and 'savages' – an absurd and impossible scenario, he said, not least because they were too physically weak – but he said they could self-consciously improve themselves by living moderately and exercising their bodies. Tragically, Tissot said, the affluent had all the means to live a long and healthy life, but they chose to wallow in filth and depravity. They then wanted remedies to suppress their symptoms but they never treated the underlying cause. Doctors could not help their patients when they refused simple health advice. He concluded:

> Leave me, like others, to behold with regret, that persons who, by their birth, station, and education, ought to give essential examples to society, and whose health is as important as their influence might be powerful, are precisely those who give the worst, because they continuously labour to destroy it, by following a mode of life which is directly opposite to it, and which is so far from increasing their pleasures, shortly deprives them of the very power of enjoying them, by throwing them into that state which excludes all.[88]

When Tissot attacked the upper crust and fellow men of letters for their unhealthy lifestyle, he was also attacking libertinism in general, both as a system of sexual free-living and philosophic freethinking. These views appeared, most dramatically, in his notorious book *Onanism*, which he first published in the vernacular in 1760. The book was an instant bestseller and was translated into all major European languages.[89] Usually, historians claim that Tissot's book sparked the Enlightenment's 'great fear' over masturbation, a panic that reflected a rising bourgeois asceticism or even a general crisis of the self.[90] But it should be emphasized that Tissot was also responding to specific concerns about degeneracy and decline among fashionable elites, and this concrete agenda directly informed his text. He wrote *Onanism* as a polemic against all sexual excess; he wanted to reform the bawdy and cheeky world of the mid-Enlightenment, with its sly mix of eroticism, materialism and philosophic scepticism.[91] By showing readers 'the influence of regimen upon the manners', doctors could teach 'medical morality' and cure libertine vices. Tissot promised,

---

87 Ibid., pp. 83, 162–63.

88 Ibid., pp. 83, 161–62.

89 See L. J. Jordanova, 'The Popularisation of Medicine: Tissot on Onanism', *Textual Practice* 1 (1987): 68–79.

90 See Jean Stengers and Anne Van Neck, *Histoire d'une grande peur: la masturbation* (Brussels, 1984); and Thomas W. Laqueur, *Solitary Sex: A Cultural History of Masturbation* (New York, 2003). For a recent overview, see Michael Stolberg, 'An Unmanly Vice: Self-Pollution, Anxiety, and the Body in the Eighteenth Century', *Social History of Medicine* 13 (2000): 1–22.

91 On the erotic underside of Enlightenment culture, see especially Darnton, *Forbidden Best-Sellers*; and Lynn A. Hunt (ed.), *The Invention of Pornography: Obscenity and the Origins of Modernity, 1500–1800* (New York, 1993).

'this would be the surest means of preventing that decay which is complained of in human nature, and perhaps of restoring to her, in a few generations, the strength and power of our ancestors'.[92]

For Tissot, masturbation epitomized everything that was wrong in French society. As he saw it, the masturbator sinned 'by violating all laws, [by] trampling upon all the sentiments and designs of nature'. The disease was spreading like wildfire, infecting schools and whole communities; once the doctor had learned the signs and symptoms, he could spot this 'internal disorder' everywhere. Masturbators were 'sallow', 'pale', 'effeminate', 'lazy' and 'base'. They went blind or insane or became consumptive. They could no longer have normal sex and semen constantly dripped from their genitals. Some even ejaculated blood. The men descended into an 'intense melancholy' whilst women fell into 'hysterical fits' or 'shocking vapors'. For adolescents, early sex experiences stunted their growth and Tissot doubted whether they could 'ever become vigorous and robust'. As they became addicted to their habit, they turned into 'lascivious brutes' and 'less resembled a living creature than a corpse'. The end was bleak, as the masturbator descended into madness and death; it was an end filled with an anguish that extended beyond any known pain.[93]

In this book, Tissot did not just deal with masturbation: all non-procreative sex, he stressed, could disrupt mind and body, and he presented cutting-edge medical science to support this claim. Like prominent physiologists, Tissot believed that semen was a concentrated form of the animal spirits that filled the nerves and acted as medium to communicate between soul and body. During sex, blood filled the pericranium and distended the nerves. The body became 'enfeebled' and could not resist nervous 'impressions'; the person then experienced 'irregular perspiration', 'depraved digestions' and 'weakness of the brain, and of the nervous system'. In extreme cases, sex could cause apoplexies, convulsions, insanity and epilepsy. Indeed, there was little difference between an orgasm and insanity. Listing example after example, Tissot said, 'The violent palpitations, which sometimes accompany coition, are always convulsive symptoms'.[94]

In all his writings, Tissot denounced the social breakdown and anomie caused by modern life. In the debate between the ancients and moderns, the moderns had won, but at a terrible price to health and morality. Tissot bemoaned that his compatriots had lost moral and civic virtue; individualism and self-interest had overturned faith in God, family and country. These problems were exemplified by men of letters, people of fashion and libertines: they pursued their own desires until they lost all sense of values and shut themselves from their community. Like masturbators, they only cared about themselves. They consumed but they did not create. They took but did not give back. They indulged their desires and poisoned their bodies until they lost all reason and 'plunged [themselves] in a sea of misery, and without perhaps the hopes of a single plank to escape upon'.[95] Masturbation, for Tissot, literally

---

92   S.-A. Tissot, *Onanism, or, A treatise upon the disorders produced by masturbation* (London, 1766), pp. xii, 150.

93   Ibid., pp. 5, 25, 41–42, 85, 145, 152–53.

94   Ibid., pp. 59, 61–62; for specific case studies, see pp. 38, 40, 142.

95   Ibid., p. 76.

embodied mental and economic solipsism. In an astonishing passage, Tissot drew out this analogy by comparing habitual masturbators to intellectuals:

> Nothing so much weakens as that continual bent of the mind, ever occupied with the same object. The masturbator, entirely devoted to his filthy meditations, is subject to the same disorders as the man of letters, who fixes his attention upon a single question; and this excess is almost constantly prejudicial. That part of the brain, which is then occupied, makes an effort similar to that of a muscle, which has been for a long time greatly extended; the consequences of which are such a continued motion in the part as cannot be stopped, or such a fixed attention, that the idea cannot be changed: this is the case with masturbators; or else an incapacity to act at all. Although exhausted by perpetual fatigue, they are seized with all the disorders incident to the brain, melancholy, catalepsy, epilepsy, imbecility, the loss of sensation, weakness of the nervous system, and a variety of similar disorders.[96]

In this manner, Tissot took all the fears about physical and moral degeneracy and boiled them down to one simple maxim: Don't masturbate. Like consumerism and rakishness, everyone was doing it. Everyone knew about it. But no one talked about the dangers. For Tissot, the cure was simple. He told readers: Stop it. Take control of your life. In a world of self-indulgence, this is where self-discipline began. By not masturbating, a person took the first step towards leading a healthy and responsible life, a life in which they were happy and self-satisfied because they could distinguish between real needs and phantasmagoric desires. He wrote, 'It is nevertheless of great consequence in physic, as well as morality, to know how to sacrifice the present for the future; by neglecting this rule, the world is overrun with unhappy objects and valetudinarians'.[97] Tissot thus urged a kind of godly asceticism and work ethic that finds an analogy in Benjamin Franklin's homespun almanacs; but in this case, he spoke less to his own social class than to upper-class patients and patrons.

If masturbators couldn't stop themselves, then others had to do it for them. Unlike his books on men of letters and people of fashion, Tissot became much more controlling and paranoid when he dealt with masturbators, and these concerns were echoed by other moral hygienists.[98] Doctors could try to cure the masturbator, but more often than naught an 'enlightened father' needed to put his house in order. Fathers must diligently control their children and their servants, and needed to watch 'what is done in the darkest recesses of his house'. Tissot exhorted them '[to] use that vigilance which discovers the coppice where the deer has taken shelter, when it has escaped all other eyes: this is always possible when it is earnestly pursued'.[99] Other doctors agreed. As they saw it, young people learned to masturbate in the unsupervised and shady margins of daily life, whether from the domestic servants or from their friends at school. Masturbating was a dangerous byproduct of commerce

---

96   Ibid., p. 75.

97   Ibid., 133.

98   SRM 124, d. 10, Marigues, 'Observations sur quelques effets de la masturbation sur l'oeconomie animale', 21 May 1782; and SEM, 'Mémoires et observations', c. 4,Thillaye, 'Rapport sur des modèles de ceintures destinées à empêcher les enfants de se livrer à la masturbation' [post-1800].

99   Tissot, *Onanism*, pp. 44–45.

and sociability. These intimate spaces faded into a twilight of loss and addiction, beyond which lay only madness and death.[100] Doctors must seize these evils and bring them into the light; in a transparent world, public and private vices could not last. By rooting them out, doctors could regenerate society and make their patients healthy and happy again.

Vaporous women and the moral cure

For moral hygienists like Le Camus, Brouzet, Vandermonde and Tissot, patients must balance real needs and personal desires; if not, people became alienated from their own bodies and fell into sickness and degeneracy. Their message was simple: individuals must learn to control themselves in a luxurious and libertine world; personal hygiene, they promised, could strengthen mind and body and helped individuals navigate the decadent world of old regime France. In this sense, individuals became personally responsible for their own regeneration: presumably, concerned citizens would apply moral hygiene in their daily lives after doctors had opened their eyes to the dangers of luxury and libertinism. This was all fine for literate and affluent men, men upon whom doctors could count upon to use their reason and to understand their own self-interest. But what of those groups, asked some doctors, who could not reason for themselves and who lacked the requisite self-control?

Doctors saw this an acute problem for one group of people: women. By the mid-century, moral crusaders started to blame the perceived morbid crisis upon elite urban women, and thereby plunged into acrimonious debates about women's participation in public culture, especially within court networks and fashionable salons.[101] This debate appeared in a variety of contexts, from philosophic treatises like J.-J. Rousseau's *Émile* (1762) to J.-L. David's neoclassical images.[102] These moral critics rejected *philosophes* such as Voltaire, Denis Diderot and G.-L. de Buffon, who had defended feminine sociability and who believed that the salon and polite society had advanced civilized behaviour. By contrast, moral critics claimed that sociable women had undermined family values and were thus making themselves and their country sick.[103]

Of course, doctors had long believed that women were inherently sick. These views originated in Hippocratic and Aristotelian teachings, which had emphasized a woman's wet and humid temperament, her wandering womb and periodic hemorrhaging. These natural qualities served a teleological goal: for theologians and

---

100 Nicolas Chambon de Montaux, *Des maladies des filles* (2 vols, Paris, 1785), vol. 2, pp. 92–93.

101 See Sylvana Tomaselli, 'The Enlightenment Debate on Women', *History Workshop*, no. 20 (1985): 101–24.

102 On this literature, see Madelyn Gutwirth, *The Twilight of the Goddesses: Women and Representation in the French Revolutionary Era* (New Brunswick, 1992).

103 On debates over female sociability and the salon, see Goodman, *The Republic of Letters*, pp. 12–51, 233–80.

doctors, God had made women weak and fickle so they could serve men, procreate and raise children.[104]

The Enlightenment really hadn't changed these attitudes, especially within medical circles. When discussing the female body and disease, doctors usually focused upon problems involving menstruation, pregnancy, childbirth, breast-feeding and menopause, and they attributed all sickness to the womb and feminine weakness.[105] Often, these doctors then moved from obstetrical and gynecological issues to generalize about female nature and ideal gender roles, claiming the female body suggested a particular social and biological destiny. For Dr Nicolas Chambon de Montaux – who later became the mayor of Paris during the French Revolution – woman's flesh was 'humid and flaccid' and the cellular tissue was very fatty and 'engorged with liquids'. The bones and muscles seemed less 'solid', the pulse was frail, and the blood vessels were weak.[106] For these reasons, Dr Coutouly wrote in a 1786 manuscript, female diseases were more deadly and difficult to cure than those of men.[107] As a consequence, Dr Jean Astruc – who composed a sprawling six-volume work on women's health – claimed that the best preventive medicine was marriage itself, because a woman could only alleviate her obstructed body through conjugal duties and motherhood.[108]

Medical attitudes reflected shifting cultural values. As several historians have argued, Enlightenment thinkers – despite their token promises of liberty, equality and the pursuit of happiness – actually degraded women and lowered their social and cultural status. According to Londa Schiebinger and Thomas Laqueur, modern ideas about sex difference first emerged sometime during the eighteenth century. In this period, science and medicine shifted from a 'one-sex model' to a 'two sex model' of sexual dimorphism.[109] Doctors and naturalists no longer saw men and women as anatomically homologous, distinguished simply by humoral qualities: rather, they thought men and women were sexually distinct beings and inscribed sexual difference all over the body, from the genitalia to the skeleton.[110] At the same time, doctors and naturalists moved from the old Galenic model of conception, which

---

104 See Yvonne Knibiehler and Catherine Fouquet, *La femme et les médecins: analyse historique* (Paris, 1983), pt 1; and Londa Schiebinger, *The Mind Has No Sex? Women in the Origins of Modern Science* (Cambridge, MA, 1989), pp. 161–70.

105 FMP, ms. 5192, fol. 572, Jean Astruc, 'Traité des maladies des femmes en général' (n.d.); FMP, ms. 5087, 'Extrait des leçons de Mr. Astruc' (1737); SRM 201, d. 14, Gautier, chirurgien à Saint-Hilaire, 'Mémoire sur les règles des femmes', 4 Sept. 1788; Gérard Fitzgerald, *Traité des maladies des femmes* (Paris, 1758), pp. 60–63, 235–39, 304–08.

106 Chambon de Montaux, *Des maladies des filles*, vol. 1, pp. 3–7, and *Des maladies des femmes* (2 vols, Paris, 1784), vol. 1, pp. xxvi–xxx.

107 ANM, ms. 1025, fol. I, Coutouly, 'Des maladies des femmes en général' (1786).

108 Jean Astruc, *Traité des maladies des femmes* (6 vols, Paris, 1761–65), vol. 1, pp. 122–23.

109 Thomas Laqueur, *Maxing Sex: Body and Gender from the Greeks to Freud* (Cambridge, MA, 1990), pp. 149–92.

110 Thomas Laqueur, 'Amor Veneris, vel Dulcedo Appeletur', in M. Feher (ed.), *Fragments for a History of the Human Body* (New York, 1989), pp. 90–131; Londa Schiebinger, 'Skeletons in the Closet: The First Illustrations of the Female Skeleton in Eighteenth-Century

emphasized that both partners contributed to procreation, to a new ovist model, which devalued sexual activity in generation. In so doing, doctors elided female orgasm from medical texts and now claimed that women were sexually passive and frigid beings.[111] As François Azouvi has put it, doctors effectively turned women into a 'model of pathology'.[112]

What is often overlooked in these accounts is the social and cultural forces that changed medical beliefs. In the old regime, pervasive fears about degeneracy and decline largely shaped these attitudes about women. Here again, doctors used ideas about the sensibility to frame a model of social pathology. This approach characterizes Louis de Lacaze's *Idée de l'homme* (1755) and Victor de Sèze's *Recherches phisiologiques* (1786). According to Lacaze, male sensibility was concentrated in three areas: the brain, the gastric regions and the so-called phrenic centre, the diaphragm. Health occurred when one region balanced the other. The diaphragm anchored the whole system because it was connected to the entrails and nervous system. As a consequence, it moderated the phrenic forces as 'the first cause that determines the necessary interplay of functions in the animal economy'.[113]

For Lacaze, women posed special physiological problems. In women, the uterus disturbed this bodily equilibrium, averting the phrenic forces directed towards the diaphragm. In this sense, the womb accumulated excessive energy until it spasmodically discharged its waste in its monthly crisis. To stay healthy, women must balance the forces of the womb and diaphragm; otherwise, the body suffered what he called 'revolutions', which 'must, by consequence, produce distressing accidents'. Unfortunately, the phrenic centre needed to counteract the womb's sepulchral hunger; therefore, women constantly needed to revitalize 'through [the medium of] sensation, the action of [the diaphragm]'. In other words, she must *increase* her sensibility to keep herself healthy, but this increase exposed her to nervous disease.[114]

Like Lacaze, Victor de Sèze argued that sensibility and weakness marked women as 'a being apart', with their unique 'passions, morals, temperament, health and illnesses'.[115] She was weak because nature had marked her for a 'sedentary lifestyle' of maternity; but her inconstant mind kept children from consuming her 'tenderness'. In theory, sensibility supported woman's corporeal 'revolutions' and diminished morbid threats: 'Nature is always just in how she dispenses her gifts.' Though nature subjugated women to disease and 'devour[ed]' them in pain, it still gave them ways

Anatomy', in Catherine Callagher and Thomas Laqueur (eds), *The Making of the Modern Body: Sexuality and Society in the Nineteenth Century* (Berkeley, 1987), pp. 83–106.

111 Thomas Laqueur, 'Orgasm, Generation, and the Politics of Reproductive Biology', in Callagher and Laqueur, *Modern Body*, pp. 1–41.

112 François Azouvi, 'Woman as a Model of Pathology in the Eighteenth Century', trans. Michael Crawcour, *Diogenes*, no. 115 (1981): 22–36.

113 Louis de Lacaze, *Idée de l'homme physique et moral* (Paris, 1755), pp. 74, 124. My overview of Lacaze follows Azouvi's lucid analyis.

114 Ibid., 280-81, 282; see also SRM 116, d. 2, Balthagard Laugier, 'La névropathie, ou mémoire sur les maladies nerveuses, proprement dites', 7 Mar. 1786.

115 Victor de Sèze, *Recherches phisiologiques et philosophiques sur la sensibilité ou la vie animale* (Paris, 1786), pp. 217–18.

to dull these impressions. But like men of letters and people of fashion, modern life had imbalanced these physical qualities, demonstrating how 'social institutions have corrupted that equitable distribution of goods and evil; laws, morals and, above all, [public] opinion weigh ceaselessly upon this lovable sex, [and] aggravate the natural yoke under which she is subordinate'.[116]

Doctors returned to the theme already explored by Tissot – that modern life made people sick – but they found this was doubly true for women. In the 1750s and 1760s, these fears exploded in the hysteria ('vapors') panic, which suddenly consumed the medical scene and touched off an unprecedented public discussion.[117] It began in 1756 when C.-A. Vandermonde and Pierre Hunauld warned that hysteria had become 'à la mode' in high society and other doctors quickly jumped on the bandwagon.[118] For them, hysteria exemplified a deeper physical and moral degradation, and they were horrified that hysteria manifested itself in convulsive display but left no lesions on the body.[119] By 1783, the Royal Society of Medicine believed the epidemic was serious enough to ask for opinions from their correspondence networks. In response, provincial practitioners fervently responded to the call, claiming that nervous disorders were spreading in the countryside.[120]

Traditionally, physicians believed that uterine miasma caused hysteria; but Enlightenment doctors, armed with new physiological models, quickly blamed it upon hypersensibility. According to Joseph Raulin, 'The sensibility attached to the essence of women, or to particular constitutions that are more susceptible than others, assures that their fibers, often taken to the highest point of delicacy, are affected by the least accident; here is the source of an infinite number of hysterical symptoms and often the most violent vapors'.[121] The body degenerated into contractions and spasms and thus caused syncopes, apoplexy and apparent death. The attack was intensified by factors such as menstrual suppression, spermatic retention and masturbation. In a series of well-received books, Pierre Pomme blamed hysteria

---

116 Ibid., pp. 221–25.

117 See Ilza Veith, *Hysteria: The History of a Disease* (Chicago, 1965); Paul Hoffmann, *La femme dans la pensée des Lumières*, 2d edn (Geneva, 1995), 175–81; and, most recently, Vila, *Enlightenment and Pathology*, pp. 229–238.

118 Pierre Hunauld, *Dissertation sur les vapeurs et les pertes de sang* (Paris, 1756), p. 42, quoted in Hoffmann, *La femme*, p. 181. Subsequent works include Joseph Raulin's *Traité des affections vaporeuses* (1758), Boissier de Sauvages's *Pathologia methodica* (1758), Pierre Pomme's *Traité des affections vaporeuses* (1760), J.-B. Pressavin's *Nouveau traité des vapeurs* (1770), D. T. de Bienville's *Traité de la fureur utérine* (1778), and E.-P.-C. Beauchêne's *De l'influence des affections de l'âme* (1781).

119 Marat, *De l'homme*, vol. 2, pp. 288–90; Barthez, *Nouveaux élémens*, vol. 2, pp. 174–75.

120 For responses, see SRM 138, d. 14, Estienne, letter of 8 Nov. 1786; SRM 139, d. 9, correspondence Bissout, n. p. (1790); SRM 174, d. 30, Pajot des Charmes, report to S.R.M., Paris, 7 Mar. 1788; and SRM 178, d. 6, Destrapière, 'Mémoire sur la topographie du pays d'Aunis', 19 Dec. 1777.

121 Joseph Raulin, *Traité des affections vaporeuses du sexe* (Paris, 1758), p. xix.

upon a dryness [*racornissement*] of the nervous system, which ought to be treated by intensive bathing and humidifying techniques.[122]

In their writings, doctors blamed nervous degeneracy upon luxury and libertinism, contrasting upper-class debauchery with a sentimental image of rural life and rustic virtue.[123] According to E.-P.-C. Beauchêne, rural women avoided hysteria because they did hard physical work and didn't overuse their simple minds. Quite simply, they lacked 'abstract' or 'metaphysical' ideas – they only cared about religious faith and moral duties – and they rarely wandered from their 'prescribed' roles. Unlike fashionable elites, country women did not drift in permissive social circles; instead, they only cared about the simple 'needs of nature'. Daily chores, seasons and festivals gave country women a good mental outlook and a hearty endurance, attributes that were lost in upper-class life. This was because urban living produced an insatiable appetite for pleasure, 'that tyrant of the large cities' – and these unnatural desires exhausted the body's sensibility, predisposing it to nervous disorder.[124] According to prominent hysteria experts, the most disturbing element was that urban decadence had also effeminized men, making them hysterical as well.[125] For all these reasons, Dr Lurde wrote that nervous diseases were 'so commonplace, that except for women of the countryside, for whom luxury and idleness are unknown and who live a hard and labourious life, there are very few who, from one time to another, do not experience some form of attack'.[126]

Given the shocking prevalence of the vapors in high society, women thus needed moral hygiene to regenerate them. This more 'natural' lifestyle, in short, meant submitting to male authority and embracing domestic duties. Happy submission meant a healthy life. For Raulin, domestic hygiene could decrease feminine sensibility and strengthen their temperaments. Women must follow a direct regimen – preferably supervised by the doctor – because they were too weak and 'stupid' to take care of themselves. He complained, 'It is after having ruined her health and destroyed her temperament by excess and abuse, she lacks sufficient courage to practice the means of self-conservation.'[127] In a notorious passage, Beauchêne assumed a more violent tone:

> I will say to men: barricade otherwise your homes, change your lifestyle, assure the morals and happiness of your women, by occupying them in a useful and agreeable manner, by leaving no time for them to form their own desires. Destroy your theatres, or at least drive

122 SRM 200, d. 1, 'Mémoire sur les maladies nerveuses', 7 Mar. 1786; SRM 200, d. 1, Dr A.G.F.D.S.B., 'Question de la Société royale de médecine qui exige de déterminer quels sont les caractères des maladies nerveuses proprement dites; telles que l'hystéricisme et l'hipochondria [*sic*]' (1786); Pierre Pomme, *Nouveau recueil de pièces relatives au traitement des vapeurs* (Paris, 1771), p. 177.

123 E.-P.-C. Beauchêne, *De l'influence des affections de l'âme dans les maladies nerveuses des femmes* (Montpellier and Paris, 1781), p. 9; Pierre Pomme, *Traité des affections vaporeuses des deux sexes*, 2d edn (Lyon, 1765), pp. 14–15.

124 Beauchêne, *De l'influence*, pp. 1–4.

125 Raulin, *Traité*, p. 44; Pomme, *Traité*, pp. 15–16; Beauchêne, *De l'influence*, pp. 24–25.

126 SRM 200, d. 1, Lurde, 'Mémoire sur les maladies nerveuses', 7 Mar. 1786.

127 Raulin, *Traité*, p. xxxii.

away dramas or modern tragedies. Burn those little books, where the stylistic affection, the unrealistic content and the exaggeration of sentiments are the least faults. Incessantly call your children to the feet of their mother: her affection for them will soon become the most lively of her affections; and this pure sentiment will no longer cause her migraines, vapors or melancholia. Recall for her those happy times when a mother was honoured by her fertility, and when the most agreeable spectacle for her was a numerous family that she was happy to form for virtue's sake.[128]

Within this context, Pierre Roussel first published his *Système physique et moral de la femme* in 1775. In this important book, Roussel tried to explain women's true nature and set out the guidelines of good health and hygiene. With good reason, Roussel has interested recent historians and literary critics. A Montpellier graduate who moved through Parisian high society, Roussel was the first physician to explore sensibility as it related to sex. His *Système de la femme* rapidly became a classic Enlightenment book: it went through five editions by 1809, earning him the epitaph as the 'Buffon of the fair sex', and it was constantly cited by doctors and *philosophes*.[129] In 1815, the authoritative *Dictionnaire des sciences médicales* still recommended that doctors read him.[130] Although historians have criticized Roussel for his misogyny, both Elizabeth A. Williams and Anne C. Vila have recently analyzed his work within its medical context, arguing that historians should understand him within the evolving discourse on sensibility rather than debates over female incommensurability.[131] Nevertheless, my analysis here underscores another of Roussel's themes: his overwhelming desire to regenerate women. Despite the existing books on female physiology and pathology, Roussel believed he was literally rediscovering the truth of female nature. In his view, his work gave readers an alternative image of the physical and moral qualities of women, one that considered their normal roles beyond their current degeneracy. He promoted, in part, an agenda of moral reform and he clearly wanted his book to be the medical counterpart to Rousseau's educational writings about women.[132]

Roussel contended that doctors should study women as a whole being and not just focus upon her anatomical or pathological peculiarities. Moreover, doctors should consider more than her ideal attributes or her current degradation; rather, they must study her in 'the state of perfect health' to understand her natural and civil roles. In Roussel's hands, human sexuality assumed an ontological dimension, something that went to the very heart of what it meant to live and to be human. For him, all living things could preserve themselves, but they could not reproduce. As a result, nature created a sexual division of labour: hence, in biological and social

---

128 Beauchêne, *De l'influence*, pp. 7–8.

129 Hoffmann, *La femme*, pp. 141–52; and Yvonne Knibiehler, 'Les médecins et la "nature féminine" au temps du code civil', *Annales: E.S.C.* 31 (1976): 824–45.

130 'Femme', *Dictionnaire des sciences médicales, par une société de médecins et chirurgiens* (60 vols, Paris, 1812–22).

131 See Elizabeth A. Williams, *The Physical and the Moral: Anthroplogy, Physiology, and Philosophical Medicine in France, 1750–1850* (Cambridge and New York, 1994), pp. 54–56; Anne C. Vila, 'Sex and Sensibility: Pierre Roussel's *Système physique et morale de la femme*', *Representations*, no. 52 (1995): 76–93.

132 Pierre Roussel, *Système physique et moral de la femme* (Paris, 1775), pp. iii–iv.

terms, men and women were interdependent, since 'one only sees in the other the means of happiness and the complement of their being'. But this sexual difference transcended the anatomical parts of the body. On the contrary, sex penetrated every part of a woman's body. As he said, sexuality 'extends by more or less sensible nuances to all her parts, so that woman is not a woman by all the facets by which she can be envisaged'.[133]

For Roussel, sensibility inscribed sexual difference upon the organism, saturating each anatomical and physiological detail. In this manner, he rejected philosophers who believed that a person's environment nurtured mind and body, and he particularly dismissed the sensualist thinker C.-A. Helvétius, 'who regards the mind as the sole result of education'. As Roussel saw it, women contained 'a radical, innate difference' within them that transcended all educational and environmental forces. Any reasoned observer could discern the pleasing forms of the female body and 'this difference' in form and matter, he said, 'also extends to all parts lost to sight'. Women had a soft and fat cellular tissue and rapid pulse. They were more vocal, mobile and nimble than men. Moreover, their bodies were excessively sensible; they were besieged by catastrophic impressions, not just from menstruation, pregnancy and menopause, but from everything else they experienced in their daily lives.[134]

Sex difference unfolded throughout the female life course. Though Roussel, much like Vandermonde, believed in an epigenetic form of generation, he did not recognize sexual difference in the human embryo, as Lazarro Spallanzani and J.-L. Moreau de la Sarthe later claimed in the 1780s and 1790s. For Roussel, children demonstrated few signs of sexual distinction: they were similar in appearance and possessed the same delicate organization. But as the child approached puberty, the body was radically transformed. The male body became denser, darker and forceful, as his mind and body acquired the traits he needed to protect and provide for his weaker sexual partner. By contrast, women hardly developed at all. 'Woman', Roussel wrote, 'in advancing toward puberty, seems to differ less than man from her primitive constitution. Delicate and tender, she always conserves something of a temperament more proper to children.'[135] Of course, women's ontogenic growth was appropriate for the biological and social role they assumed when mature – that is, motherhood – but they remained, when compared to men, childlike and dependent.

Roussel dismissed other doctors and moralists who believed that a woman's body kept her from being useful and happy. When one considered that the natural causes of misery were few, human suffering had to originate from moral causes. He noted, 'We shall see that woman, for whom the same variation of sensations resists continuance, and which save [her] from that focus of reflection that torments so many thinking beings, is perhaps less removed than man from the happiness that human nature comports'. Woman's sensibility tempered male cruelty and spared her the deeper agony of a reflective life, but it prohibited her from intellectual labour and cultural visibility.[136]

---

133 Ibid., pp. 1–2, 143–44.
134 Ibid., pp. 16–17, 19 n. 1, 21 n. 1.
135 Ibid., p. 6.
136 Ibid., pp. 28–29, 31–32.

These were the ideals, but all was not well in the upper-class household. For Roussel, women had infiltrated political and aesthetic spaces. As a result, they shattered sexual complementation, uprooted healthy domestic roles and caused physical and moral degeneration. He distinguished natural sexual roles – pregnancy and breast-feeding – from the coquettish and sentimental world that women now lived in. Indeed, menstruation ('the sign [and] measure of health') measured this dislocation. Roussel assured that women menstruated less in the countryside than in the city; rural women could even conceive 'without ever having menstruated'. Here, he followed J.-J. Rousseau who asserted – like many travel writers – that women in the state of nature did not menstruate: '[T]here must have existed a time when women were not subordinate to this uncomfortable tribute, and the natural flux, far from being a natural institution, is an artificial need contracted [outside] the state of nature.' Leisure and luxury caused an overabundance of humoral blood and made women menstruate. As evidence, he argued that nervous and effeminate men also had periodical hemorrhaging, as seen with nosebleeds and hemorrhoids.[137]

Like Tissot with intellectuals and fashionable elites, Roussel advocated moral hygiene, and he later wrote a two-volume book, for women, on this subject.[138] Nevertheless, he never spoke as a legislator or moralist; rather, he was a physician, whose primary concern was preventive and therapeutic responses. However, his *Système de la femme*, ostensibly a tool for moral reform, did not speak to women readers; rather, he wrote the book for male doctors and philosophers, who would use it as a weapon to reform social abuses. This is an important point. As Roussel told male readers, a woman's proper place was in the home; when she left it, she caused disease and disruption.

Significantly, doctors such as Roussel ignored female mortality as it related to pregnancy and childbirth (about 11.5 deaths per 1000 women in the first sixty days after childbirth).[139] Rather, they generally criticized libertinism, luxury and, above all, women's visibility in public life. There was another paradox: several physicians, while arguing that 'very sensible subjects rarely attain a long life', admitted that the demographic evidence, compiled by natural historians, showed that women had lower mortality than men.[140] Nevertheless, most medical writers consigned women to morbidity and pain, and they believed that aristocratic and bourgeois women were utterly degenerate. These attitudes were also shared by women reformers. For example, Marie Thiroux d'Arconville and Anne de Miremont believed contemporary women were frivolous and degenerate, and that they were partially responsible for

---

137 Ibid., pp. 178–79, 196–97, 370–71.

138 Pierre Roussel, *Médecine domestique, ou moeurs simples de conserver la santé* (3 vols, Paris, 1790–92).

139 Hector Gutierrez and Jacques Houdaille, 'La mortalité maternelle en France aux XVIIIe siècle', *Population* 38 (1983): 975–83. Demographers usually attribute the increase of female deaths over men among the 25–40 age group to maternal mortality. See Alain Bideau, Jacques Dupâquier and Hector Gutierrez, 'La mort quantifiée', in *Histoire de la population française* (Paris, 1995), vol. 2, pp. 222–43.

140 Barthez, *Nouveaux élémens*, vol. 2, pp. 251, 298; de Sèze, *Recherches*, p. 229.

their sorry state.[141] In their *De l'éducation physique et morale des femmes* (1779), Riballier and Cosson thought that poor physical education caused women to degenerate; but should they learn good hygiene they would become better mothers and educators.[142]

By the 1770s, then, medical practitioners had moved from intellectuals and libertine rakes and had made upper-class women largely responsible for physical and moral degeneracy. As women neglected their natural family values, they became sick and infertile and dragged down the family and all of society with them. To make this point, doctors drew upon one chilling image: the unheeded cries of the infant child, murdered by maternal neglect. For this reason, women must control their health and hygiene at all costs. This was particularly true for pregnant mothers. As physicians saw it, prenatal behaviour could degrade or improve the child's inherited constitution; indeed, the expecting mothers became completely responsible for their children's health. According to Dr J.-C. Desessartz, all children – both the born and the unborn – had natural rights; maternal neglect was a form of homicide and needed to be censured by husbands, the church and the state.[143] As a consequence, pregnant women must follow a careful regimen of moral hygiene, and avoid things such as the salon, intellectual activity, dancing, singing, constraining dresses, corsets and sexual intercourse.[144] Doctors repeated this point. To cure this sickness and conflict in the body politic, women must learn a new science of manners and hygiene, one that extolled the dignity of motherhood and child education.

Conclusion: families at risk

By the time that Roussel published his *Système de la femme*, a significant element of the medical community had come to believe that the French nation was physically and morally depraved. This belief had been first invented by doctors such as Antoine Le Camus, N. Brouzet de Béziers and C.-A. Vandermonde, and it was subsequently exploited and disseminated by self-help writers such as Samuel Tissot, child hygienists such as J.-C. Desessartz and Jacques Ballexserd, and self-appointed hysteria experts such as Joseph Raulin, Pierre Pomme and E.-P.-C. Beauchêne. Generally, doctors believed that people could regenerate society through self-help; therefore, mothers and fathers must learn personal hygiene to improve their minds, bodies and progeny. Personal virtue and patriotic sentiment demanded this awareness. To avoid these diseases, patients must liberate themselves from debased desires and return to traditional family values. Indeed, for a number of these medical activists, moral degeneracy had become somewhat of an article of faith, a lens through which

---

141 Lindsay Wilson, *Women and Medicine in the French Enlightenment: The Debate over 'Maladies des Femmes'* (Baltimore, 1993)., pp. 95–96, 194 n. 43.

142 Riballier and Cosson, *De l'éducation physique et morale des femmes* (Paris and Brussels, 1779), p. 67.

143 J. C. Desessartz, *Traité de l'éducation corporelle des enfans en bas-âge*, 2d edn (1760; Paris, Year VII), p. 17.

144 Ballexserd, *Dissertation sur cette question*, pp. 12–15, and *Dissertation sur l'éducation physique* (Paris, 1762), pp. 5–11; Nicolas, *Le cri*, p. 38.

they looked at the world and demanded social and moral reform. As Dr Delaporte passionately wrote, 'By cutting the illness at its source, the murderous germ will fade forever; and all will lead to a future age where we shall observe those natural laws to which our fathers had owed their existence'.[145]

Yet, as doctors suggested, diagnosing the problem was not enough, because society had not cured the underlying causes. At first, they berated fathers for not disciplining their wives and children and for forgetting their domestic and patriotic patrimony.[146] However, they soon looked for other ways to treat society. Therefore, health activists put less faith in individual initiative and asked public authorities to make physical and moral hygiene into public policy. For example, Dr Coffinières hoped that the government would soon cure the moral and physical degeneracy experienced by people of fashion, intellectuals, women and children. He believed that public officials would soon create mandatory health councils to examine all prospective couples and recommend healthy marital matches. Following moral hygiene insights, the state could stop degeneracy and breed enough 'beaux hommes' to fill a 'beau royaume'.[147] Coffinières is an extreme example, but his ideas are telling. In less fanciful ways, other health crusaders also looked for institutional support to regenerate the sick nation. As we shall see, what they learned about health conditions in rural and urban France shocked and perplexed them. Physical degeneracy might be spreading through the body politic, but it did so for markedly different reasons.

---

145 SRM 120, d. 2, Delaporte, 'Mémoire sur l'éducation physique des enfans' (1783).

146 SRM 193, d. 13, Martin, 'Réflexions et observations sur un point rélatif à l'éducation physique, et au traitement des maladies des enfans' (n.d); and Desessartz, *Traité*, xxi.

147 SRM 200, d. 2, n. 5, Coffinières, 'Les maladies héréditaires' (1788).

CHAPTER TWO

Depopulation and Institutional Response, *c.* 1776–1789

Between 1750 and 1770, medical crusaders created a new model of health activism to respond to widespread fears about moral decline and physical degeneracy. According to these practitioners, a number of people – fashionable elites, intellectuals, women and children – were at high risk for deadly nervous diseases. But good hygiene, they hoped, could give debauched elites the tools they needed to reform their morals and manners and thus lead more virtuous and healthier lives. Crusaders adopted the mantle of moral values, telling upper-class patrons and patients that they could not justify their social and political authority if they continued to lead such depraved and dissolute lives. In this manner, they turned simmering class resentments into questions about personal morality: they demanded that fashionable elites conform to a new moral code, but it was a code sanctioned by their middle-class inferiors. Physicians thus cast themselves as the true defenders of civic and moral virtue, saying they best understood the present and future health needs of the French nation. In this discourse, they often made one particular group scapegoats: women. By playing upon long-standing prejudices about women and sexual propriety, medical practitioners tried to enlist elite men into their moral crusade by asking them to control their wives and children.

In the 1770s, medical activists opened a new front in their crusade to regenerate the nation, as they turned their focus upon the health of the urban and rural poor. This activism was driven by new policy initiatives that stemmed from the royal government. Between 1776 and 1778, two major proponents of bureaucratic and medical reform – the controller-general A.-R. Turgot and comparative anatomist Félix Vicq d'Azyr – formed the Société Royale de Médecine to advance medical science and improve public health.[1] The immediate stimuli were a series of rinderpest outbreaks and public disturbances after grain provisioning collapsed. In the wake of these disasters, the royal government asked the Royal Society to study epidemics,

---

1   On the Royal Society of Medicine, see Jean Meyer, 'L'enquête de l'Académie de Médecine sur les épidémies, 1774–1794', in *Médecins, climat et épidémies à la fin du XVIIIe siècle*, by Jean-Paul Desaive et al. (Paris, 1972), pp. 9–20; Caroline Hannaway, 'Medicine, Public Welfare, and the State in Eighteenth-Century France: The Société Royale de Médecine of Paris (1776–1793)' (PhD thesis, Johns Hopkins University, 1974); Charles C. Gillispie, *Science and Polity in France at the End of the Old Regime* (Princeton, 1980), pp. 194–203; and Jean-Pierre Peter, 'Le corps du délit', *Nouvelle revue de psychoanalyse*, no. 3 (1971): 71–108, and 'Médecine, épidémies et société en France à la fin du XVIIIe siècle d'après les archives de l'Académie de médecine', *Bulletin de la Société d'histoire moderne* 14th ser., no. 14 (1970): 2–9.

epizootics, mineral waters, proprietary remedies and all other matters relating to public health. According to the founding members, the old medical guilds had failed to meet public needs; and many medical reformers hoped that the Royal Society would reform abusive privileges, increase health activism and regenerate society.[2] To help these activities, Louis XVI gave the Royal Society a generous budget, meeting offices at the Louvre and, most importantly, direct access to bureaucratic networks through the Ministry of Finance and the Maison du Roi.[3] In turn, the regional intendants selected local doctors to correspond with the Royal Society and act as part of their 'medical police' apparatus. Ultimately, the Royal Society boasted over a thousand correspondents – including celebrities ranging from Antoine Lavoisier to Benjamin Franklin – who saw the Royal Society as a national health bureau, and engaged it on all matters pertaining to health.[4]

As the pioneering studies by Caroline Hannaway and J.-P. Peter have shown, the Royal Society constituted a watershed in the history of public health. In global terms, it was the first national health agency created by a modern state and it brought together a staggering amount of medical talent, allowing medical practitioners to redefine their self-image both as professionals and as engaged citizens. They were no longer Molière's buffoons but rather proud members of a bona fide science and – perhaps just as significantly – members of the enlightened vanguard. As this chapter shows, however, the Royal Society also allowed medical crusaders to expand their health programme.[5] In its works, the Royal Society conducted a number of studies about population decline, nervous disease, sexual hygiene and child education. These studies were sometimes alarmist in tone and prognosis, and they helped spread the belief, amongst doctors, intellectuals and public officials, that the kingdom was declining in health and fertility. In this correspondence, an important change emerges. According to reformers, the problem was no longer limited to the upper classes; rather, physical degeneracy was spreading within the general population, and the ultimate signs were depopulation and economic decline. Doctors catalogued

---

2   Félix Vicq d'Azyr, *Pièces concernant l'établissement fait par le Roi d'une commission ou société de médecine* (Paris, n.d.), 3–4; AN F[17]1246, n. 186, 'Projet d'arrest', Versailles, 29 Apr. 1776; and SRM 148, d. 22, Varnier, médecin à Vitry, 'Mélanges/Pratiques', 1783.

3   AN F[17]1246, 'Commission de médecins établie par arrêt du conseil du 19 avril 1776 (1773–77)': n. 169, 'Projet de lettre à Messieurs les Intendants sur les maladies épidémiques', 22 Aug. 1775; and n. 292, *Arrest du Conseil d'État du Roi, qui établit une commission de médecins à Paris* (Paris, 1776).

4   For good examples, see especially SRM 168, d. 3 (no. 1–11, 11 *bis*), correspondence Amelot (intendant at Dijon); SRM 168, dos 3, n. 12–22, correspondence Ballainvilliers (intendant at Languedoc); SRM 168, d. 4, Boucheparu (intendant at Béarn), letter of 30 Jan. 1787. The Royal Society carefully cultivated these official contacts.

5   For provincial views, see SRM 177, d. 1, C.-L. Dufour (in St Fargeau), 'Topographie médicale de la ville de St Fargeau et du pays de Puisaye, suivie de quelques observations de médecine et de chirurgie, et des réflexions sur les changements que l'état actuel de la médecine et l'administration laissent à désirer' (n.d.); SRM 193, d. 13, Martin (in Narbonne), 'Maladies qui ont régné dans l'hôtel-Dieu de la ville de Narbonne en Languedoc, généralité de Montpellier (pendant les mois de juin et juillet 1783)'; and SRM 141, d. 43, [anon.], 'Topographie médicale du dépôt de la mendicité de Bourg-en-Bresse' (n.d.).

the causes: epidemics, poverty, rural backwardness, bad health and bad urban planning. Now, more than ever, doctors saw health as a national security problem, and demanded that authorities improve health and hygiene. Doctors thus pioneered new medical research and set out an ambitious programme of health-care reform. In so doing, they invented a bold new idea: social medicine.

Health activism, depopulation and rural reform

These ideas about social medicine stemmed from new attitudes towards preventive medicine and a new desire to collaborate with public authorities. Unlike the traditional hygiene inherited from Galenic-Arabic medicine, which dealt with individual regimen, social medicine dealt with the health of large-scale populations: instead of an individual patient, the doctor treated everyone on the aggregate level. Medical practitioners wanted to do more than cure disease: for them, this approach seemed too reactive, even passive. Rather, they should become more proactive by calculating health risks and then building new policies and institutions. Following upon the example set by the moral hygienists (as seen in Chapter 1 above), physicians redefined their role as medical activists. They now saw themselves as the principal authorities on health matters and wanted to be equal partners with the government when it made health policy.

As a consequence of these new beliefs, social medicine broke with older policy approaches to public health. Before the 1770s, hygiene was only one component of the absolutist state's bureaucratic system, a system that contemporaries called 'the police'. For eighteenth-century thinkers, the word 'police' meant something different from what it means today. When they spoke of a 'police state', they meant a 'civilized state' – that is, it was a society that enjoyed the rule of law and could thus cultivate commerce, the arts and the sciences.[6] According to this view, hygiene was a law-and-order issue, as sickness could disrupt commerce and the social peace.[7] Combining humanitarianism and social control, public officials focused upon three things: they wanted to contain sickness and death amongst the very poor; they wanted to clean up the towns and cities, removing the filth and debris that caused disease; and, most importantly, they wanted to contain epidemic diseases such as the plague by imposing quarantines. In these activities, as Jan Goldstein points out, doctors played a decidedly 'ancillary' role in making health policy. Though the royal government appointed regional *médecins des épidémies* during the 1750s, medical personnel rarely worked with public officials nor did they advise health policy. At

---

6   'Police', *Encyclopédie méthodique ou par ordre des matières: jurisprudence* (10 vols, Paris, 1782–91), vol. 10, pt 2, pp. 578–88, at p. 578. For discussion, see Marc Raeff, *The Well-Ordered Police State: Social and Institutional Change Through Law in the Germanies and Russia* (New Haven, 1983), p. 31; and Lucien Febvre, '*Civilisation*: Evolution of a Word and a Group of Ideas', trans. K. Folca, in Peter Burke (ed.), *A New Kind of History and Other Essays* (New York, 1973), pp. 219–57.

7   See the classic articles by George Rosen, 'Cameralism and the Concept of Medical Police', *Bulletin of the History of Medicine* 27 (1953): 21–42, and 'Mercantilism and Health Policy in Eighteenth-Century French Thought', *Medical History* 3 (1959): 259–77.

this point, public hygiene didn't constitute an independent sphere of medical study and action.[8]

During the 1770s, all this changed, as medical practitioners now interested themselves in public health issues and authorities encouraged them to plan health policies. This new attitude was influenced by several factors, and it built upon the kind of health crusading pioneered by Antione Le Camus, N. Brouzet de Béziers, C.-A. Vandermonde, Samuel Tissot, and others. On one level, public authorities hoped that science and technology could improve the kingdom's power and make the population more productive and happy – an ideology that sociologists usually refer to as 'scientism'.[9] Following this ideological impetus, the royal government created a number of schools, learned academies and institutes to promote the theoretical and practical sciences, especially those relating to agriculture, manufacturing, mining and engineering. This list includes impressive institutions such as the Académie des Sciences, the Collège de France and the Jardin des Plantes, to name just a few.[10] By the mid-century, medicine became an obvious candidate for institutional reform, because doctors wanted to advance medical science and public officials wanted to improve the nation's health.[11] Both parties saw opportunity.

On a second level, physicians believed that health activism allowed them to advance more specific professional and humanitarian interests: improving one, they thought, would improve the other. They had good reasons to want change. Medical reformers deplored the current state of medical education and hung their heads when major *philosophes* complained that medicine was a medieval guild still stuck in scholasticism and formal rationalism. Health institutions, reformers continued, were in a worse state. Critics pointed out that hospitals and charitable services were inadequate for health needs: hospitals, in particular, were death traps for the poor and a drain on the public treasury.[12] But here practitioners saw opportunity: by reforming schools and hospitals, they could improve their skills and the nation's health.

In this case, physicians were motivated by both professional and moral impulses. Medical reformers believed that medicine could change society because physicians could alleviate pain and sickness and thus transform the human condition. Progress was immediate and tactile. Nowhere could Enlightenment ideas touch people so intimately in mind and body. But the emphasis is important. Doctors offered not cures, but prevention. The key was hygiene. The doctor must leave the bedside and treat society as a whole. Where the old-fashioned doctor had failed, the modern

---

8   Jan Goldstein, *Console and Classify: The French Psychiatric Profession in the Nineteenth Century* (Cambridge, 1987), p. 21.

9   Joseph Ben-David, *The Scientist's Role in Society: A Comparative Study* (Engelwood Cliffs, 1971), p. 82.

10   Roger Hahn, *The Anatomy of a Scientific Institution: The Paris Academy of Sciences* (Berkeley, 1971), chap. 5.

11   See the analysis in Harvey Mitchell, 'Politics in the Service of Knowledge: The Debate Over the Administration of Medicine and Welfare in Late Eighteenth-Century France', *Social History* 6 (1981): 185–207.

12   AP 711 Foss 1, 'Mémoire sur la mendicité, par M. le Arch. de Toulouse' (n.d.).

hygienist would go: but a hygienist armed with Enlightenment knowledge and a deep sense of civic virtue.[13]

This new health activism was also driven by another concern: depopulation. This issue exploded on the public scene in the late 1750s and pushed the discourse about luxury and libertinism into public policy circles. The fear of population decline was a European-wide phenomenon – parallel cases appear in Sweden and the Dutch Netherlands – but it had specific consequences in France. Depopulation fears provoked a veritable craze amongst public authorities and intellectuals, forcing discussion about welfare and charity reforms that could increase fertility and decrease mortality. The irony here is that these fears were unfounded, because France was actually experiencing unprecedented demographic growth. But this mirage might as well have been reality and it inspired unprecedented public action.[14]

The reasons for the depopulation panic are difficult to explain, stemming from long-standing apprehensions about royal centralization, extensive warfare, failed administrative reform and strained charity resources. Beginning with C.-L. de Montesquieu's *Lettres persanes* (1721), social critics charged that the Sun King's ruinous domestic and foreign policies had jeopardized France's great power status, eating away at its underlying demographic and economic strength. Though these writers first targeted absolutist policies, they began to criticize luxury, philosophic free-thinking and sexual free-living.[15] These ideas resonated in intellectual and administrative circles. In the 1760s and 1770s, even demographers who had correctly established that France's population was not declining, such as the Abbé Expilly, Louis Messance and J.-B. Moheau, still sympathized with the depopulationist social agenda, believing that invisible pathologies were rotting the body politic from within.[16] According to Moheau, 'we cannot be persuaded that we live in a century

---

13   J.-E. Gilibert, *L'anarchie médicale, ou la médecine considérée comme nuisible à la société* (3 vols, Neuchâtel, 1772), vol. 1, pp. 172–76, 185–86.

14   Joseph J. Spengler, *French Predecessors to Malthus: A Study in Eighteenth-Century Wage and Population Theory* (Durham, NC, 1942), pp. 78–103; James C. Riley, *Population Thought in the Age of Demographic Revolution* (Durham, NC, 1985), pp. 52–57; Robert Favre, *La mort dans la littérature et la pensée françaises au siècle des Lumières* (Lyon, 1978), pp. 275–331; Harvey Chisick, *The Limits of Reform in the Enlightenment: Attitudes Toward the Education of the Lower Classes in Eighteenth-Century France* (Princeton, 1981), pp. 185–97; Carol Blum, *Strength in Numbers: Population, Reproduction, and Power in Eighteenth-Century France* (Baltimore, 2002).

15   C.-L. de Montesquieu, *Lettres persanes* (1721; Paris, 1964), p. 182; Victor de Mirabeau, *L'ami des hommes, ou traité de la population* (7 vols, The Hague, 1758), vol. 6, pt 2, p. 88.

16   Louis Messance, *Recherches sur la population des généralités d'Auvergne, de Lyon, de Rouen et de quelques provinces et villes du royaume* (Paris, 1766), pp. 270–71; *Dictionnaire universel des sciences morales, économiques, politiques et diplomatiques, ou bibliothèque de l'homme d'état et du citoyen*, ed. J.-B. Robinet (London, 1777–83), s.v. 'Dépopulation' and 'Population'; Pierre Lefebvre de Beauvray, *Dictionnaire social et patriotique, ou précis raisonné des connoissances relatives à l'économie morale, civile et politique* (Amsterdam, 1770), s.v. 'Population'.

people have called Enlightened, in one of the most civilized countries of Europe, and in a nation where the word humanity is known'.[17]

Depopulation, critics said, was caused by an underlying physical degeneracy. For instance, the Chevalier de Cerfvol claimed that 'incontinence' had 'enervated the better part of what remains in us'; according to him, the debased libertine communicated 'the corrupt virus that resides within him' to his children and thus spawning degenerate and sterile offspring.[18] Other social critics, such as abbé Pierre Jaubert, alleged that upper-class women had stopped nursing and educating their children because they were overly attached to fashion and manners.[19] Some political economists suggested that the police should regulate lower-class women in the cities: if poor women could not attest to gainful, moral employment they should be expelled, lest they become prostitutes and ensnare men in the cycle of degradation.[20]

By the early 1760s, other social thinkers had picked up the banner of physical and moral hygiene. The most astonishing work is Joachim Faiguet de Villeneuve's *L'econome politique: projet pour enricher et pour perfectionner l'espèce humaine* (1763), in which he argued that the government should study plant and animal breeding and then apply these insights to the human species. In his view, the elite classes urgently needed sexual hygiene, because their 'excessive weakness' spawned 'a feeble and delicate temperament, which becomes hereditary for their descendants'. Directly citing Vandermonde, he argued that the government should forbid marriages between people who were 'feeble, thin and delicate', the 'diminutive' and the 'deformed', and others who were 'vitiated in heart and spirit'. In addition, administrators should put these degenerates in health compounds. He concluded: 'Our political writers incessantly celebrate the advantages of a large population; everyone claims it is the proof of a perfect administration. However, if population increase is important, then regulating and perfecting it is still more necessary'.[21]

By the 1760s, doctors also joined the depopulation panic and pushed health activism beyond the earlier works by Le Camus, Brouzet de Béziers and Vandermonde. According to them, the depopulation crisis needed the expertise that only a trained doctor could provide. Moral values and patriotism were dying away in men's hearts, but public authorities could revive it by using hygiene to give the body strength and discipline. Not surprisingly, the first major medical crusader to explicitly join this public debate was the tireless Tissot, in his best-selling health manual, *Avis au peuple sur sa santé* (1761). In the introduction to this text, he announced that: 'The diminution in the number of inhabitants in this land is a striking fact for everyone, and which is proven by population inquiries.' For him, population decline stemmed from a variety

---

17   J.-B. Moheau, *Recherches et considérations sur la population de la France* (1778; Paris, 1994), p. 237.

18   Chevalier de Cerfvol, *Mémoire sur la population* (London, 1768), pp. 7, 9–10.

19   Abbé Pierre Jaubert, *Des causes de la dépopulation et des moyens d'y remédier* (Paris, 1767), pp. 9–10, 49.

20   Henri le Goyon de La Plombaine, *L'homme en société, ou nouvelles vues politiques et économiques pour porter la population au plus haut degré en France* (2 vols, Amsterdam, 1763), vol. 1, pp. 70–87.

21   Joachim Faiguet de Villeneuve, *L'econome politique: projet pour enricher et pour perfectionner l'espèce humaine* (London and Paris, 1763), pp. 118–19, 125, 145–7.

of possible causes – such as conscription, commerce, labour migrations, hereditary disease, libertinism, debauchery, abortion, infanticide and child abandonment – but he also added an important new factor: '[T]he way in which the people are treated in the countryside when they are sick.'[22]

Tissot expressed an emerging belief – that depopulation was a rural phenomena – and his rural colleagues passionately agreed. In letters to medical authorities and administrators, country doctors reiterated three major problems in the countryside: quackery, inadequate health services and, above all, epidemic disease.[23] For example, Dr Carrère argued that epidemics 'depopulated' the countryside and annihilated 'a considerable and precious portion of our citizens, and spread consternation in the realms where they strike'.[24] In Marseilles, Dr Raymond blamed depopulation on the 1720 plague, poverty and inadequate hospitals and charities.[25] In Gascogne, Dr Dufau thought that epidemic disease and indigence caused depopulation, and he insisted central authorities ought to subsidize health measures, since local elites in Auch seemed uninterested in reforms.[26] In other instances, physicians used parish records to quantify demographic patterns, and forwarded this data to public officials and learned societies, hoping that it might cause the government to act.[27] In rural France, depopulation rhetoric undergirded substantial calls for health and welfare reform.

Country doctors weren't exaggerating about health conditions. In the countryside, disease came and went with grim seasonal regularity: autumn dysentery and digestive fevers; winter colds and pulmonary pneumonia; spring influenza; and a brief summer break before the cycle started all over again.[28] Country people suffered heavily from other sicknesses, such as tuberculosis, typhus, typhoid fever, malaria, smallpox, scarlet fever, measles, chronic diarrhoea, scurvy and venereal disease.[29] Recent epidemic outbreaks had been disastrous: in 1775–76, there was a continental influenza; in 1779, dysentery hit northern France; in 1782, a 'sweating

---

22 S.-A. Tissot, *Avis au peuple sur sa santé* (Lausanne, 1761), pp. 1, 13.

23 SRM 120, d. 2, Delaporte, 'Mémoire sur l'éducation physique des enfans'; SRM 178, d. 6, Destrapière, 'Mémoire sur la topographie du pays d'Aunis', 19 Dec. 1777; SRM 120, d. 2, Amoreux, 'Quels sont en France les abus à réformer dans l'éducation physique, et quel est le régime le plus propre à fortifier le tempérament et à parvenir les maladies des enfans', 15 Mar. 1784; and SRM 120, d. 3, Pujol, 'Mémoire sur les maladies héréditaires', 1790.

24 Carrère, 'Mémoire sur un moyen de se préserver des maladies épidémiques contagieuses', *Histoire de la Société Royale de Médecine* (10 vols, Paris, 1779–98), vol. 4, pt 2, p. 215.

25 SRM 180, d. 7, Raymond, 'Mémoire sur les causes de la dépopulation de quelques contrées de la Provence', 15 Jan. 1787, and 'Mémoire sur la topographie médicale de Marseille et de son territoire, et sur celle des lieux voisins de cette ville', *Histoire de la Société Royale*, vol. 2, pt 2, pp. 111, 119, 123.

26 SRM 169, d. 11, Dufau, La Basti de d'Armagnac, letter of 5 July 1776.

27 SRM 167, d. 7, Poma and Renaud, 'État de la population de ville et du baillage de Saint-Dié en Lorraine', 1786; SRM 177, d. 1, Bonnot, 'Topographie historique médicale de Toulon sur d'Arcoux . . . rédigé de concert avec M. Guyton le jeune d'Autun', 11 June 1786.

28 SRM 179, d. 23, Rouard, 'Topographie médicale'.

29 SRM 156, d. 12, no. 1–11, Boutellier de Lisle (in Cholet), correspondence; Madier, 'Mémoire sur la topographie médicale de Bourg-Saint-Andéol', *Histoire de la Société Royale*, vol. 4, pt 2, p. 138.

illness' appeared in Languedoc; and in 1781–85, an infectious pneumonia swept the kingdom.

To complicate matters, the countryside lacked trained medical personnel. When public authorities tried to count the number of country doctors, they discovered that the doctor–patient ratio was alarmingly low: there was about one doctor for 3,242 persons and about 40,000 barber-surgeons total in France.[30] In the countryside, ordinary people usually consulted a quack or a priest because there were few university-trained physicians and surgeons and costs were prohibitive. According to Harvey Mitchell, physicians who did take up a country practice did so for complex reasons: either they didn't want to compete in the towns, or they lacked proper training and skills, or they were responding to a humanitarian vocation.[31] Urban doctors knew some of these realities, but they didn't know the depth of the problem. So country doctors used medical and bureaucratic networks to tell this story and push for reform.

For these reasons, rural practitioners were excited about the creation of the Royal Society of Medicine. They hoped that this new agency would raise awareness about rural health and that the government would push welfare reform. A typical voice was Pierre Nicolas, a doctor who had achieved some national recognition with his venomous anti-wetnursing tract, *Le cri de la nature en faveur des enfants nouveau-nés* (1775). A native to Grenoble, Nicolas wrote constantly about degeneracy and depopulation, hoping to push local authorities to change health conditions.[32] In letters to the Royal Society, Nicholas denounced local poverty and rural backwardness and he demanded that the king create a national policy on health care and poor relief. He decried local hygiene and complained that local doctors resisted change: the town's medical school was 'good for nothing' and showed 'no signs of life'; meanwhile, the province was flooded with barber-surgeons, quacks, mountebanks and other itinerant healers. At times, though, Nicolas's passionate commitment to health reform caused him to embrace dubious medical fads and he even dabbled in occultism, as seen in his interest in mesmerism.[33]

Beginning in September 1776, Nicolas forwarded the Royal Society a series of ambitious projects that outlined how to create a national system of medical police. The French kingdom, he said, urgently needed health reform because the population was

---

30 Cf. the doctor-patient ratio of 1–869 in 1965; see Jacques Léonard, *Les médecins de l'ouest au XIXe siècle* (3 vols, Lille, 1978); Jean-Pierre Goubert (ed.), *La médicalisation de la société française, 1770–1830* (Waterloo, 1982). For detailed studies, see Toby Gelfand, 'The Decline of the Ordinary Practitioner and the Rise of a Modern Medical Profession', in Martin S. Staum and Donald E. Larson (eds), *Doctors, Patients, and Society: Power and Authority in Medical Care* (Waterloo, 1981), pp. 105–29; Jean-Pierre Goubert, 'The Extent of Medical Practice in France Around 1780', *Journal of Social History* 10 (1976–77): 410–27. For a contemporary accounting, see the incomplete FMP, ms. 221, 'État des médecins et chirurgiens de la province' [ca. 1780].

31 Harvey Mitchell, 'Rationality and Control in French Eighteenth-Century Medical Views of the Peasantry', *Comparative Studies in Society and History* 21 (1979): 81–112.

32 SRM 199, d. 13, n. 15, letter of 11 Feb. 1780.

33 ANM, ms. 33, fol. 128, letter of 20 Sept. 1784; SRM 199, d. 13, n. 12, letter of 10 Oct. 1776.

degenerating and poverty was rising. Past policies offered only failures.[34] Beginning in the early eighteenth century, authorities had tried to control the homeless and migrant poor in the so-called 'Great Confinements', imprisoning the transient poor or deporting them back to their native parishes to keep them from draining charitable relief. But this move had proven disastrous. Local charities couldn't support the deserving poor and the hospitals siphoned the able-bodied. Nicolas warned that 'mendacity is just as dangerous for the moral order, as pleurisy, for example, is for the physical order'.[35]

Nicolas wanted action. As a physician, he wanted to ameliorate disease and poverty, not engage in abstract discussion about political economy. To reform society, he said, the Royal Society needed to create a new Paris agency specifically dedicated to health reform, an agency that he called 'a Royal Commission on Public Health'. This commission would be the central office for a network of local bureaus across the country. Inspired by the state-appointed *médecins des épidémies* of the 1750s, Nicolas thought that the Paris commission should employ district inspectors who would work with intendants and investigate local conditions.[36] The inspectors would receive salaries, official uniforms and even, upon retirement, noble privileges. They would send their reports to the regional bureaus, who would sort the data and send them to the central commission in Paris. In turn, the regional bureaus would provide health services on a local level. They would treat venereal diseases and teach first-aid, especially in cases of drowning and asphyxia. During epidemics, they would direct sanitary responses and transport personnel and supplies to afflicted areas.[37]

Like other medical reformers, Nicolas hoped that one day a central agency such as the Royal Society could systemically coordinate health care and welfare throughout the kingdom. He thought in big terms. In every local *arrondissement*, authorities should establish a charity agency for the sick, which would be staffed by salaried physicians, surgeons and a steward for 'valid poor of the district'. Authorities would put the poor and homeless in these charities, and they would also dispense medical care and treatments to supplicants. Following his previous publications on wet-

---

34   SRM 199, d. 13, n. 11, letter of 10 Sept. 1776. On the poor and poor relief, see especially Olwen Hufton, *The Poor in Eighteenth-Century France, 1750–1789* (Oxford, 1974); Robert Schwartz, *Policing the Poor in Eighteenth-Century France* (Chapel Hill, 1988); and T. M. Adams, *Bureaucrats and Beggars: French Social Policy in the Age of Enlightenment* (Oxford, 1990).

35   SRM 132, d. 57, Nicolas, 'Mémoire sur la nécessité et les moyens d'améliorer les hôpitaux de la province de Dauphiné, d'en fonder les nouveaux, sous une dénomination moins humiliante pour le pauvre, et d'y occuper les mendians valides, sans recourir à des nouveaux impôts, sans avoir besoin de faire aucune dépense' (n.d.).

36   Other doctors thought along similar lines; see SRM 116, d. 5, Massie, 'Mémoire sur l'état de la médecine dans les campagnes', 23 July 1776; and SRM 169, d. 11, Dufau, La Basti de d'Armagnac, 'Mémoire concernant l'établissement d'un médecin inspecteur des épidémies de la généralité d'Auch présenté à Monseigneur de Bertin, Ministre et secrétaire d'État' (n.d.).

37   SRM 132, d. 58, Nicolas, 'Mémoire sur la nécessité et les moyens d'établir une police médicale en France, et les avantages qui en résulteroient pour l'État et pour les sujets', 4 Mar. 1777.

nursing and midwifery, Nicolas thought that pregnant women should also receive free prenatal and obstetric care. But he acknowledged that it was difficult to finance these institutions, particularly given the kingdom's chronic financial difficulties. So instead of raising taxes, he modestly suggested that religious orders could maintain girl schools and sell licensed pharmaceuticals.[38]

Nicolas identified another cause of sickness and depopulation: quackery. Nicolas promised that his medical police could bring the huge world of folk healers and barber-surgeons under foot. Like most educated doctors, he looked down upon these healers and hated to compete against them – and he wanted public authorities to act with all legal powers at their disposal. To eradicate folk healers, he urged, local health bureaus must license all medical personnel and make them take qualifying exams. The best applicants would receive national marks. But if a doctor or surgeon failed, they must go back to medical school and hone their skills; if they refused and continued to practice, they would be punished by whipping and imprisonment (ostensibly, to keep the system fair, failed practitioners could appeal against the test results). In this discussion, Nicolas showed a particular malevolence towards midwives. He had already published a polemic against Madame de Coudray, the famous 'king's midwife' who had received a brevet from Louis XV to train midwives throughout the kingdom, and he used his contacts in the Royal Society to push his agenda. Instead of women like Coudray, he wanted his new health bureaus to instruct and license midwives; and each year, he said, medical authorities needed to examine midwives and keep them certified.[39]

In this discussion, Nicolas tapped into medical concerns about the flourishing proprietary remedy trade, and demanded that public authorities regulate drug sales. He was not alone in his criticism. Then as today, French people favoured self-medication over calling a doctor and they consumed large numbers of remedies. As a consequence, eighteenth-century France boasted a enormous market for all sorts of drugs, and medical reformers despaired that the underground remedy trade provided a huge opportunity for quacks and renegade apothecaries. For some reformers, the problem seemed so acute that regulating drugs and quackery became one and the same thing.[40] In one manuscript, a provincial doctor named Robin de Kiavalle (or Kériavalle) claimed that most patients simply wanted remedies, so they avoided qualified doctors and consulted apothecaries or herbalists instead. Infants and young children suffered most from this abuse, since parents called the doctor only after the disease had become lethal. To deal with these problems, Kiavalle wanted to create his own 'lieutenant general' of medical police, who would repress all irregular abuses. Like Nicolas, Kiavalle wanted a network of health bureaus to police

---

38　Nicolas, 'Les moyens d'améliorer les hôpitaux'.

39　Nicolas, 'Police médicale en France'. See Nina Rattner Gelbart, *The King's Midwife: A History and Mystery of Madame du Coudray* (Berkeley, 1998), pp. 203–04.

40　SRM 115, d. 9, Virard, 'Observations sur les moyens de favoriser les progrès de la médecine dans les provinces', 10 May 1781. On the proprietary remedy trade, see Pascale Gramain-Kibleur, 'Le monde du médicament à l'aube de l'ère industrielle: les enjeux de la prescription médicamenteuse de la fin du XVIIIe et au début du XIXe siècle' (thèse du doctorat, Université de Paris–VII, 1999).

traditional corporate privileges and he asked public authorities to imprison irregular practitioners.[41] This rhetoric was typical in these kinds of health manifestoes. For example, Vicq d'Azyr accused charlatans of malpractice and murder; and Dr Touret even said that the government should 'totally extirpate that destructive vermin of the human species': that is, all quacks, sorcerers and cunning-folk.[42]

Still, it is possible to overemphasize elite animus towards popular medicine, as real and angry as it was. Reformers saw quackery as but one part of a larger problem, and the Royal Society ignored local doctors who did nothing but carp about folk healers and who dwelled on turf battles between jealous medical guilds. Instead, medical crusaders dreamed of regenerating the whole of French society through more utopian plans of public hygiene, which would allow them to obliterate the twin evils of degeneracy and depopulation. As Nicolas put it, 'it is in the greatest interest of the sovereign to preside over the increase of the population and to prevent it from ruin. Conditioned by these principles, the government must fix its gaze on all the objects that interest its citizens.'[43] The Royal Society of Medicine, in particular, had ambitious dreams for dealing with the health concerns of the French population, and it needed doctors across the kingdom to coordinate their skills and efforts in order to turn this dream into reality.

Medical topography and rural health

Before the Royal Society could set out on its reform project, it first wanted to know, as much as possible, the kingdom's actual state of health. Its members needed reliable empirical data on health and sickness throughout France, and needed them in a format that allowed doctors to study and apply them. Obviously, these health data did not exist and no public authority had yet tried to compile them. To meet these needs, the Royal Society launched a vast inquiry into health conditions in rural and urban France. It wanted to know everything about health and sickness: who got sick, when they got sick, what caused their sickness, and whether or not there were adequate resources to deal with these sick people. Once the Royal Society had collected this mountain of vital statistics, it was hoped, doctors could study the data and then draft sound health policy.[44]

To compile these data, the Royal Society promoted a new genre of medical study, something medical practitioners called 'medical topography'. Ideally, a medical topography studied the exact relations between health and environment, identifying

---

41 SRM 184, d. 27, Robin de Kiavalle, 'Projet pour la destruction du charlatanisme en France', 8 Oct. 1784.

42 Vicq d'Azyr, 'Rapport sur les inconvéniences de l'opération de la castration, pratiquée pour obtenir la cure radicale des hernies', *Histoire de la Société Royale*, vol. 1, pt 1, p. 295; SRM 179, d. 26, Touret, letter to S.R.M. (n.d.). On folk medicine, see Matthew Ramsey, *Professional and Popular Medicine in France: The Social World of Medical Practice* (Cambridge, 1987).

43 Nicolas, 'Police médicale en France'; also Massie, 'Mémoire sur l'état de la médecine'.

44 'Préamble', *Histoire de la Société Royale*, vol. 4, pt 1, p. 18.

the local factors that influenced sickness.[45] This medical environmentalism, as James C. Riley has called it, was an ancient idea, one that dated back to the Hippocratic text, *On Airs, Waters and Places*. Originally, Hippocrates argued that doctors must consider local conditions when they treated patients, because disease was caused by environmental factors such as terrain, climate, seasons, winds, local waters and town location. This belief was deeply rooted in humoral theory. Accordingly, the humours regulated individual health, whilst outside forces – especially the air – shaped disease predisposition and aetiology. In cases of endemic or epidemic disease, these environmental forces acted in a more or less uniform manner, thus causing the same disease symptoms to appear amongst a large number of persons.[46]

During the Enlightenment, doctors put these Hippocratic teachings into a more empirical context. They were strongly influenced by the new philosophy of the Scientific Revolution and the Enlightenment, and looked to Robert Boyle's studies on chemistry and meteorology and C.-L. de Montesquieu's geographical theories about human societies. These ideas inspired a new generation of medical thinkers, such as Thomas Sydenham and François Boissier de Sauvages, to study disease and environment in more exact terms by coordinating climatic and clinical observations.[47] In France, these interests culminated in the sophisticated studies by Louis Lépecq de Cloture, a Rouen physician who wrote two major topographies on disease in north-western France. In these books, Lépecq said that doctors must study sickness in its natural habitat before they could treat large-scale health issues. The Royal Society enthusiastically supported his work and included him in their correspondence network. For them, Lépecq embodied a new kind of health activist who looked beyond the patient's bedside and thought about the broad environmental factors that shaped human disease.[48]

The Royal Society pushed these interests to a new level. Inspired by doctors like Lépecq, the Royal Society announced that, as one its primary goals, it would create a comprehensive medical topography of France, and it invited all its affiliates and correspondents to participate in the project. In this endeavour, the society hoped to exploit all its contacts in the royal bureaucracy and its extensive network of correspondents. Practitioners would use this administrative authority to

---

45 For discussion, see SRM 118, d. 108, Gontare, 'De la contagion' (n.d.); and Raymond, 'Mémoire sur les épidémies', *Histoire de la Société Royale*, 4, pt 2, pp. 2, 37, 78.

46 On environmental medicine, see L. J. Jordanova, 'Earth Science and Environmental Medicine: The Synthesis of the Late Enlightenment', in L. J. Jordanova and Roy S. Porter (eds), *Images of the Earth: Essays in the History of the Environmental Sciences* (Chalfont St Giles, 1979), pp. 119–46; and, above all, James C. Riley, *The Eighteenth-Century Campaign to Avoid Disease* (London, 1987), pp. xv–xvi. For a recent survey, see Nicolaas A. Rupke (ed.), *Medical Geography in Historical Perspective* (London, 2000).

47 'Topographie médicale', *Encyclopédie méthodique ou par ordre des matières: médecine*, ed. Félix Vicq d'Azyr (13 vols, Paris, 1782–1832), vol. 13, p. 278. See also the entries under 'Air' (vol. 1, pp. 488–92), 'Airs, eaux et lieux' (vol. 1, p. 590), 'Climat' (vol. 4, 878–79), and 'Lois topographiques' (vol. 8, pp. 185–93).

48 Louis Lépecq de la Clôture, *Observations sur les maladies épidémiques* (Paris, 1776), and *Collection d'observations sur les maladies et constitutions épidémiques* (2 vols, Rouen, 1778).

conduct their local investigations and then remit their studies back to Paris, where the Royal Society would assemble a national disease map, putting together these local snapshots like pieces of a puzzle. To achieve their goals, the Royal Society gave correspondents leading questions, standardized forms, instruments such as thermometers and barometers and even copies of its latest publications, which presumably served as a model. These doctors were to be like detectives, sifting the evidence and distinguishing the real clues from the red herrings – as though they could materialize the disease by putting it on the map. Once the Royal Society had collected all these facts and figures, it would have a panoramic view of health and disease in the kingdom.[49]

The Royal Society instructed its correspondents to compile specific geographic, anthropological and epidemiological data. In geographic terms, the doctor should pinpoint the area's latitude and longitude, tabulating the physical terrain, water sources and meteorological trends.[50] In anthropological terms, the doctor should describe the local peoples and community, identifying all the physical and moral factors that moulded local temperament, and indicate how this local temperament shaped local disease patterns. These details included sex, occupation, average age, diet, morals, lifestyle, housing and sanitation. Finally, in epidemiological terms, the doctor had to create a local disease profile, charting disease and seasonal regularity. Doctors should overlook no detail, even if it seemed insignificant, which might influence health patterns.[51]

Overall, provincial doctors, surgeons and apothecaries responded enthusiastically to the Royal Society's call. From the provinces and colonies, medical personnel sent the Royal Society over 300 topographies (indeed, authorities later confessed that the project had turned into a daunting, if not impossible, task).[52] These topographies gave the Royal Society an unexpected and sometimes astonishing sketch of provincial life. Medical practitioners set aside private practice and family life and recorded the rich tapestry of rural France – kinship ties, village life, fields, marketplaces, workshops, festivals, local history and ancient monuments – and some encapsulated a lifetime's experience of medical practice.[53] On the surface, many doctors hoped

---

49   SRM 151, d. 4, 'Questionnaire', 6 Oct. 1775; and SRM 129, d. 3, Pujol, 'Topographie médicale, séance du 9 novembre 1776'.

50   SRM 189, d. 7, Limousineau, 'Tableau des maladies qui ont regné tant dans la ville et marquisat d'Airvault qu'aux environs en l'année 1789 avec la description topographique de laditte ville et celle de la paroisse de Sud-Lièvre qui vient d'éprouver une maladie épidémique' (n.d.); and SRM 163, d. 9, Ayrault, 'Maladie de la paroisse de St Chartres en Anjou avec la description topographique de l'endroit', 17 Feb. 1789.

51   SRM 168, d. 3, Marre, report of 6 Sept. 1787; SRM 168, d. 3, Trinque, 'Mémoire sur une maladie épidémique qui règne à Balagué', 18 Aug. 1786; SRM 177, d. 1, Geny, 'Topographie de la Plaine du Forez et observations sur les maladies qui affectent particulièrement les habitans' (n.d.).

52   AAFM, carton 1, 'Rapport de la commission nommée d'après la lettre du Ministre de l'Intérieur, en date du 26 Prairial, portant invitation à l'École de s'occuper de la topographie médicale de la France', 19 Messidor, Year VIII.

53   SRM 179, d. 23 (pièces 'a–j'), Roaurd, 'Topographie médicale de la ville d'Embrun, son territoire, et production de la nature des vents qui y dominent, des maladies épidémiques

to please the Royal Society simply by saying what it wanted to hear. They dutifully reported that rural society had significant health problems which needed to be fixed through some kind of national policy, thereby justifying the Royal Society's activities (especially since the new society was criticized by traditional medical faculties). Doctors also affirmed the Royal Society's environmental approach to epidemic disease, and convinced its leading members that they were on the right aetiological track. Nevertheless, the Royal Society wasn't always satisfied with the results. Privately, members complained about the quality of rural topographies, and despaired about the poor skills of country doctors and surgeons. More often than not, rural practitioners ignored clinical and statistical data, preferring to use case studies, private observations and other forms of anecdotal evidence.

At the same time, medical topographies challenged elite ideals about the rural environment in important ways. During the eighteenth century, writers and artists had celebrated the countryside as more natural in its bucolic and rustic simplicity, seeing it as 'a form of liberation and flight' from the affected world of courtly and urban life.[54] These ideas emerged in the painted pastorals and *fêtes champêtres* of J.-A. Watteau and J.-J. Fragonard, or in the novels of J.-J. Rousseau and J.-H. Bernardin de St Pierre. These beliefs influenced urban doctors, who in turn believed that the primitive, less affluent life in the country made people healthier in body and spirit. Medical writers sometimes made extravagant claims. For example, Dr Jean-Joseph de Brieude wrote, 'The poverty under which [the peasant] lives makes him free. By habituating himself to every privation, he is happy.' A. P. Jacquin added, 'Happy [are] the labourers and inhabitants of the country! They find in their condition constant exercise!'[55]

By contrast, provincial topographies told society members something quite different: the countryside was pathological to the core. According to Harvey Mitchell, doctors never relinquished their belief that the peasant lived in a pristine world that had been corrupted by ignorance, superstition and prejudice. In medical opinion, this potentially healthful world was constantly menaced by the 'grotesque' aspects of folk culture, and they signalled out excessive festivals, bouts of drinking and gorging, carnal familiarity and lackadaisical disposal of bodily wastes. They bemoaned how peasants used dirt and excrement to mark bodily boundaries, and denounced the practice of shaping corporeal features, especially the baby's skull, right after birth.[56]

---

et endémiques, de leurs causes, de leurs signes, et de leur temps', 10 Nov. 1781; and SRM 137, d. 12, Picqué, letter of 31 Dec. 1780, which forwarded a topography written by his recently deceased father.

54   Luigi Salerno, 'La pittura di paesaggio', *Storia dell'arte* 24/25 (1975): 113.

55   J.-J. de Brieude, 'Topographie médicale de la Haute-Auvergne', *Histoire de la Société royale de médecine*, vol. 5, p. 301; A.-P. Jacquin, *De la santé, ouvrage utile à tout le monde*, 2d edn (Paris, 1763), p. 243.

56   See Mitchell, 'Rationality and Control'; F. Loux and M.-F. Morel, 'L'enfance et les savoirs sur les corps: pratiques médicales et pratiques populaires dans la France traditionelle', *Ethnologie française* 6 (1976): 309–24; and Jacques Gélis, 'Refaire le corps: les déformations volontaires du corps de l'enfant à la naissance', *Ethnologie française* 14 (1984): 7–28.

In letter after letter, doctors insisted that peasants had terrible hygiene and character. In Viellevigne, Dr Baudrey found the peasants 'weak, lax, indolent and drunken'. They were uncouth and dressed in poorly-made rags, and lived in appalling poverty.[57] In Lamballe, Dr Delaverge complained that peasants built their homes upon damp ground and kept them poorly ventilated.[58] In Lorraine, the surgeon Didelot described peasant housing as 'very reprehensible'. During the winter, he continued, the family and their animals huddled together in a single room to avoid the cold, closing the doors and windows to keep out the purifying air. Peasants collected refuse by their wells and front doors, as though they were insensible to 'the terrible smell that exists there'.[59] Many country doctors shared Didelot's disgust and stressed that excremental odours caused 'putrid fevers' (usually gastroenteritis or gangrene) – which oftentimes became epidemic.[60] In St Fargeau, for example, Dr Dufour said that the harsh climate, soil and work had deformed the local peasants in mind and body, and even hardened their hearts against their own children. He wrote:

> The inhabitant … carries the particular imprint of the land: he is small, phlegmatic and pale; his body is neither slender nor robust and his fibres are flaccid and his character indolent. Forced to work so he might earn his daily bread, he does so with neither dexterity nor agility. The barren earth demands a labourious and sustained harvesting, providing only that which cannot be absolutely refused. Hardly given to affection, he loves life not and leaves it without regret. One watches with difficulty the little interest that he takes from the existence of what is most dear to man, that of his children. Far from helping them in their infirmities, he wants to see them leave a world in which treasury exaction and the despondency that it creates only prepares a long suite of privations and pain. For the labourer, the birth of a child is the greatest misfortune; his death, only a negative joy, or a trifling disturbance.[61]

As country doctors made clear, the peasants were abandoned to nature's worst elements, and this fact alone should give sentimental writers pause. Nature did not always promote the good and harmonious. The best example was disease.[62] In an insightful essay, Dr Berthe rejected the idea that nature alone healed disease, instead emphasizing the doctor's ameliorative powers and responsibility (presumably, he

---

57   SRM 179, d. 2, Baudrey, 'Topographie médicale de Vieillevigne', 26 Aug. 1788.

58   SRM 177, d. 1, n. 11, Delaverge, 'Mémoire sur une fièvre catarrhale-bilieuse, souvent inflammatoire, putride et maligne, qui a régné à Lamballe et lieux circonvoisons, surtout d'une manière épidémique dans la paroisse de Plénée-Jugon, depuis la fin de février 1785 jusqu'au commencement de juin de la même année', 27 Feb. 1787.

59   'Description topographique et médicale des montagnes de la Vôge (extrait de la correspondance de M. Didelot, chirurgien à Remiremont en Lorraine)', *Histoire de la Société Royale*, vol. 2, pt 1, pp. 128–9.

60   SRM 147, d. 1, Deberge, 'Maladies épidémiques qui ont été régné dans la généralité de Soissons depuis l'automne 1786 jusqu'à pareille époque 1787'.

61   SRM 177, d. 1, Dufour, 'Topographie médicale'. Not all doctors shared Dufour's bleak assessment: cf. SRM 177, d. 1, Camparau, 'Topographie de la ville et de l'hôpital de St Gaudens' (n.d.); and SRM 137, d. 12, Picqué, 'Matériaux pour servir à la description topographique et médicale du lieu d'Avezac' (n.d.).

62   SRM 179, d. 26, Touret, letter of 17 Oct. 1787.

targeted figures like Rousseau and Tissot). Sentimental writers, he said, wanted to personify nature and give her an active intelligence. But these beliefs were phantasmagoric; nature, he noted, was simply 'the ensemble of phenomena relating to life'. To demonstrate this point, Berthe then outlined the lifestyle of an average peasant to show that 'nature' was potentially dangerous and unhealthy. The 'back to nature' sentimentalists, he said, believed that the country promoted health because it hadn't been corrupted by civilization. But this wasn't true. The peasants lived in abject poverty and squalid conditions. They were ignorant and superstitious and lived their lives according to obscure proverbs and folk sayings. They toiled endlessly to earn their daily bread, and this suffering hardened body and mind. Like Dufour, Berthe argued that the peasants were strangers to their own bodies and could not understand their own health and well-being, which made them refuse medical help unless they were totally exhausted or close to death. But people in the towns and cities didn't know any of this. For escapist fantasy, fashionable readers bought into 'ingenious fictions' that celebrated the fertile earth and the 'pleasures of the happy cultivator'. In order to destroy these pernicious beliefs, Berthe said, doctors must inform these readers of the 'true situation' in the countryside.[63]

Berthe's ideas were shared by other doctors. In 1779, a nation-wide dysentery epidemic gave many urban doctors their first taste of rural health and set the stage for a confrontational encounter. During this outbreak, the Royal Society directed all its energies to help local authorities, mobilizing its network of correspondents and coordinating government relief. Though doctors celebrated the government's zealous action and philanthropic spirit, they vociferously complained about the country dwellers they encountered in the relief operations. According to one physician, public charity 'often found insurmountable obstacles in the errors, prejudices and indocility of that class of men'.[64] These beliefs emerge in the correspondence of Dr Chifaliou, a physician who practiced in St Malo in Bretagne. On 3 September 1779, the local intendant requested that Chifaliou and several other doctors assist at a dysentery outbreak in a small town called Clos Poulet. In his subsequent report, Chifaliou denounced rural hygiene and lifestyle. For example, he said that women and girls thought that bathing was 'dishonourable' and uncouth, and they did it 'only with regret'. Peasants ate like gluttons, drank heavily and abused their children. But Chifaliou was particularly upset because the peasants mistrusted doctors and often became impatient with their therapeutic regimens. 'In their eyes', he complained, 'the only good remedy is the one that heals promptly.' So when the doctors could no longer reason with the peasants, they tried to manipulate them. Local priests exhorted peasants to submit to medical authority, and municipal authorities bribed them with free food and extra drugs. But whenever a particular cure stopped working, the peasants chafed. Chifaliou wrote, 'Imbibed on the chimerical idea of predestination … [the peasants] rejected the monarch's gifts and refused to take the remedies'.

63 SRM 143, d. 2, Berthe, 'Réflexions sur cette question: Les maladies peuvent-elles être guéries par les seules sources de la nature?' (n.d.).

64 Caille, 'Précis historique de l'épidémie dysentérique qui a régné pendant l'automne de l'année 1779, dans la plupart des provinces du royaume', *Histoire de la Société Royale*, vol. 3, pt 2, pp. 32–4.

Gorging themselves on wine and spirits, the peasants said they'd rather die 'with a glass in their hand than with an enema in their behind'.[65]

Writing from Josselin, Dr Robin de Kiaville related similar experiences. According to him, dysentery killed more people in the countryside than in the towns. He blamed this high mortality upon peasant stupidity, obstinacy and dirtiness, intimating that the peasants were ultimately responsible for their own sicknesses. In particular, he emphasized the prevalence of rural filth:

> When we enter a village afflicted by dysentery, our olfactory sense is assaulted by a most disagreeable odor ... [and] we enter the homes and feel suffocated by an intolerable aroma. Usually, one finds three quarters of the house's inhabitants lying close together and reciprocally infecting one and the other. The air never circulates nor is it purified. Even the excrement is not removed; it is usually tossed on top of the other droppings in the stable ... . Is it not surprising that the least dangerous diseases promptly degenerate into pestilential epidemics?[66]

In all of these reports, medical practitioners such as Dufour, Berthe and Kiavalle underscored one capital point: social status determined health. In this case, doctors distinguished between the affluent, tradesmen, and the peasantry, claiming that each class which had a particular temperament shaped by affluence, occupation and habitat.[67] Here, doctors did not study health in terms of traditional estates and orders, as officially recognized in old regime law and custom, but rather by occupation and physical characteristics. According to them, social status, blood, soil and climate combined to shape the temperament of entire classes or peoples, and these differences seemed almost of a biological or racial kind. These beliefs emerge in provincial topographies. In Marseilles, for example, Dr Raymond saw class differences in biological terms, saying that environmental factors and racial interbreeding combined to make 'great varieties in the complexion and form' of the town dwellers. Whilst praising some local occupations – notably sailors and fishermen – he complained that the peasantry were physically degenerate because of hard work and a hot climate, appearing 'shrivelled, worn and bowed over as early as age fifty'. At the same time, the affluent town dwellers lived a luxurious and decadent lifestyle, which was manifest in their pale bodies and delicate, sickly children. Like moral hygienists, Raymond believed that a 'hunger for riches' drained virility and health – and the children suffered most.[68]

Similar views emerge in Dr Brieude's medical topography of Haute-Auvergne, which also emphasized biological qualities amongst local residents – though in this case, his views were of the local people were more positive. As he saw it,

---

65   SRM 124, d. 4, Chifoliau, 'Préjugés opposées aux sages précautions du gouvernement, aux efforts des ministres de la santé et à la voix de la nature', 22 Mar. 1780.

66   SRM 184, d. 27, Kiavalle, 'Constitution de l'année 1783', 7 Jan. 1784.

67   SRM 182, d. 1, n. 8, Luce, 'Topographie médicale des cantons d'Antibes, Cannes, Biot, Mougères, etc.', 19 Mar. 1791.

68   Raymond, 'Mémoire sur la topographie médicale de Marseille', vol. 2, pt 2, pp. 103–05.

the provincial people 'perfectly' embodied 'that race of white and blonde Gauls of which Caesar spoke'. They had 'strong, massive and little-irritable fibres', and this brute strength appeared in their rough-and-tumble world of games, dances and festivals. Given this 'vigorous constitution', the men were extremely virile and this sexual prowess persisted until their early sixties. For this reason, the mountain villages had families with ten, twelve and even fourteen children. But once Auvergnants left their native region, their health declined and they degenerated into 'a new race of men'. In particular, young women became overly sensible and thus suffered from the vapours.[69]

Given fears over degeneracy and depopulation, the Royal Society also asked correspondents to investigate women's health and child mortality. Predictably, doctors either praised local women for their moral rectitude and personal virtue, or they bemoaned that luxury and libertinism had corrupted provincial morals. These differing views notwithstanding, provincial doctors generally emphasized that poverty caused female disease.[70] In St Fargeau, Dufour claimed that hard work and an unforgiving climate had caused local women to degenerate, rendering them infertile. In Alsace, Dr Belz claimed that women overworked themselves in the open fields and forests, which apparently caused the elevated maternal mortality in his region. According to him, few women lived past fifty years and many local men had been married three or four times, whilst their children were raised by a succession of stepmothers. In St Jean d'Angély, Dr Fusée-Aublet studied female sicknesses within specific social classes. Upper-class women often nursed their newborn children and did not suffer from the kinds of nervous diseases described by the self-appointed hysteria experts. By contrast, women who worked in factories and cottage industries were less healthy and suffered from irregular menstruation and 'pale colours' or green sickness. More seriously, amongst the peasants, 'old and barbarous' midwife traditions made child mortality particularly high.[71]

In these rich and far-ranging topographies, then, medical practitioners provided a bleak and sometimes shocking exposition of rural health conditions, attacking the sentimental pastoralism *en vogue* amongst urban elites. Doctors, surgeons and apothecaries were shocked by peasant filth and grotesque traditions, and they complained about their superstitious and ignorant character. The peasants, it seemed, were not ideal candidates for enlightened reform. At the same time, rural practitioners emphasized that 'excessive work and profound poverty' actually caused the common people to be mired in filth and disease, and that they simply couldn't afford learned doctors.[72] Ironically, they were so successful in imparting these views that the Royal Society itself became rather pessimistic about the opportunities for rural improvement. Given the information supplied by the medical topographies,

---

69　Brieude, 'Topographie de la Haute-Auvergne', pp. 288–99.

70　SRM 139, d. 17, La Borde, 'Abrégé de topographie médicale de la Gascogne' (n.d.).

71　SRM 177, d. 1, Beltz, 'Remarques topographiques sur les environs de la ville de Soultz en Haute Alsace', 27 Feb. 1787.

72　SRM 177, d. 1, Fusée-Aublet, 'Topographie médicale de la ville de St Jean d'Angély en Saintonge' (n.d.); SRM 177, d. 1, n. 1, Boncerf, 'Topographie médicale de la ville d'Étampes', 30 Aug. 1785.

members and correspondents concluded that public officials lacked the manpower and resources needed to make the countryside clean and healthy. Quite simply, the royal government couldn't afford to build a comprehensive health system, or to fix every shanty town, or to magically transform the physical environment itself. For these reasons, medical reformers had to look elsewhere to regenerate the kingdom. Hoping to find more realistic targets, they now turned to urban tradesmen and urban planning.

Urban trades

Although the Royal Society wanted to improve rural conditions, its members saw this as but one part of a larger programme to regenerate the kingdom. Medical practitioners also worried about urban health and hygiene, and in the mid-1780s, the Royal Society launched an ambitious campaign to clean up the towns and cities. Members and correspondents focused largely upon issues relating to urban trades, housing and design – particularly insalubrious trades, cesspools, cemeteries, hospitals, prisons and roadways.[73] In these efforts, medical practitioners approached urban health challenges differently from those in the countryside. In the country, doctors had often reduced the complexity of rural life – with all its diversity in social structure, kinship, work, religious practice and local culture – to one amorphous mass called 'the peasantry'. By contrast, doctors saw city life and tradespeople in more complex ways, and were sometimes more sympathetic with the plight of urban dwellers. Moreover, medical practitioners were joined by other professional groups and academic institutions, like royal architects and members of the Académie Royale des Sciences. Working together, this diverse group of intellectuals turned the city into a scientific and aesthetic problem, one that warranted the attention of Enlightened professionals and bureaucrats.

In this discussion of moral and physical hygiene, doctors first concerned themselves with urban tradesmen and workers.[74] From its first meetings, the Royal Society called upon its correspondents to study the urban trades and the diseases and hazards that afflicted artisans. To stimulate research, in 1777, the doctor and chemist Antoine Fourcroy translated the classic book by Bernardino Ramazzini, *De morbis artificum* (1700), which had first pioneered the study of occupational disease. According to Ramazzini, working conditions potentially made people sick and he studied a number of manual trades in their actual work environment to catalogue the disease risks particular to each. Here, he identified two kinds of occupational disease: the first was caused by diet and living conditions; the second was caused by the work itself.[75] Though reviewers generally praised Ramazzini for his hard work

---

73 *Histoire de la Société Royale*: 'Histoire de la Société Royale de Médecine', vol. 1, pt 1, p. ii; and 'Préamble', vol. 8, pt 1, pp. 8–9.

74 See the brief comments in Arlette Farge, 'Les artisans malades de leur travail', *Annales: E.S.C.* 32 (1977): 993–1006; Harvey Mitchell, 'The Political Economy of Health in France, 1770–1830: The Debate over Hospital and Home Care and Images of the Working-Class Family', in Martin S. Staum and Donald E. Larson (eds), *Doctors, Patients, and Society*, pp. 90–92.

75 Bernardino Ramazzini, *De morbis artificum* (Multinae, 1700), pp. 1–3.

and insights, his successors failed to expand upon his research (except in the most general terms) or, more importantly, to implement any of his projected reforms. For his part, Fourcroy – who was a major figure in medical reform efforts and who would later engineer far-reaching professional and educational changes during the French Revolution – wanted to fill this lacuna by giving Ramazzini a modern translation and thus inspire new research into occupational health.

In his new edition, Fourcroy offered a programmatic essay that introduced readers to the current knowledge about occupational health. In this text, he connected occupational health to fears about degeneracy and decline, saying the study of work diseases and hazards contributed to the Royal Society's mission to regenerate society. He thus saw occupational health as a humanitarian and epidemiological problem. On a humanitarian level, urban tradesmen were becoming more and more sick as the leisured classes demanded more and more luxury goods. In this analysis, Fourcroy did not advocate an anti-luxury programme; nor was he a physiocrat, in that he classified manufacturing as a 'sterile' form of production (unlike agriculture, which physiocrats believed was the sole thing that generated wealth). Nevertheless, he believed that trade and manufacturing contributed to socioeconomic well-being and he feared that disease and dearth threatened productivity.[76] On an epidemiological level, he wanted to know why epidemics left some tradespeople unscathed but devastated other groups, and thus asked what exercises, what vapours and what substances left some people immune to contagious diseases.[77]

As a consequence, Fourcroy urged correspondents to discuss artisan disease within their medical topographies. Following Ramazzini, doctors should study working conditions first-hand in the shop floor and correspond with manufacturers, guild masters and employers, asking them about potential health conditions and health measures. At the same time, Fourcroy encouraged doctors to forge stronger bonds between the medical community and manufacturing leaders. The Royal Society thus approached occupational health in a 'top down' fashion, rather than 'from below'.[78]

The Royal Society was not alone in its concern about occupational hazards and disease. In 1782, for example, the prestigious Academy of Sciences picked up this issue after one of its patrons denoted £12,000 to establish a yearly essay award on occupational disease.[79] In contrast to Fourcroy's health programme, the Academy of Sciences hoped to use technological advances to prevent occupational disease and hazards. As a number of respondents claimed, manufacturers could stop work-related diseases by changing production techniques – for instance, by no longer putting lead in paint mixtures and by substituting other substances instead.[80] But above all, the Academy of Sciences underscored that occupational disease and hazards posed moral problems for consumers. As academicians put it, consumers could not fully

---

76 A.-F. Fourcroy, 'Introduction', in Ramazzini, *Essai sur les maladies des artisans ... avec des notes et des additions*, trans. and ed. A.-F. Fourcroy (Paris, 1777), pp. viii–ix.

77 Fourcroy, ibid., pp. l–li.

78 Ibid., pp. lii–liii.

79 ARS, Procès-verbaux, vol. 101, 17 Apr. and 21 Dec. 1782.

80 ARS, carton 2 (prix), d. Broyeurs de couleurs (1789), n. 6 and n. 7.

enjoy a commodity when they were aware of the real conditions under which it had been made. Consequently, they felt guilty for buying the item because they knew they were promoting an industry that hurt the people who worked in it. But learned societies could focus scientific attention upon the problem and alleviate occupational hazards. Science could thus absolve consumer conscience, and thereby increase productivity and consumerism. As the Academy explained:

> What a sad consequence of industry! Our buildings are cemented with blood, our clothes are tainted with it, our pleasures are infected by it. There isn't a day where money doesn't cause murders, and human life is bartered and sold like any other commodity. However, because we don't actually see these deaths ... we tell ourselves that we aren't being inhuman.[81]

In their topographies and reports, correspondents described hazards created by both traditional manufacturing and the new factories and cottage industries that were spreading throughout France.[82] In some ways, medical practitioners described occupational health in straightforward terms. Like the peasants, most tradesmen and women worked too hard and this exertion drained the body's vital energy. The humours degenerated and the body lost its strength. Bad diet and miserable living conditions intensified this decline and kept the body from replenishing itself. The result was sickness and death. Beyond these basic observations, however, doctors began to raise troubling questions about the relation between work and sickness. First, they wanted to know whether the work itself – like a repetitive manual task – made people sick, or whether sickness was caused by dangerous materials or an unsanitary workplace. Second, doctors wondered whether forces outside the workplace caused disease – especially immorality or poverty – and considered lifestyle a factor in disease risk. Finally, doctors asked about the ethical issues posed by occupational disease, debating whether they were morally responsible for helping the sick worker, or whether they should represent the manufacturer's socioeconomic interests. On all these questions, doctors were unable to draw firm conclusions.[83]

These concerns appear in the reports written by Honoré Flaugergues. In a series of manuscripts, Flaugergues studied a vast textile factory and putting-out system in southern France, owned by the prestigious Auresche family, which stretched across Viviers and part of the Dauphiné – a massive industry that provisioned the army with over 50,000 uniforms each year. In his report, Flaugergues described the Auresche factories as a mixed blessing. Although the factory system had lowered regional

---

81   ARS, Prochettes de séance, 17 Apr. 1782.

82   On the world of work in the old regime, see William H. Sewell, Jr., *Work and Revolution in France: The Language of Labor from the Old Regime to 1848* (Cambridge, 1980); and Michael Sonenscher, *Work and Wages: Natural Law, Politics, and the Eighteenth-Century French Trades* (Cambridge, 1989).

83   On this ambivalence, see Destrapière, 'Mémoire sur la topographie d'Aunis', which claimed that local artisans were so affluent that they were often mistaken for the town's 'premiers citoyens'; whilst La Borde, 'Topographie de la Gascogne', complained of worker poverty and poor dietary habits. Others emphasized an unsanitary working environment: see SRM 168, d. 3, Legrand, 'Observations sur les maladies épidémiques de la Picardie', 13 June 1786; and SRM 146, d. 9, Hassenfratz, 'Mémoire sur les maladies des fondeurs' (n.d.).

unemployment and brigandism, it had also undermined traditional morals and health by creating a new taste for luxury. As a consequence, the young workers had become more libidinous and luxurious: they indulged in evening escapades on Sundays and festive events, and they recklessly wasted their hard-earned wages (six or seven *sols* per day) on puerile distractions.

At the same time, the Auresche factories posed physical hazards to the workers. For example, the workers treated the wool with chemicals in the local river that the poor used as their only water supply. On the looms and spinning machines, sharp instruments protruded and posed obvious dangers to extremities. Inside the mill, workers treated the wool with oil and urine solutions that filled the environment with noxious miasma. Consequently, employees experienced recurring respiratory infections and the younger workers regularly coughed up blood. The women suffered from irregular menses, jaundice and a melancholy disposition (no doubt from spending long hours in an enclosed work place). In general, nine out of fifteen workers died from respiratory infections – and tuberculosis was the leading cause of death in the Dauphiné. Still, he insisted, neighbouring localities suffered even worse.[84]

Not all observers criticized factory conditions. One mirror manufacturer, named Deslandes, wrote to the Royal Society to describe the health conditions of his nearly 2,500 workers at the great St Gobain factory. As he made clear, every job had its own risks and dangers, and factory work was no exception. In terms of manufacturing, workers became sick because they passed their days in hot sweatshops, performed monotonous physical tasks, and breathed miasma and vitiated airs. But fortunately, a well-meaning and paternalistic manufacturer could keep them healthy. To achieve these ends, Deslandes had made his workshops into a sanitary showcase. The factory ovens purified the air, and he did not put arsenic in the local water. Believing that laziness made workers sick, Deslandes made them exercise regularly and eat their meals outside in the fresh air. Therefore, worker diseases were caused either by climatic factors or by a lack of personal hygiene. Whereas poverty, diet and living conditions might sometimes influence sickness, these factors were beyond the owner's personal control. So if workers got sick, they should blame fate or blame themselves – but, he implied, not his factories.[85] In typical ways, Deslandes reflected how eighteenth-century commentators often disassociated work from the real conditions of production. A good example of this thinking appears in the lavish plates of Diderot's *Encyclopédie*, which portrayed artisanal manufacturing quite anonymously and without reference to the worker's milieu.[86]

Unlike Deslandes, many observers struggled between class interests and genuine empathy for the labouring poor. A good example of this ambivalence appears in the correspondence of Pajot de Charmes, who was a government inspector of glass factories at Abbeville. After surveying working conditions, he concluded

---

84 SRM 131, d. 21, Flaugergues fils, 'Observations sur l'influence des travaux relatifs à la fabrication des étoffes de laine sur la santé des ouvriers qui y travaillent dans les manufactures de la ville de Viviers en Vivarais', 10 Dec. 1779.

85 SRM 196, d. 8 (no. 1–2), Deslandes, directeur de manufacteur des glaces de St Gobain, 'Mémoire' (n.d.).

86 Mitchell, 'The Political Economy of Health'.

that mineral poisons and mephitic air found within the glass factories directly caused the high levels of pulmonary and nervous disorders. As he described it, many workers fell into syncope and had to be resuscitated on the shop floor, whilst others suffered apoplectic or hysterical seizures. Clearly, the manufacturers had to alter the production process.[87] Yet most observers avoided placing direct blame upon owners and managers, even when they identified significant problems in the work environment itself. Instead, these medical observers often preferred to wax philosophical about the cosmic meaning of work and the timeless plight of the poor. According to Dr Bertrand, a physician who tended patients at the glass works at Sainte-Catherine in Nivernais, the labouring arts proved a mixed blessing. Although work elevated the human spirit, it also caused health problems because it sapped the body's vital energies and left a pathological imprint upon the animal economy. In this case, Bertrand believed that factory conditions contributed to the high levels of disease amongst the glass workers – but he also blamed their high morbidity because of 'their way of life, in their pernicious habits, but, above all, in the indifference and the absolute contempt they demonstrate in general'. According to him, workers could potentially reduce predisposing morbid causes through private hygiene, and he particularly stressed daily bathing, clean clothing and a more sensible diet.[88]

In some instances, public officials and manufacturers asked doctors to mediate in labour disputes over occupational health. For example, in the early 1770s, municipal authorities in Marseilles became alarmed when journeymen and apprentices in the hat making guilds went on strike to improve health conditions. The hat makers said they suffered more than other manufacturing trades from sickness, including tremors, pain, paralysis, bloody coughing, paleness, blackened teeth, salivation and sensory loss. Town elders followed the strike closely because hat making was Marseilles's primary luxury export and it employed a high percentage of the urban work force. In 1774, town officials summoned four physicians (Raymond, Magnan, Mingaud and Montagnier) to investigate the journeymen's complaints, and two years later they published their results in the *Journal de physique*.[89]

These doctors took the municipal order seriously and applied the method outlined by Ramazzini and Fourcroy. In their investigation, they directly observed the hat makers at home and at work, and even interviewed masters, journeymen, apprentices and wage-earners. In their report to the city elders, the physicians suggested that a so-called *eau de composition* caused occupational diseases. Masters made this chemical solution in secret to treat skins and fabrics, and it often contaminated the workers' bodies and their food. After work, journeymen and apprentices carried this deadly substance back to their homes, causing the family to get sick as well.

---

87 SRM 174, d. 30, no. 14, Pajot de Charmes, 'Mémoire sur les maladies et incommodités auxquelles sont exposées les ouvriers de verrerie et particulièrement ceux de glacerie' (1787).

88 SRM 182, d. 2, Bertrand, 'Mémoire sur les maladies les plus fréquentes des verriers, et la manière de les traiter; où, à plusieurs observations relatives à cet objet, l'on a joint quelques remarques importantes sur les moyens de conserver leur santé', 28 Dec. 1787.

89 SRM 139, d. 35 *bis*, Magnan, 'Mémoire sur les accidents auxquels sont exposés les garçons chapeliers de la ville de Marseille et sur les moyens de les prévenir' (n.d.).

When interrogating the trade masters, the doctors discovered the compound's secret substance: mercury.[90] Fortunately, as they found, comparative experiences in Paris taught that well-ventilated workshops decreased hazards related to mercury poisoning. For these reasons, doctors recommended that owners implement more stringent health precautions on the shop floor, promising that these new regulations would not interfere with manufacturing costs. According to the physicians, owners should make sure that the air circulated freely in the workplace; they should use less mercury in the *eau de composition*; they should remove unnecessary chemical compounds; and journeymen and apprentices should not associate with the masters who made the chemical solutions. In addition, the shop owners and masters must provide clean water in the shop, so workers could wash their hands after handling contaminating agents; and labourers should avoid inhaling chemical miasma.[91]

At least one tradesman joined this medical discussion. On 18 March 1789, a master craftsman named Santini wrote a letter to the Academy of Sciences that described his general health and health regimen. That year, the Academy had posed its yearly essay question on the dangers of lead smelting. Santini was a lead caster who worked near Versailles and supplied the king and his court with hunting goods. He did not want to compete for the prize but simply wanted to tell the Academy about his own health experiences, which he felt were relevant to the proceedings. As Santini described it, he did well for himself in economic terms, but his success also offered dangers, because he had to work everyday in his shop and was constantly surrounded by deadly fumes from the molten lead. As was well known, many tradesmen and manufacturers who worked around lead – such as smelters, painters, potters and paint makers – suffered from 'terrible colics' after they had inhaled or ingested the substance. To avoid poisoning, Santini thus urged workers to adapt a sober, ascetic regimen. Unlike other tradesmen, he avoided drinking spirits and undiluted wine. Every morning, he began his day by eating a slice of buttered bread. Throughout the workday, which he described as 'long and hard', he only drank water coloured with red wine and raw milk. This regimen, he believed, had preserved his health through forty-eight years as a lead smelter. As a result, he required his fourteen-year old son and all his journeymen and apprentices to follow the same diet, which was then approved by Dr Malloin (a physician attached to the royal court). One wonders, of course, whether Malloin had encouraged him to write to the Academy or whether Santini did it on his own cognizance. Revolution was in the air: Louis XVI had just convened the Estates-General, and maybe Santini was emboldened enough by the events to speak directly to elites on matters regarding his personal health.[92]

The medical concern about occupational diseases is significant. Not only does it highlight doctors' anxieties about labour sedition and industrial change, but it also shows how they understood disease in terms of group behaviour, whether sexuality,

---

90 SRM 139, d. 6 (3 pièces), Achard, 'Essai sur les maladies des chapeliers' (1781).

91 Magnan, 'Mémoire sur les accidents'; Achard, 'Essai sur les maladies'.

92 ARS, carton II (prix), 1789, Broyeurs de couleurs: Santini, letter of 18 Mar. 1789, Versailles.

physical constitution, community, geography or – in this case – occupation.[93] Medical practitioners wanted to understand shared health experiences – women, children, people of fashion, intellectuals, artisans, peasants, workers, soldiers and sailors – *and* the habitat in which they lived – schools, universities, convents, ships, barracks, prisons, factories, workshops and the private household. At this time, physicians thought that workers also formed a distinct community that deserved to be studied and observed. In his study of women lacemakers, for example, Dr Claude-Denis Balme appealed to this reasoning, stating that 'it is about them, about the indisposition they have acquired by this labour or by their manner of life'.[94] By approaching health problems in group terms, practitioners could better study social pathologies and thereby regenerate the sick kingdom. They were applying, on an even broader scale, the methodological and ideological concerns first raised about the health of fashionable elites, intellectuals, women and children during the 1750s and 1760s.

Urban sanitation

Health activists moved from urban trades to the city itself. As with their writings about the countryside, these doctors saw urban life in complex and ambivalent ways, and they often contradicted the negative views found in Enlightenment philosophy and sentimental literature.[95] These anti-urban attitudes are well-known. For example, L. S. Mercier's *Tableau de Paris* and Nicolas Restif de la Bretonne's *Les nuits de Paris* had sketched a terrifying and hallucinatory vision of the city: its streets were filled with excrement and human effluvia, its polluted air choked inhabitants, and its private and secret spaces were home to moral horrors – much like Giovanni Battista Piranesi's haunting prisons or the Marquis de Sade's gothic castle of Silling.[96] Not surprisingly, several prominent physicians claimed that urban life made people sick. For example, in his *Domestic Medicine* – a work translated and much admired in France – Dr William Buchan talked about cities in tandem with words such as 'contagion', 'contaminate', 'dirty', 'excrement', 'filth', 'infection', 'pollute' and

---

93   On the continuity of these fears, see the detailed analysis in Steven Kaplan, 'Réflexions sur la police du monde du travail, 1700–1815', *Revue historique* 256 (1979): 17–78.

94   SEM, carton A-B, d. Balme (no. 1), Claude-Denis Balme, 'Recherches sur la santé de quelques communautés d'artisans', 20 Apr. 1788.

95   See SRM 147, d. 1, Bouillet, 'Exposition des maladies les plus fréquentes qui ont été observées à Béziers et dans plusieurs autres lieux soit en France, soit dans les pays étrangers, depuis le commencement de l'année 1746 jusqu'à la fin de 1769 (séance du 24 décembre 1776)'; SRM 168, d. 3, Weguelin, 'Sur les principes, progrès, nature et cause de la maladie épidémique, qui a régné à Mieleshiem', 12 Aug. 1786; and SRM 168, d. 3, Tallibon, 'La fièvre putride épidémique de Mesrobert', 16 July 1786.

96   On eighteenth-century images of the urban environment, see Pierre Saddy, 'Le cycle des immondices', *Dix-huitième siècle*, no. 9 (1977): 203–14; and P.-D. Boudriot, 'Essai sur l'ordure en milieu urbain à l'époque pré-industrielle: boues, immondices et gadoue à Paris au XVIIIe siècle', *Histoire, économie et société* 5 (1986): 515–28.

'putrid', all which encapsulated how the unsanitary milieu rendered city dwellers 'effeminate', 'weak' and 'deformed'.[97]

Small-town doctors saw the city with different eyes. For them, the towns offered great opportunities to improve health – not least because townspeople had access to learned physicians – but they cautioned that urban living offered another set of health hazards. Whereas doctors believed poverty, ignorance and superstition had corrupted the countryside, they also believed that libertinism and luxury ruined urban health.[98] With Balzacian relish, Dr Brieude described a world of bourgeois mediocrity, petty desire and creature comfort that ultimately degenerated the health of town dwellers. '[The townspeople] are constantly preoccupied with their neighbours' lifestyle', he complained. '[T]hey are jealous of them, deliberately provoke anxieties and commit malicious deeds. From this is born an incessant hate [and] ruinous affairs … . In these small towns there are only liaisons of convenience: one doesn't understand that true happiness consists in doing good for one's neighbour'.[99] This vacuous lifestyle, contended Dr Bogreau de la Fon, caused nervous exhaustion, madness, sterility and early death.[100]

Although French doctors enthusiastically responded to the Royal Society's call to make a national medical topography, the members were astonished that correspondents had neglected that spiritual, intellectual and political centre of France: Paris.[101] For if cities were laboratories of collective experience, then Paris must embody these tendencies on the highest level; but encapsulating her social and physical conditions warranted an exacting medical mind. Only two physicians rose to this challenge: J.-J. Ménuret de Chambaud and Jacques Dehorne.

In 1786, Ménuret de Chambaud, a Montpellier graduate and contributor to Denis Diderot's *Encyclopédie, ou dictionnaire raisonné des sciences, des arts, et des métiers* (1777–79), published the first medical topography of Paris. Written in form of an epistolary novel, Ménuret outlined an empirical method, much like Lépecq's magisterial topography of the Norman landscape, for studying the Paris environment. His conclusions were mixed. In Paris, he claimed, bad city planning had subverted an otherwise favourable geography: the city walls and tall buildings, he emphasized, kept clean air from circulating. For example, the areas of Harpe, Huchette, Saint-Jacques, Saint-Denis and Les Halles were so filthy and narrow that one could hardly see the sky above; and slaughterhouses, cesspools, cemeteries and hospitals belched miasma into the air and created an 'atmospheric cesspool'.[102]

---

97   William Buchan, *Domestic Medicine, or, a Treatise on the Prevention and Cure of Diseases by Regimen and Simple Medicines* (London, 1772), pp. 37–38, 93, 125.

98   SRM 177, d. 1, Gerey, 'Topographie médicale de la ville de Pont à Mousson'; and Pierre Berthelon, *De la salubrité de l'air des villes et en particulier des moyens de la procurer* (Montpellier, 1786), p. 4.

99   Brieude, 'Topographie de la Haute-Auvergne', 301–02.

100 SRM 177, d. 1, Bogreau de la Fon, 'Topographie des paroisses d'Availles, Limouzine et Pressac' (n.d.).

101 AN F[17]1148, d. 8, no. 30, 'Extrait des registres de la Société Royale de Médecine', 12 Apr. 1785.

102 J.-J. Ménuret de Chambaud, *Essais sur l'histoire médico-physique de Paris*, 2d edn (Paris, Year XIII), pp. 28–29.

When emphasizing these factors, Ménuret highlighted a paradox in urban life: by assembling in urban communities, man had followed his sociable instincts and obtained clear political and cultural advantages. In the cities, he learned to communicate, hone his reason and exercise his sense. But Ménuret wondered whether people were happier on account of these 'new and artificial qualities' – as he confessed, 'I wouldn't dare decide'.[103] The cities promoted science, art, manners and progress, but they also sapped physical and moral vitality, destroyed man's original bond with nature, and increased desire and imagination. This was particularly true in Paris. Paris, he concluded, was a place where 'everything is modified, altered and denaturalized', and its inhabitants scarcely retained 'their primitive character'. Whilst charitable by impulse, Parisians loved luxury, extravagance and spectacle – indulgences that overly irritated their nerves.[104]

But Ménuret also said good things about Parisian health. Despite urban blights, Parisians lived in a favourable climate and they naturally had a moderate and gay temperament. Overall, Parisians were bilious, pituitous and sometimes melancholic; they boasted a healthy constitution, an 'advantageous' height and a light-brown, white complexion. Left to its own devices, the population naturally expanded; and the racial intermixture in the city rendered its children vibrant and virile. Unfortunately, Parisian children were precocious and prodigious and sometimes they wasted their vital energy and become degenerate libertines instead.

According to Ménuret, Parisian women and the labouring classes abused their health. Women, in particular, were luxurious and indulged in libertine debaucheries. They refused to nurse their children – 'a duty', he fumed, 'which seems like the *corvée* for them' – and they suffered from uterine maladies and convulsions. By contrast, artisans and merchants breathed poisoned air and lived in cramped, unsanitary conditions. He wrote, 'The people are piled and pressed together; a room without windows serves as a sanctuary for twenty sweepers and porters. Within these filthy quarters and amongst the inferior classes the disadvantages of humanity and atmospheric alteration are multiplied'.[105]

Whereas Ménuret gave his readers a travelogue of Paris disease, Dr Jacques Dehorne, one of the Royal Society's prominent associates, offered a series of manuscripts to the Royal Society and official administrators to reform urban health conditions; his extensive topography was part method, part action.[106] Dehorne praised the Royal Society's studies on occupational and environmental sickness and boasted that a medical topography of Paris would be academy's crowning achievement. Here, questions about space and population overlapped, and his topography left few stones unturned.[107] Like Ménuret, Dehorne felt ambivalent about Parisian health and he criticized health conditions. In particular, he insisted that authorities should

---

103 Ibid., pp. 7–9.
104 Ibid., pp. 63–64.
105 Ibid., pp. 98, 121.
106 ANM, ms. 10, Procès-verbeaux de la SRM, séance publique, 30 Aug. 1785.
107 AN F¹⁷1148, d. 8, n. 29, Jacques Dehorne, 'Plan de la topographie médicale de la ville de Paris, présenté à Monseigneur le Baron de Breteuil, Ministre et Secrétaire d'État au département de Paris, par M. Dehorne, docteur en médecine' (n.d.).

remove fish markets, butcher shops and slaughter houses from the centre of Paris; and the cemetery of St Innocents, situated north of the Seine in the heart of the city, was an insufferable urban blight.[108] But Dehorne also identified social factors that caused disease, and he saw poverty as an acute cause of morbidity and mortality. As he wrote, 'The government must do everything for this [lower] class of people, one of the most useful for societal maintenance, to give Paris all the healthy conditions it is capable of and to destroy the greatest number of potential infectious causes'.[109]

Given his neo-Hippocratic sensibilities, Dehorne offered predictable reforms. The blights associated with poverty, he thought, would be best alleviated through environmental engineering, which would promote urban health. To help the air circulate, city authorities should pave the roads, build new quays alongside the Seine and put in new sewers and drains because the river banks were often clogged with excrement and filth. Finally, Dehorne hoped that the Academy of Sciences' recent inquest into prison and hospital conditions would provide important suggestions for removing institutional sources of contamination. Of course, the government lacked the resources and will to implement these reforms, but Dehorne shows a new utopian emphasis in environmental engineering.[110]

In many ways, Ménuret and Dehorne built upon recent ideas about urbanism and urban renewal that were spreading in intellectual circles. In the 1760s, for instance, abbé Laugier and Pierre Patte published major architectural tracts, in which they argued that authorities should improve air circulation in Paris. These architects argued that the government should widen and pave thoroughfares; construct supplementary cesspools and cemeteries; and commission public squares and fountains. Following these works, the Académie Royale d'Architecture sponsored competitions on urban design: the participants underscored rational spatial management, neoclassical sensibilities and public propriety. As a consequence, even renowned architects, such as Marie-Joseph Peyre and Jean-Claude Delafosse, saw water works and slaughterhouses as objects for serious design studies.

Following these aesthetic interests, physicians joined public discussion about urban reform, as well. In 1767, Dr Léopold de Genneté proposed mechanized ventilation systems for private and public buildings, and four years later, Dr Oliver of Montpellier advocated making new 'air reservoirs' (city squares) in his *Sépultures des anciens, où l'on démontre qu'elles étaient hors des villes* (1771). After the devastating Paris *hôtel-Dieu* fire on New Year's Eve of 1773, Dr Antoine Petit began thinking about hospital design in his *Mémoire sur la meilleure manière de construire un hôpital de malades* (1774), whilst Mathieu Géraud designed cesspools in his *Essai sur la suppression des fosses d'aisance et de tout espèce de voiries* (1786). In the 1780s, A.-L. Lavoisier and Baron L.-A. Breteuil at the Academy of Sciences

---

108 AN F[17]1148, d. 8, n. 28, Jacques Dehorne, *Mémoire sur quelques objets qui intéressent plus particulièrement la salubrité de la ville de Paris* (Paris, 1788).

109 AN F[17]1148, d. 8, n. 31, Jacques Dehorne, 'Observations sur les moyens d'augmenter la salubrité de Paris' (n.d.).

110 Ibid.

studied prison and hospital conditions, and in 1783 the royal government adopted new building codes in Paris.[111]

In all these examples, observers considered urban pollution with greater care. At this stage, lay people seemed less interested health planning and urban aesthetics than articulating tolerable levels of cleanliness for the entire community. In the 1770s and 1780s, debates about air quality demonstrate this new sensitivity. For contemporaries, as Alain Corbin has demonstrated in his pioneering history of smell, the air ultimately embodied agents of purity and danger.[112] After Lavoisier discovered oxidation, physicians identified gaseous pollutants (whether mephitic, acidic, alkaline or 'hepatic') and how they affected the animal economy.[113] They even hoped to develop an empirical language to describe the elusive world of smell and to discover remedies to alleviate gaseous dangers.[114] In one memorable example, the hygienist J.-N. Hallé conducted a series of walks alongside the Seine, recording all the smells he came across. In other works, Hallé tested 'anti-mephitic' remedies (such as vinegar and snow), proving their advertised efficacy remained dubious at best.[115]

Contemporaries soon turned to the smelliest places in urban Europe: cesspools and cemeteries. Throughout France, doctors and administrators studied graveyards and septic pits with new scientific rigor. For them, the link between disease, excrement and death was apparent. Dead bodies, decaying plants, and human and animal excreta filled the air with fetid substances, which suffocated, poisoned and degenerated everything in their path. Moreover, the dangers grew in large urban areas. The Royal Society warned: 'It is necessary to have travelled through those infected places to know what residues and products can be called the excrement of a large city, and to know, for science, the incommensurable augmentation of filthiness, stench and corruption that follows the confluence of people in cities with an immense population.'[116]

But these dangers were also recognized by royal administrators. In 1781, Parisian officials closed the antiquated cesspool in the centre of the city, 'la voirie de l'Enfant-Jésus'. But now this meant that waste and refuse had to be taken to the northern dump at Montfaucon, which also doubled as a site for public executions. As a consequence, the government turned to the Royal Society to help design a new

---

111 See the excellent overview in Richard A. Etlin, *Symbolic Space: French Enlightenment Architecture and Its Legacy* (Chicago, 1994).

112 Alain Corbin, *Le miasme et la jonquille: l'odorat et l'imaginaire social XVIIIe–XIXe siècles* (Paris, 1986); Georges Vigarello, *Le propre et le sale: l'hygiène du corps depuis le moyen âge* (Paris, 1985).

113 J.-N. Hallé, *Recherches sur la nature des effets du méphitisme des fosses d'aisance* (Paris, 1785), 74.

114 Brieude, 'Mémoire sur les odeurs que nous exhalons, considérées comme signes de la santé et des maladies', *Histoire de la Société Royale*, vol. 10, pp. xlvi–xlvii.

115 Hallé, 'Procès-verbal de la visite faite le long des deux rives de la rivière de Seine, depuis le Pont-neuf jusqu'à la Rapée et la Garre, le 14 février 1790', *Histoire de la Société Royale*, vol. 10, pp. lxxxv–xc; Dehorne, Thouret and Hallé, 'Rapport sur le prétendue propriété antiméphitique de la neige, et projet d'expérience suivies sur le méphitisme des fosses d'aisance', *Histoire de la Société Royale*, vol. 8, pt 1, pp. 173–87.

116 'Supplément au rapport précédente', *Histoire de la Société Royale*, vol. 8, pt 2, p. 226.

waste disposal system. After some research, a medical team, consisting of Dehorne, Hallé, Thouret and Fourcroy, submitted a detailed prognosis.

In this report, the doctors highlighted two problems: first, they wondered whether a single cesspool could accommodate the influx of human waste; and second, they wanted to know whether it was hazardous to transport excrement from city centre to the north. For the first point, the Royal Society voiced few objections, since the city had recently acquired new land around Montfaucon and entrepreneurs now mined solid waste for fertilizer. In addition, Montfaucon was strategically located: its peripheral location meant that wind wouldn't blow miasma back into the city.

However, practitioners worried about removing the debris. Waste, they contended, should be transported at night and the materials should be shipped in sealed containers. In this regard, they rejected a proposal by the lieutenant general of the Paris police, M. de Crosne, who wanted to strain the liquid waste into the Seine river before carting off the solid excrement. But the doctors believed that dumping solid wastes in the river was too dangerous, and they feared this policy would also encourage private citizens to engage in unhygienic acts. In this case, these doctors believed that waste disposal was now a medical matter. But the report didn't stipulate which doctors would have to inspect waste deposits, nor they did suggest how the strapped royal government could finance it.[117]

In last years of the old regime, doctors achieved one spectacular victory in their efforts to transform urban health. Starting in the 1780s, they forced municipal authorities first to close and then to actually remove all cemeteries from urban centres.[118] For years, reform-minded doctors and administrators had clamoured for the government to take this bold initiative. In truth, however, local complaints often forced municipal authorities to close down old graveyards. In public documents, city dwellers asserted that noxious airs from cemeteries and church miasma violated their 'right' to breath pure air and to enjoy a sanitary environment.[119] These concerns, in turn, were championed by Enlightenment philosophers and philanthropists. In 1737, the Academy of Sciences issued a report by Lémery, Geoffroy and Hunauld, in which they warned that authorities should be more careful when disposing of the dead. In 1745, abbé Porée followed this claim and declared that church burials defiled sacred space. By the mid-century, intellectual elites believed that it was dangerous to keep the dead near the living. They couched the language less in aesthetic than health

---

117 See *Histoire de la Société Royale*: Dehorne, Hallé, Fourcroy and Thouret, 'Premier rapport sur la voirie de Montfaucon', vol. 8, pt 1, pp. 198–221; and Thouret, 'Second rapport sur le service des voiries', vol. 8, pt 1, pp. 227–37.

118 See Madeleine Foisil, 'Les attitudes devant la mort au XVIIIe siècle: sépultures et suppressions de sépultures dans le cimetière parisien des Saints-Innocens', *Revue historique* 510 (1974): 303–30; Owen Hannaway and Caroline Hannaway, 'La fermature du cimetière des Innocents', *Dix-huitième siècle*, no. 9 (1977): 181–92; Philippe Ariès, *The Hour of Our Death*, trans. Helen Weaver (New York, 1981), pp. 475–507; and Riley, *Campaign to Avoid Disease*, pp. 108–11.

119 See Thouret, 'Rapport sur les exhumations de cimetière de l'église des Saints-Innocens', *Histoire de la Société Royale*, vol. 8, pt 1, p. 239; and also the later complaints voiced by Paris inhabitants: AN F^{8}92, d. 11B (f), 'Cimetière sous Montmartre, 1806–07'.

terms. As one doctor explained, the smell caused by decaying flesh could infect an entire locality with disease.[120]

The urban legends grew. In elite and popular circles, people told horrible tales of grave diggers and sewage workers who, upon opening grave pits, crypts, or septic tanks, were attacked by mephitic gas and fell into states of apoplexy, hysteria and syncope – often fatal. The most widely read book was Dr Henri Haguenot's *Sur le danger des inhumations* (1746), a short piece that recounted stories of people who had been miraculously revived after suffering miasmic poisoning. These stories about 'resuscités' appeared in popular literature throughout France and terrified the general public.[121] At this point, cemeteries had begun to haunt administrators, doctors and architects alike. In the words of one commentator: 'For quite some time, the truth has been known that those places in which the dead are disposed exhale putrid emanations that slowly kill the living or infect the air they breathe and the food they eat. Such is the opinion of doctors, juriconsults and savants'.[122]

By the 1770s, urban cemeteries were causing a major administrative headache, and provoked fights between enlightened reformers and church authorities. At first, the clergy opposed the Paris parlement's 1765 order to remove all cemeteries and prevent future burials within city walls. Soon after, however, a number of writers revived the issue and warned against the dangers of burying people in churches and town cemeteries. From its first meetings, the Royal Society concerned itself with cemetery relocation; and Vicq d'Azyr dug up Scipion Piattoli's Italian treatise on the topic, which he translated as *Essai sur les lieux et les dangers des sépultures* in 1778.[123] Outside the major cities, country doctors were also animated about 'the danger posed by inhuming cadavers in the midst of the living' and they thought that local cemeteries posed grave hazards.[124] In Toulouse, archbishop Loménie de Brienne took the first step and prohibited church burials. The new king Louis XVI finally put the matter to rest when he outlawed burials in churches and town cemeteries throughout the kingdom.[125]

Still, as doctors complained, the existing graveyards hadn't moved themselves. But the costs and logistics seemed insurmountable. In Paris in 1779, the situation came to a head. That year, mephitic vapours began leaking from the common graves of St Innocents, the oldest and most venerable cemetery of Paris. Cellars were infected,

---

120 P.-N. Navier, *Réflexions sur les dangers des exhumations précipitées, et sur l'abus des inhumations dans les églises* (Amsterdam and Paris, 1775), p. 7.

121 J.-J. Bruhier d'Ablaincourt, *Dissertation sur l'incertitude de la mort et l'abus des enterremens et embauments précipités*, 2d edn (2 vols, Paris, 1749), vol. 1, pp. 594, 601.

122 AN F⁸92, d. 11A(b), 'Mémoire tendant à l'établissement d'un cimetière général hors de Paris' (n.d.).

123 Richard A. Etlin, *The Architecture of Death: The Transformation of the Cemetery in Eighteenth-Century Paris* (Cambridge, MA, 1984), pp. 3–39.

124 SRM 168, d. 3, Legrand, 'Observations sur les maladies épidémiques de la Picardie', 13 June 1786.

125 AN F⁸92, d. 11A (b), 'Précis sur l'établissement de nouveaux cimetières hors de Paris et sur la nécessité d'un dépôt général des régistres des personnes décédées à Paris, dans les hôpitaux militaires, dans les colonies, dans l'Inde, dans les voyages maritimes et dans les pays étrangers', 4 Oct. 1787.

and public pandemonium followed. In 1781–82, therefore, the Paris police officially closed all local cemeteries, including St Innocents, Chaussée-d'Antin (St Roch), St Joseph (St Eustache), St Sulpice and the Île St Louis. Unfortunately, these actions could not stop the mephitic contamination at St Innocents; after all, the cemetery was still stuffed with rotting bodies. On 5 November 1785, the royal government took the extraordinary step and ordered authorities to demolish the ancient cemetery. Between 1786 and 1788, the Paris police razed the church and its graveyard and transported the decomposing bodies and polluted soil to the Catacombs, once a famous hideaway for thieves. In place of the cemetery, the government built a fruit market and fountain square. The dead were now buried in four major cemeteries: Clamart, Vaugirard, Montmartre and Ste Marguerite (the last of which was replaced in 1804 by Père-Lachaise). This landscape of death still dominates Paris.[126]

Though the Royal Society was dissolved during the French Revolution, it could claim a distinguished history in the service of public health. But for all of the society's medical police endeavours, it congratulated itself, above all, on how it moved the cemetery of St Innocents. In many ways, this act summarized the Royal Society's entire mission to cure a sick and declining nation. Fearing popular resistance against violating this sacred space, as well as the threat of local infection, the academy took every imaginable precaution to honour the dead, maintain tranquillity and preserve propriety – whilst all along doctors privately celebrated the clinical opportunities afforded by exhuming such an enormous number of corpses.[127] Public authorities dismembered the cemetery at night and tried to clear the air by using copious douses of lime, streams of purifying water, ventilating machines and bonfires. Louis Héricaut de Thury described the spectacle:

> The work was carried out with the greatest deliberation and the setting frequently took on a pictorial quality. The many torches and the circles of fires which surrounded the scene, spread a funereal light whose flickering reflections disappeared into the surrounding objects; the outline of the crosses, the tombs and the epitaphs, the silence of the night, the thick cloud of smoke which cloaked the work-site, in the center of which the workers moved like shadows, their various tasks being indistinguishable, the different ruins caused by the demolition of the buildings, the upturned soil from the exhumations; all of these gave the scene an impressive but lugubrious aspect. The religious ceremonies only added to this spectacle. The carrying of the coffins, the solemnity which accompanied the removal of the graves of the most distinguished people, the hearses and catafalques, the long trains of funeral chariots loaded with bones slowly wending their way, at the close of the day to the new catacombs, outside the walls of the city, which had been prepared to receive these sad burdens … . The ministers of the church officiated at these various

---

126 For earlier plans, see AN F^{8}92, d. 11A (b), Pérard, 'Plan de nouveaux cimetières' (n.d.); and 'Mémoire tendant à l'établissement d'un cimetière général hors de Paris' (n.d.). See also Ariès, *Hour of Our Death*, pp. 495–96; and Etlin, *Architecture of Death*, pp. 33–4.

127 See *Histoire de la Société Royale*: Thouret, 'Rapport sur les exhumations de cimetière', vol. 7, pt 1, p. 241, and his 'Mémoire sur la nature de la substance du cerveau, et sur la propriété qu'il paroît avoir de se conserver long-tems après toutes les autres parties, dans les corps qui se décomposent au sein de la terre', vol. 8, pt 1, pp. 302–19.

operations. Thus, amidst the great bustle of work, the respect owed to the remains of the dead were never lost sight of.[128]

Conclusion: actor-network systems at work

As this chapter has shown, the Royal Society opened a new front in the battle to regenerate the kingdom, consciously picking up the cause to improve rural and urban conditions. In the late Enlightenment, this crusade formed part of the broader exchange between science and politics. In one sense, the Royal Society extended the central government's 'territorial ambitions' to mould France into a uniform and coherent polity. These ambitions dated back to the seventeenth century, when Louis XIV's mercantile policies – usually associated with Jean-Baptiste Colbert – used geographic science to extend military and administrative control over a diverse and fragmented kingdom. According to sociologist Chandra Mukerji, royal authorities linked land and bureaucracy in order to create a 'single material culture dedicated to the accumulation of power'. The best example was the Versailles gardens: here, the absolutist state transformed the physical landscape to make absolutism seem like a natural part of the earth itself.[129]

As recent historians and sociologists of science have shown, science played an important role in these territorial politics – both at home and in the colonies. In colonial ventures, especially, naturalists and doctors joined a parade of explorers, soldiers, settlers, missionaries and bureaucrats, helping to map out conquered space and provide public officials with the tools to expand and control their territories.[130] In this process, learned societies and scientific networks played a formative role by connecting practitioners and explorers from far-flung regional and socioeconomic backgrounds, and were sometimes just as important as print media in disseminating scientific knowledge and skills.[131] These networks could also push political and ideological agendas, as central authorities used dependency and patronage to control local practitioners and influence their activities. According to Bruno Latour, scientific networks managed how scientific practitioners exchanged data and specimens across vast differences, functioning as 'centres of calculation' that collected empirical data and put them in larger classificatory systems. In particular, these centres also allowed public officials and colonial enterprisers to survey non-European territories

---

128 Louis Héricaut de Thury, *Description des catacombes de Paris, précédé d'un précis historique sur les catacombes de tous les peoples de l'ancien et du nouveau continent* (Paris, 1815), pp. 170–72, quoted in Hannaway, 'Medicine, Public Welfare, and the State', p. 397.

129 Chandra Mukerji, *Territorial Ambitions and the Gardens of Versailles* (Cambridge and New York, 1997), p. 38.

130 Peter Hulme, *Colonial Encounters: Europe and the Native Caribbean* (Cambridge and New York, 1987); Michel de Certeau, *Heterologies: Discourse on the Other*, trans. Brian Massumi (Minneapolis, 1985), p. 67.

131 J. L. Pearl, 'The Role of Personal Correspondence in the Exchange of Scientific Information in Early Modern France', *Renaissance and Reformation* 8 (1984): 106–13; Anne Secord, 'Corresponding Interests: Artisans and Gentlemen in Nineteenth-Century Natural History', *British Journal for the History of Science* 27 (1994): 383–408.

and ultimately conquer and control them.[132] The best-studied are examples are the networks established by André Thourin at the Jardin du Roi and Joseph Banks at the Royal Society of London – two figures who both kept vast naturalist networks that spanned the globe.[133]

It is tempting to characterize the Royal Society's health activities – especially its topographic project – as part of these broader territorial ambitions associated with the absolutist state. Seen in this light, society members were engaged in a process of internal colonization, diligently mapping spaces and communicating health information to control local populations in metropolitan France. In this case, public officials and doctors used physical and moral hygiene to impose a standardized, homogenous culture upon in France – and they started with the basic and most intimate thing: the individual body. Ideological 'hegemony', in this interpretation, was the final goal.

Nevertheless, I must emphasize that government and scientific interests did not always neatly correspond. As Anne Secord and Emma Spary have shown in their work on naturalist exchanges in France and England, Latour's actor-network system fails to explain how scientific practitioners can use networks to push their own agendas and thus change beliefs and policies in the centre itself. In this manner, local correspondents could either refocus or subvert agendas first established by elite scientific bodies and their members.[134] These insights, I would argue, also apply to medical networks in old regime France. This is particularly true with medical topographies. In these reports, medical correspondents used the Royal Society to make their ideas about physical and moral hygiene into broader public concerns. In so doing, practitioners helped spread the belief, within official and medical circles, that the kingdom faced nervous degeneracy and depopulation, and forced new administrative interest into urban and rural health conditions. At the same time, correspondents gave urban doctors and public authorities a shocking – and sometimes unwanted – insight into rural conditions, forcing many doctors to explore the relationship between dearth and disease.

This is not to suggest, however, that medical crusaders were entirely able to force government to act upon their campaign for physical and moral hygiene. In some ways, correspondents were only too effective in convincing elite doctors and public officials about the problems facing rural health and hygiene. Faced with daunting circumstances, doctors abandoned their hopes to improve the countryside and instead advocated sanitary engineering in the towns and cities. Indeed, only war and revolution turned these concerns into a broader public debate about national regeneration. As the next chapter shows, these radical ideas about physical and moral hygiene first developed in the colonial context.

---

132 Bruno Latour, *Science in Action: How to Follow Scientists and Engineers through Society* (Cambridge, MA, 1987), pp. 215–57.

133 Emma C. Spary, *Utopia's Garden: French Natural History from Old Regime to Revolution* (Chicago, 2000), pp. 49–98; and David Philip Miller, 'Joseph Banks, Empire, and "Centers of Calculation" in Late Hanoverian London', in David Philip Miller and Peter Hanns Reill (eds), *Visions of Empire: Voyages, Botany, and Representations of Nature* (Cambridge, 1996), pp. 21–37.

134 Secord, 'Corresponding Interests'; and Spary, *Utopia's Garden*, pp. 96–98.

CHAPTER THREE

Colonial Bodies and Hygiene in the Antilles, *c.* 1750–1794

In Western thought, people have long associated contact and conquest in the torrid and desolate climates of the New World, Africa and the Near East with disease and death. In the eighteenth century, these themes habitually appeared in travel accounts such as Père Labat's *Nouveau voyage aux isles de l'Amérique*, Abbé Raynal's *Histoire des deux Indes*, Moreau de Saint-Méry's *Description de la partie française de l'isle de Saint-Domingue*, and M.-C.-F. Volney's *Voyage en Syrie et en Égypte*. According to these writers, colonial encounters invariably caused disease: Labat's lengthy narrative, for instance, began with his brethren missionaries' struggle against sickness and the grave, all which emphasized the daring and dangerous nature of the colonial project.[1]

This travel literature created two powerful and long-standing myths about disease and colonialism. On one level, contemporaries believed that epidemic diseases originated outside the Occident's clean and temperate lands and, like other commodities, they followed colonial trade and contact.[2] Therefore, European ports and colonial trading centres – such as Toulon and Marseilles – constantly worried about contamination and developed elaborate sanitary techniques to stop diseases from entering the mainland.[3] On another level, these travelogues spawned yet another myth: only doctors could heroically overcame colonial disease and dangers and thus bring European civilization to exotic – albeit pathological – lands and their native populations.[4]

---

1 Jean-Baptise Labat, *Nouveau voyage aux isles de l'Amérique, contenant l'histoire naturelle de ces pays, l'origine, les moeurs, la religion et le gouvernement des habitans anciens et modernes* (8 vols, Paris, 1742), vol. 1, pp. 1–22.

2 SRM 146, d. 1,Gennotte, 'Mémoire sur les maladies contagieuses', 1 Sept. 1789; SRM 118, d. 108, Gontare, 'De la contagion' (n.d.); and 'Voyage dans les échallelles du Levant, avec des détails sur les maladies qui y règne, sur la nature du sol, et sur le tempérament des habitans', *Histoire de la Société Royale de Médecine* (10 vols, Paris, 1779–98), vol. 2, pt 1, pp. 303–12. See also C.-F. Volney, *Voyage en Syrie et en Égypte, pendants les années 1783, 1784, et 1785* (2 vols, Paris, 1787), vol. 1, pp. 221–24.

3 After the traumatic Marseilles plague outbreak of 1720, doctors and public officials always worried about extra-European contacts and quarantines. For examples, see the documents in AN F⁸7, d. 2–3 and F⁸1, d. 1, 'Épidémies et trafic maritime, particulièrement en Provence', and d. 2, 'Épidémies et trafic maritime en Provence, Bretagne, Languedoc'; and SRM 180, d. 7, n. 9, Raymond, 'Mémoire sur le charbon de provence, les bubons et la peste' (n.d.).

4 See especially Daniel R. Headrick, *The Tools of Empire: Technology and European Imperialism in the Nineteenth Century* (New York, 1981); Philip Curtin, *Death by Migration:*

In this chapter, I explore how French doctors and social commentators responded to the different health experiences of the European and African slave populations in the French West Indies. Specifically, the analysis delineates the extent to which physicians used categories of race and class, and ideas about pollution and purity, to explain the incidence of disease among Europeans and Africans in the Caribbean tropics.[5] In the Antilles, I show, deplorable health conditions challenged how medical practitioners traditionally understood health and hygiene, and opened powerful debates about slavery, race and public health during the early stages of the French Revolution.

In the colonies, medical personnel were exposed to a bewildering array of lethal pathogens. French doctors and surgeons observed that two outsider population groups – Africans and Europeans – responded quite differently to the tropical setting, and they tried to explain these variations by using prevailing ideas about disease aetiology and prevention.[6] In contrast to doctors in Europe (who, as we have seen, often emphasized differences in class), colonial doctors often stressed differences of

---

Europe's Encounter with the Tropical World in the Nineteenth Century (Cambridge, 1989); and also William H. McNeill, *Plagues and Peoples* (New York, 1976). William B. Cohen first questioned these assumptions, pointing out that medical advances, particularly uses of quinine, actually followed imperial conquest and the implementation of colonial administration; see his 'Malaria and French Imperialism', *Journal of African History* 24 (1983): 23–36.

5   See Nancy Stepan, *The Idea of Race in Science: Great Britain 1800–1960* (London, 1982); and Seymour Drescher, 'The Ending of the Slave Trade and the Evolution of European Scientific Racism', *Social Science History* 14 (1990): 415–50. For variations on this theme, see especially Carminella Biondi, *Mon frère, tu es mon esclave! Teorie schiaviste e diabtti antropologico-razziali nel Settecento francese* (Pisa, 1973); and Pierre H. Boulle, 'In Defense of Slavery: Eighteenth-Century Opposition to Abolition and the Origins of a Racist Ideology in France', in Frederick Krantz (ed.), *History from Below: Studies in Popular Protests and Popular Ideology in Honor of George Rudé* (Montreal, 1986), pp. 221–41. On eighteenth-century racism, see Michèle Duchet, *Anthropologie et histoire au siècle des Lumières: Buffon, Voltaire, Rousseau, Helvétius, Diderot*, 2d edn (Paris, 1995); William B. Cohen, *The French Encounter with Africans: White Response to Blacks, 1530–1880* (Bloomington, 1980), ch. 3 and 5; Richard H. Popkin, 'The Philosophical Basis of Eighteenth-Century Racism', in Harold E. Pagliaro (ed.), *Racism in the Eighteenth Century*, vol. 3, *Studies in Eighteenth-Century Culture* (Cleveland, 1973), pp. 245–62; Ann Thomson, *Barbary and Enlightenment: European Attitudes towards the Maghreb in the Eighteenth Century* (New York, 1987), 64–93; and Harvey Mitchell and Samuel S. Kottek, 'An Eighteenth-Century Medical View of the Diseases of the Jews in Northeastern France: Medical Anthropology and the Politics of Jewish Emancipation', *Bulletin of the History of Medicine* 67 (1993): 248–81.

6   On colonial medicine and general disease aetioloigy, which focus primarily upon the nineteenth and early twentieth centuries, see James E. Paul, 'Medicine and Imperialism', in John Ehrenreich (ed.), *The Cultural Crisis of Modern Medicine* (New York, 1978), pp. 271–86, and the methodological considerations in David Arnold, 'Disease, Medicine, and Empire', in Arnold (ed.), *Imperial Medicine and Indigenous Societies* (Manchester, 1988), pp. 1–26. On the development of tropical medicine as a distinct specialization, see Michael Worboys, 'The Emergence of Tropical Medicine: A Study in the Establishment of a Scientific Specialty', in Gerard Lemaine, Roy MacLeod, Michael Mulkay and Peter Weingart (eds), *Perspectives on the Emergence of Scientific Disciplines* (The Hague, 1976), pp. 75–98; and Anne Marcovich, 'French Colonial Medicine and Colonial Rule: Algeria and Indochina', trans. A. J. Grieco and S. F. Matthews, in Roy MacLeod and Milton Lewis (eds), *Disease,*

a racial type. But when doctors tried to improve black health conditions, they opened a powerful debate on the ways that slavery affected African health and hygiene, as observers concluded that abuse and oppressive conditions caused the high rates of death and disease among the slave population.

These controversies resonated in the broader sphere of French political culture. On the eve of the French Revolution, abolitionist writers, such as Abbé Grégoire, Daniel Lescallier and Lecointe-Marsillac, widely denounced African slavery as causing excessive morbidity and mortality, and they seized upon physical and moral hygiene as a means to regenerate and assimilate the potentially liberated African body. In this manner, French abolitionists appropriated earlier medical concerns about the physical and moral constitution of the African body to advocate a political programme of regeneration and social rebirth. As this chapter concludes, both proslavery and antislavery discourses were inflected with two contradictory agendas: one aimed at reforming the 'peculiar institution' and the other aimed at rationalizing colonial production. These agendas caused reformers to treat slave health as a technical problem, one they could solve without threatening the dominant planter class.

Settlers and acclimatization

Though eighteenth-century Europeans worked within long-standing traditions of conquest, administration and proselytism, there were a number of broad political and cultural shifts during the Enlightenment that made them look at colonial exchanges with a new perspective.[7] In France, a combination of cultural and territorial transformations helped change collective attitudes. On the cultural level, James Cook's and Louis-Anne de Bougainville's recent voyages of discovery in the Pacific Ocean caused some observers to reflect critically upon the European colonial past, especially conquest in the Americas. As a result, some intellectual and public authorities criticized European bigotry and colonial policies and called for more humane and philanthropic attitudes when dealing with non-European peoples.

This cultural sensibility also corresponded with significant geostrategic changes. On a territorial level, the Seven Years War forced many French elites to reconsider their global status and policies. Because of this humiliating defeat, France ceded her North American possessions and Indian interests to Britain and her claims in Louisiana to Spain. The war reduced the French overseas empire to Guadeloupe and Martinique in the West Indies, French Guinea and Cayenne in South America, an outpost in the Indian Ocean at the Mascarene islands near Madagascar and a contact in India in Pondicherry.

As a consequence, French authorities and settlers began to reconceptualize colonial policies and practices, in the hope of capitalizing on what remained of the colonial empire. This was because, despite all the imperial setbacks, France did keep the jewel of her New World possessions: Saint Domingue (present-day Haiti). The

---

Medicine, and Empire: Perspectives on Western Medicine and the Experience of European Expansion (London, 1988), pp. 103–17.

7   See Edward Said, *Culture and Imperialism* (New York, 1993), pp. 62–63; cf. Duchet, *Anthropologie au siècle des Lumières*, passim.

island made an enormous profit with sugar, coffee, indigo, cotton and cacao; and over 10 per cent of the French population was attached to Saint Domingue trade in one way or another.[8] After the Seven Years War, public authorities and colonial enterprisers wanted to increase economic productivity in the Caribbean even more and thus directly compete with British commerce. Consequently, they focused upon the great slave plantations in Saint Domingue, a system that Sidney Mintz has described as 'agroindustry' because it united 'field and factory'.[9] In this new ideology of colonial development, public authorities, enterprisers and intellectuals took metropole precedents of absolutist rationalization and Enlightenment scientism and applied them to the European and African populations in the Antilles.[10] Doctors participated in this project.

As doctors saw it, disease impeded conquest, control, and productivity.[11] To be sure, their concerns were well-founded. Both European settlers and African slaves were decimated by a bewildering array of diseases such as yellow fever, malaria, typhoid fever, dysentery, tetanus, neonatal tetanus, yaws, scurvy and scrofula (tuberculosis) – clearly, demographers and medical historians cannot call the West African coasts and Caribbean islands as only the 'white man's grave'.[12] Not surprisingly, however, colonial authorities first focused upon European health. Mortality rates among European seamen, for example, were so staggering that Kenneth Kiple and

---

8   As Médéric Louis Élie Moreau de Saint-Méry put it, 'La Partie Française de l'île Saint-Domingue est, de toutes les possessions de la France dans le Nouveau-Monde, la plus importante par les richesses qu'elle procure à son Métropole et par l'influence qu'elle a sur son agriculture et sur son commerce'; see *Description topographique, physique, civile, politique et historique de la partie française de l'isle Saint-Domingue*, eds Blanche Maurel and Étienne Taillemite (3 vols, Paris, 1958), vol. 1, p. 25.

9   Sidney Mintz, *Sweetness and Power: The Place of Sugar in Modern History* (New York, 1985), pp. 51–52.

10   Philip D. Curtin originally observed a similar transformation in British thinking about West Africa in the wake of the loss of the North American colonies; see *The Image of Africa: British Ideas and Action, 1780–1850* (Madison, 1964), pp. 58–119. For similar views expressed toward west Africa in French colonial thought at the turn of the century, see especially the detailed analysis in François Manchuelle, 'The "Regeneration of Africa": An Important and Ambiguous Concept in Eighteenth and Nineteenth-Century French Thinking about Africa', *Cahiers d'Études Africaines*, no. 144 (1996): 559–88. I owe an enormous debt to Professor Manchuelle, who shared this manuscript with me shortly before his tragic passing.

11   On eighteenth-century French tropical medicine, see Pierre Pluchon (ed.), *Histoire des médecins et pharmaciens de marine et des colonies* (Toulouse, 1985), pp. 89–129; James E. McClellan, *Colonialism and Science: Saint Domingue in the Old Regime* (Baltimore, 1992), pp. 75–107; and Paul Brau, *Trois siècles de médecine coloniale française* (Paris, 1931). For the doctor as an agent of colonial authority, see Frantz Fanon, 'Medicine and Colonialism', in Ehrenreich, *Cultural Crisis of Modern Medicine*, pp. 229–51.

12   Mark F. Boyd, 'Introduction', in Boyd (ed.) *Malariology: A Comprehensive Study of all Aspects of this Group of Disease from a Global Standpoint* (2 vols, Philadelphia, 1949), vol. 1, p. 228, cited in Kenneth F. Kiple and Virginia H. King, *Another Dimension to the Black Diaspora: Diet, Disease and Racism* (Cambridge, 1981), p. 12. See especially Philip Curtin, '"The White Man's Grave": Image and Reality, 1780–1850', *Journal of British Studies* 1 (1961): 94–110.

Virginia King have suggested that only poor information-networks allowed slave traders to recruit West African ship hands from Europe with any consistency. Troops fared no better in the Americas: of 1,500 French occupying forces that landed in Saint Lucia in 1685, for instance, only eighty-nine survived an onslaught of what was apparently yellow fever.[13] Pierre Barrère, the royal physician at the island of Cayenne, sardonically noted in 1743 that the ravages of typhoid fever had turned the islands of Martinique and Saint Domingue into a veritable 'graveyard' for the French forces.[14]

Understandably, settlers wanted to avoid tropical disease. But for doctors, administrative myopia and inadequacies in the educational curriculum itself frustrated health-care provision. In 1788, physician and naval surgeon J.-B. Dazille, a Saint Domingue correspondent for the Royal Society of Medicine, complained that doctors neglected colonial health care, practice and instruction, and he urged the government to reform colonial hospitals and teach tropical medicine within the continental medical faculties.[15] In truth, New World and African disease had troubled doctors since the seventeenth century, as evinced by a substantial body of literature, primarily in English, on health conditions in the southern American and West Indies colonies. Many of these works reflected the Sydenham school of neo-Hippocratic teachings and emphasized the environmental factors that caused disease.[16] As Karen O. Kupperman first pointed out, colonial physicians used this literature to teach English settlers how to manage their lifestyle and accommodate the demands of a foreign, but not necessarily pathogenic milieu.[17] In his well-received book on the 'state of health' in Jamaica (written in 1679), Dr Thomas Trapham claimed that colonial migration at first caused discomfort, but later settlers found diseases such as scurvy, plague, fevers and consumption to be rare in the tropical environment. In his view, the tropical climate sometimes alleviated venereal disease.[18]

---

13   Kiple and King, *Another Dimension*, pp. 12–14, 37.

14   Pierre Barrère, *Nouvelle relation de la France équinoxiale* (Paris, 1743), pp. 61–62. The English physician, Robert Jackson, noted that 'The climate of the West Indies has been fatal to the European constitution, ever since its first discovery by Columbus'; *A Treatise on the Fevers of Jamaica, with some Observations on the Intermitting Fever of America* (London, 1791), p. 391.

15   J.-B. Dazille, *Observations sur le Tétanos, ses différences, ses symptômes, avec le traitement de cette maladie et les moyens de prévenir* (Paris, 1788), pp. 10, 13–14, 19, and *Observations sur les maladies des climats chauds, leurs causes, leurs traitements et les moyens de les prévenir* (Paris, 1785). Dazille compiled perhaps the largest bibliography on tropical medicine during the eighteenth century; see McClellan, *Colonialism*, pp. 140–42.

16   For colonial developments, see J. H. Cassedy, 'Meteorology and Medicine in Colonial America: Beginnings of the Experimental Approach', *Journal of the History of Medicine and Allied Sciences* 24 (1969): 193–204.

17   See Karen O. Kupperman, 'Fear of Hot Climates in the Anglo-American Colonial Experience', *William and Mary Quartlery* 41 (1984): 213–40; and Gary Puckrein, 'Climate, Health and Black Labor in the English Americas', *Journal of American Studies* 13 (1979): 179–93.

18   Thomas Trapham, *A Discourse on the State of Health in the Island of Jamaica* (London, 1679), pp. 9–10, 50–51, 87–88. Similar views were expressed by physician Hans Sloane, who also doubted the unique morbid conditions of the tropics. See especially Mark

In the eighteenth century, medical attitudes changed, as trade and military ventures caused a greater awareness of tropical sickness and death. Consequently, French physicians and travel writers often emphasized that the tropical climate was not at all healthy and was instead filled with pathological and destabilizing forces. In their eyes, the greatest threat was the biological process of acclimatization or tropical 'seasoning'.[19] A good example of this belief appears in the famous study of Saint Domingue by Médéric-Louis-Élie Moreau de Saint-Méry. In this book, Moreau de Saint-Méry insisted that the island's stifling heat and humidity menaced health, but he cautioned that not everything in the tropical environment was dangerous. Like Thomas Trapham, he believed that the torrid climates sometimes improve overall health and bodily physique: because the atmosphere was charged with damp electricity, it sometimes calmed nervous degeneracy found among sedentary or convalescent peoples.[20] Yet, he stressed, colonial health was never consistent. The biggest factor, he said, was race, and he indicated that whites, blacks and mulattos all experienced health in different ways.

According to Moreau de Saint-Méry, the environment of Saint Domingue (especially the northern city of Cap François) was particularly lethal for white voyagers and recent settlers. In a levelling fashion, all colonists must acclimate. But seasoning became less deadly as time passed and as colonists changed their habits to adapt their racial constitution to their new environment. Still, the European body was healthier in temperate climates, since seasonal changes and the winter cold toughened the fibres and allowed individuals to endure nature's relentless demands. By contrast, the hot and humid climate made the body flaccid and weak, so colonial disease could creep into daily life, suddenly manifesting itself and stealing away hope and life. He exclaimed: 'One has been cheated by death even before suspecting its appearance, and unless a chance occurrence had not accustomed the doctor to distinguish that ghastly malady from its apparent simplicity, all hope is lost. Oh! What land had greater need of talent from those who exercise the art of healing?'[21]

As Moreau de Saint Méry saw it, however, European health problems were partially self-induced. Following moral hygienists writing in metropole France, he claimed that colonial elites lived a luxurious and libertine lifestyle that aggravated the passions and caused nervous degeneracy. For him, white settlers had forgotten how to conduct themselves in civil society:

> Here, one lacks familiarity with the pleasures of society, of that reunion of individuals that remains well-suited and that provides commonality to please one another and to charm

---

Harrison, '"The Tender Frame of Man": Disease, Climate, and Racial Difference in India and the West Indies, 1760–1860', *Bulletin of the History of Medicine* 70 (1996): 68–93.

19   On the idea of acclimatization, see Warwick Anderson, 'Climates of Opinion: Acclimatization in Nineteenth-Century France and England', *Victorian Studies* 35 (1992): 135–57; David N. Livingstone, 'Human Acclimatization: Perspectives on a Contested Field of Inquiry in Science, Medicine, and Geography', *History of Science* 25 (1987): 359–94; and Dane Kennedy, 'The Perils of the Midday Sun: Climatic Anxieties in the Colonial Tropics', in John M. MacKenzie (ed.), *Imperialism and the Natural World* (Manchester, 1990), pp. 118–40.

20   Moreau de Saint-Méry, *Description*, vol. 1, pp. 509–10.

21   Ibid., p. 516.

the hours of their leisure. People ignore the pleasure of surrendering to that species of abandonment where one's individuality is forgotten, so to speak, in order to better taste the relinquishment that calls and excites gaiety.[22]

By neglecting self-control and moral virtue, many colonists brought painful, frightful diseases upon themselves.

Moreau de Saint-Méry put widely shared medical beliefs into an eloquent format. As doctors and surgeons agreed, the European body began to degenerate shortly after people arrived in the Antilles. As Amable Chèze, an army surgeon and former member of the Académie des Sciences et Arts du Cap François, explained to an audience of Parisian physicians, many disembarked European travellers quickly succumbed to the ravages of tropical illness, and the established settler or slave populations euphemistically spoke of yellow fever as a lethal 'stranger's disease'.[23] In his manuscript on colonial disease and race, Dr Cassan of Saint Lucia underscored that the colonial environment was totally pathological. He contrasted European health to acclimatized non-whites:

> The effects of humidity are primarily remarkable in the phenomena that we observe in animated bodies. We know that the property of humidity is to relax all bodies that are exposed to its action, by weakening the invisible and unknown space that unites the fibres to one another. In the torrid zone, [the humidity's] excessive relaxation seizes the inhabitant's constitution. Their fibres, instead of being taunt and elastic like those of Europeans, are soft, weak, and non-energetic; this atony and natural inertia are principally observable in Negroes, Caribbean, and other peoples who originate from this climate. They are more marked by it than are the whites, because the constitution of the latter are not yet perfectly denatured … . However, the solids of the people of whom we have just spoken are absolutely without force and are deprived of that physical sensibility that characterizes Europeans and renders them active and decided in their movements.[24]

Similar beliefs were expressed by surgeon Antoine Bertin in his *Des moyens de conserver la santé des blancs et des nègres, aux Antilles ou climats chauds et humides de l'Amerique* (1768). Bertin observed that the disembarked European male suffered immediately from 'depleted' blood, maintaining that the body was then susceptible to inflammation or feverish distemper. In the colonies, the 'unexpected heat' overexcited the organism's vital properties and caused the organs and humours to decay. The body also secreted too much bile. Not only did this weaken the body; the blood could not defend the body against the 'spontaneous generation' of parasitic worms so common in the colonial environment. There was little by way of comparison. Bertin said, 'It is only in the case if sickness, when [these humours]

---

22   Ibid., p. 517. On libertism and colonial fantasies of sexuality, see Doris Lorraine Garraway, *The Libertine Colony: Creolization in the Early French Caribbean* (Durham, NC, 2005).

23   SEM, c. C, Amable Chèze, ancien chirurgien et major aux armées de terre et de mer, officier de santé à Chalon-sur-Saône, 'Fièvres de Saint-Domingue', commented on by Hallé et Chaussier, 10 Nov. 1808.

24   SRM 179, d. 7, Cassan, médecin du roi à Saint-Lucie, 'Traité de l'influence des climats chauds sur les corps animés, suivi d'un tableau des maladies particulières à la zone torride' (1790).

have been overheated by fever, or altered by the passions of the mind, that we have
seen a notable and corrosive acrimony [such as this]'.[25]

Bertin followed Hippocratic medicine and emphasized how the environment
stimulated sensibility. For him, the constitution of the body was not 'equal in all
seasons, in all places or in all people'.[26] Antoine Poissonnier-Desperrières (1722–
93), the *médecin du roi* in Saint Domingue from 1748 to 1751, also emphasized this
point. He wrote:

> The animal economy is nearly the same in all men. Whatever existing differences, in
> the dissection of subjects taken from the same nation, does not confuse an Enlightened
> anatomist [*anatomiste philosophe*], whether in the bones, the muscles and the nerves;
> whether in the vessels, the viscera, their functions or even in the fibres! These differences
> are otherwise highly expressed under the diverse climates.[27]

He further insisted that the environment caused different diseases amongst
individuals. Thus, the colonial milieu, whether humid, hot or filled with pernicious
airs, affected the body in varying levels, and it responded in unique ways.

Physicians saw that colonial disease affected not just individuals, but specific
social groups or races as well. Bertin stated that although the acclimatized populations
of the Antilles suffered heavily from physical degeneration, the hostile environment
hosted the most severe illnesses for European settlers. In the following passage, it
is not clear whether he was pejoratively comparing the European constitution to the
native-born white, black or mulatto populations:

> The Europeans who arrive come mostly with rich blood and strong, taunt fibres that the
> heat quickly slackens, but do not immediately lose their initial strength and vigour. It is
> only with time and after several years that the solids and fluids, by the constant action of
> a hot and often humid atmosphere, by the change of nutrition, or by the effects of illness,
> absolutely lose their initial constitution. They *creolize* [*se créolisent*], as we say, and the
> temperament begins to be united with the climate. (emphasis in original)[28]

'Creolization' was like death itself. Naturalists, such as Georges-Louis Leclerc de
Buffon, claimed that living and dying were reciprocal processes within the life cycle.
Death slowly rotted the human frame from within. First, the fibres, the bones and
the blood congealed and lost their earlier sensibility. In turn, the organism could
not resist the anarchic properties of sickness and death. The life course was nothing
more than a history of degeneration.[29] For physicians such as Bertin and Poissonnier-
Desperrières, the tropical climate hastened this degeneration and thus caused
sickness and death.

---

25   Antoine Bertin, *Des moyens de conserver la santé des blancs et des nègres, aux
Antilles ou climats chauds et humides de l'Amérique* (Paris, 1768), pp. 14–15.

26   Ibid., p. 15.

27   Antoine Poissonnier-Desperrières, *Traité des fièvres de l'isle de St.-Domingue*, 2d
edn (Paris, 1766), pp. vi–ix.

28   Bertin, *La santé*, pp. 15–16.

29   G.-L. Leclerc de Buffon, *Œuvres complètes*, ed. M. A. Richard (34 vols, Paris, 1825–
28), vol. 12, pp. 14–17.

The question thus arose: If the diseased body remained only a symptom of a pathological environment, how could one avoid or prevent disease in tropical climates? Responses were both collective and individual, though public authorities were slow to implement health reforms. Royal and municipal ordinances in Saint Domingue reveal that in 1708, 1736 and 1763, for instance, officials took interest in drainage and sewage, proper burial for the dead, quarantining the sick and urban air quality. By the 1770s and 1780s, both local doctors and powerful navy surgeons believed in the environmental disease theories advocated by the Royal Society of Medicine in Paris, and they stressed that environmental engineering could prevent disease. But much of the correspondence between the Antilles colonies and Versailles, however, either focused upon hospital oversight and funding, or reveals professional antipathies between jealous medical personnel.[30] In 1787, Jean-Noël Hallé (1754–1822), the future chair of hygiene at the Paris Health School, still called for authorities to 'police' habitations and regulate the public health within the French colonies.[31]

Since the colonies lacked adequate health services, doctors and surgeons thus encouraged white settlers and travellers to control their own bodies. Good health was an individual prerogative. As physicians sternly warned, one must make good use of the non-naturals. In an environment that bred the most pathogenic of all non-natural causes, perhaps the doctor could offer little more. In a bizarre contradiction, doctors suggested that the male European body, because of the superior constitution of its solids, fibres and humours, seemed more predisposed to disease. Sickness selected the best-adapted bodies. No wonder that women, with their weaker fibres and liquid substances, seemed less inclined to colonial pathogens – as though this pathological specimen found her proper ecological niche in the torrid climates.[32] Against these odds, it became the responsibility of the male individual, and more so in the colony than in the continental metropole itself, to regulate the exogenous causes of disease through personal hygiene.

Doctors warned lay readers on these points. After ten years in medical practice in Saint Domingue, Dr J.-F. Lafosse became convinced that colonial disease species were more prevalent and lethal than the sicknesses found in Europe. As a result, he composed a short book to put the appropriate health knowledge into the hands of the literate white populace. Although his clientele possessed little experience with the art of healing, they could still be taught health rudiments so they could avoid disease and prolong life and productivity *outre mer*. Following the rhetorical strategies found in continental health tracts, Lafosse claimed that physicians had long ignored the preventive (and hence most useful) aspects of medical knowledge. In his view, it was the simple abuses, prejudices and 'the lack of order in the home' that caused the majority of diseases in Saint Domingue – more so than the influences of the climate, to which many doctors ascribed too great importance. Lafosse wrote:

---

30 McClellan, *Colonialism*, pp. 75–107; Pluchon, 'La santé dans les colonies de l'Ancien Régime', pp. 126–27; Brau, *Trois siècles*, pp. 72–107.

31 J.-N. Hallé, 'Afrique', in *Encyclopédie méthodique ou par ordre des matières: médecine*, ed. Félix Vicq d'Azyr (13 vols, Paris, 1782–1832), vol. 1, pt 1, pp. 350–51.

32 J.-B. Pouppée-Desportes, *Histoire des maladies de Saint-Domingue* (2 vols, Paris, 1770), vol. 1, pp. 56–8.

It is only after having reflected that it would be possible to achieve this goal, by putting under everyone's eyes the manner that one should take to obviate an infinite number of accidents of which the first originate from simple negligence and others from ignorance of suitable procedures, that I believed it highly important to expose learned people of the consequences of their negligence and to make up for the incapacity of others.[33]

Although doctors like Lafosse extolled the unique and special character of each European body (contrasting it to the indiscriminate, stereotyped physical experiences of Africans), they still based their health-care prescriptions on normalized behavioural patterns. Jean-Damien Chevalier claimed that the individual should monitor food intake with care. Gluttony, for example, caused the humours to swell up and encouraged 'regrettable' diseases. If necessary, the body should be bled and purged, and the traveller should live soberly at all times.[34] Antoine Bertin was more explicit. He cautioned against overexposure (the body should gently perspire, not sweat copiously), and he promoted moderate eating, drinking citrus beverages, emotional self-control, carrying a parasol when out in the sun, wearing sensible clothing and engaging in sensible exercise. Colonists should avoid dancing. The individual must place themselves under a health regimen, no matter how inconvenient it might be. He warned, 'on the islands the majority of the sick die by not taking proper care of the things that do not depend on the doctor'.[35]

Doctors thought that drinking and sex also caused degeneracy. Alcohol shattered the fragile interactions between the solids and the fluids and facilitated the onslaught of disease. Tellingly, Dr George Cheyne – a major advocate for individual health and health regimen – also warned against drinking 'punch' in the English colonies.[36] Most important, however, was the careful control over one's sexuality. One should avoid 'commerce of women and, above all, that of Negresses', as Antoine Poissonnier-Desperrières cautioned. As seen in Chapter 1 above, doctors such as Achille Le Bègue de Presle and Samuel Tissot obsessed about 'spermatic loss'. Of all the excretions, the seminal liquid was the most precious and its undue expense could wreck the impressionable passions of the mind. Poissonnier-Desperrières stated:

> Now, according to this disposition in the humors, they only wait for the favourable opportunity to enter by their acrimony the entire excited nervous and vascular systems, and this opportunity presents itself after large evacuations of seminal liqueur, which, ... had it reentered the humors in a sufficient quantity, would have tempered their acrimony in such a way to render it impotent and would have kept the vessels in a state of suppleness far removed from excitability.[37]

---

33   J.-F. Lafosse, *Avis aux habitans des colonies, particulièrement à ceux de l'isle S. Domingue, sur les principales causes des maladies qu'on y éprouve le plus communément, et sur les moyens de les prévenir* (Paris, 1787), 'Avant-propos', p. 2.

34   J.-D. Chevalier, *Lettres à M. le Jean, docteur-regent de la Faculté de Medecine en l'université de Paris. I. Sur les maladies de St.-Domingue* (Paris, 1752), p. 27.

35   Bertin, *La santé*, pp. 33, 36–42; and Poissonnier-Desperrières, *Traité*, pp. 95–97, 118.

36   George Cheyne, *An Essay of Health and Long Life* (London, 1724), p. 57.

37   Poissonnier-Desperrières, *Traité*, pp. 106, 114–15.

Ordinarily, 'large evacuations' of seminal fluid caused madness or physical debility. In an environment that had thoroughly destabilized the animal economy, however, seminal loss could also cause malaria, yellow fever and death.

Physicians therefore stressed that the colonist must adopt self-regulating mechanisms to avoid disease and preserve personal health. This discussion, certainly, reflected the powerful class barriers within the colonial white population. Antoine Bertin, Jean-Damien Chevalier, Antoine Poissonnier-Desperrières and J.-F. Lafosse maintained that bourgeois values and habits allowed people to have a healthy body and live a long and productive life. But wealth and privilege alone did not prevent sickness, as Bertin stated. Rather, white settlers needed moderation, sobriety, and diligent sense.[38] Moreover, colonialists needed to control emotional passion and sexual experiences.

Slavery and sickness

If European men could avoid disease by controlling their own bodies, then the morbidity of the African slaves in the Caribbean posed new problems for the physician. Numbering some 500,000 in Saint Domingue alone on the eve of the French Revolution, here was a population that clearly had no acknowledged control over their bodies. The question of whether or not the black slave could adapt to the necessary disciplinary habits complicated this issue. As early as 1684, an anonymous author in the *Journal des Sçavans* had claimed that blacks were racially different from Europeans, and implied innate physical and moral inadequacies.[39] Following the Enlightenment stress on physical environment, doctors and natural historians (notably Georges-Louis Leclerc de Buffon and J. F. Blumenbach) speculated that blacks had degenerated because of the African climate, geographic dispersal and poor nutrition. In terms of disease pathology, however, the naturalist paradigm of degeneration became problematic. Why, for example, did some sicknesses devastate European colonists, whilst the African slave population remained curiously intact? By contrast, why did some diseases, such as dirt-eating [*mal d'estomac*], tetanus and yaws decimate the African slave population? As seen above, doctors believed that the biological inferiority of women prevented the onslaught of some tropical pathologies; unfortunately, this failed to explain why the African body languished under such diverse and shocking diseases. Doctors couldn't explain the selective nature of sickness.[40]

As a result, doctors furiously debated whether or not Africans were predisposed to disease. They wanted to know whether Africans were biologically different from

---

38 Bertin, *La santé*, pp. 18–21.

39 'Nouvelle division de la Terre, par les differentes Espèces ou Races qui l'habitent, envoyée par un fameux Voyageur … à peu près en ces termes', *Journal des Sçavans* 12 (1684): 148–53.

40 On slave morbidity and mortality, see especially Gabriel Debien, *Les esclaves aux Antilles françaises (XVIIe–XVIIIe siècles)* (Basse-Terren et Forte-de-France, 1974); and see the superb recent study by Megan Vaughan, *Creating the Creole Island: Slavery in Eighteenth-Century Mauritius* (Durham, NC, 2005).

Europeans and whether these racial differences changed how Africans experienced disease. These questions took a variety of forms. Late seventeenth- and early eighteenth-century physiologists, concerned with the process of generation, hoped to unlock the secrets of growth and reproduction by studying the black body.[41] Anatomists probed the recesses of black cadavers, searching for the causes of skin colour or innate physiological inadequacies.[42] In colonial hospitals, physicians scrutinized the morbid appearances of the black, attempting to disentangle the seats and causes of diseases. As the well-known physician and Newtonian C.-N. Le Cat declared, speculation about the African body should be a physiological undertaking, not an exercise in naturalist classification.[43]

One of the first physicians to enunciate these themes was Pierre Barrère, in his *Dissertation sur la cause physique de la couleur des Nègres* (1741). He first wanted to discover what caused African pigmentation, and he saw himself building upon the fertile contributions of the celebrated anatomist, J.-B. Winslow. When dissecting black cadavers, Barrère claimed that he had seen large amounts of black bile within the epidermal skin layer, and he thought that this morbid humour caused Africans to become black. He also linked skin colour and sexuality:

> One judges that the bile is naturally abundant in the blood of the Negroes, by the strength and the rapidity of their pulse, by their extreme lustfulness and the other impetuous passions, and especially by the considerable heat of the skin that one notices in them. Experience shows, moreover, that the heat of blood is proper to forming much bile, since one sees milk turn yellow among whites, when a nursing woman has a fever.[44]

Barrère's scalpel cut deeper. The dissected cadaver revealed that the liver, blood and vascular systems were awash in bilious matter. Even the epidermal pores released 'a disagreeable odour'. Barrère's observations seemed consistent with the morbid anatomy practised within the Antilles hospitals. Physicians who opened up colonial corpses often found bile interspersed throughout the bodies of Africans, mulattos and Europeans alike. Less obviously articulated was the notion that bodies displaying these humoral imbalances were predisposed to ill-health or caused disease.

Not all doctors agreed with Barrère. One reviewer claimed that Barrère had overemphasized bilious deposits in the skin. Blacks vomited yellow bile, suffered from jaundice and excreted the same infectious materials as whites. The reviewer did

---

41   P.-L. Moreau de Maupertuis, *Dissertation physique à l'occasion du nègre blanc* (Leyde, 1744), 93–94. See also SRM 191, d. 16, Lefevre-Deshayes, correspondant du Cercle des philadelphes, Saint-Domingue, 'Dissertation sur les nègres-blancs ou albinos (première partie)', 15 Feb. 1785; and the later comments in SEM, c. C, Chomel, 'Observation sur la coloration noir de la peau d'un homme naturellement blanc', 21 July 1814.

42   J.-B. Winslow, *Exposition anatomique de la structure du corps humaine* (Paris, 1732), p. 489; also J. B. Morgagni, *The Seats and Causes of Diseases, Investigated by Anatomy*, trans. B. Alexander (3 vols, London, 1769), vol. 3, pp. 580–81.

43   C.-N. Le Cat, *Traité de la couleur de la peau humaine en générale, de celle des nègres en particulier et de la métamorphose d'une de ces couleurs en l'autre, soit de naissance, soit accidentellement* (Amersterdam, 1765), pp. 1–4.

44   Pierre Barrère, *Dissertation sur la cause physique de la couleur des nègres, de la qualité de leurs cheveux, et de la dégénération de l'un et l'autre* (Paris, 1741), pp. 5–6.

agree, however, that some diseases caused Africans to have too much black bile.[45] In an obscure book on African skin colour, Le Cat dismissed Barrère and insisted that enlightened doctors should not consider his research seriously. Instead, Le Cat argued that an innate nervous sensibility caused pigmentation (in contrast to environmental factors) and he documented cases of female hysteria, apoplexy and syncope to show how nervous disease could discolour the skin.[46] These differences aside, the works of Barrère and Le Cat are emblematic of the broader European racial discourse that aimed at subjugating and effeminizing the African body. Moreover, the discussion of 'bilious' organisms and fragile nervous systems suggests that certain physicians believed that Africans possessed inherently morbid characteristics.

As a result, doctors told colonists that they should remove themselves from another source of disease: the African slave. As seen above, Antoine Poissonnier-Desperrières had warned that European settlers should not have sex with black females. Accordingly, he gave a case study of a subject who had a malignant fever. After diligent care and thorough purging, the patient seemed as though he would recover. But on the last day of his treatment, the patient had a severe relapse. Before dying, he confessed that he had 'caressed a Negress' the night before. Another victim, the visiting Mr. de la Haye, suffered an outbreak of bilious fever. The doctor kept the patient under strict regime for seven days and on the eighth day he began purging him. At first, the treatment appeared to work; nevertheless, Haye collapsed and soon died. Poissonnier-Desperrières noted that the patient had violated his regimen by taking wine from a black woman on three separate occasions.[47] On another level, doctors also warned that settlers should keep blacks out of the household as much as possible, lest they try to poison their masters – a threat that was a constant obsession amongst white settlers and provoked vicious reprisals against blacks.[48]

Two diseases fascinated European doctors: yaws (pians or *frambroesia*) and tetanus. Yaws is a non-venereal form of syphilis; the organism (*Treponeona pertenue*) usually penetrates the body through cuts and abrasions on the legs, below the genitalia. Heavy tissue damage can occur in extended cases, and eighteenth-century physicians often confused yaws with leprosy. Colonial doctors recognized

---

45 Review of Pierre Barrère, *Dissertation sur la cause physique de la couleur des nègres*, *Journal des Sçavans* 22 (1742): 23–45. Le Romain's article in Diderot's *Encyclopédiee, ou dictionnaire raisonné des sciences, des arts, et des métiers* (Geneva, 1777–79) follows this review; see the entry 'Nègre' (vol. 12, pp. 838–39).

46 Le Cat, *De la couleur de la peau humaine,* 73–6.

47 Poissonnier-Desperrières, *Traité,* pp. 190–91, 204–06.

48 See the comments in SRM 139, d. 17, n. 2, Geoffroy and Andry, 'Rapport d'un mémoire de M. de la Borde sur l'opinion des colons de l'Amérique qui regardent les nègres comme souvent capables d'empoisonnement' (1777); Bertin, *La santé,* pp. 18–19, 73; Dazille, *Observations sur le Tétanos,* pp. 46, 68; A.-J.-T. Bonnemain, *Régénération des colonies, ou moyens de restituer graduellement aux hommes leur état politique, et d'assurer la prospérité des Nations* (Paris, 1792), p. 16. See Pierre Pluchon, *Vaudou, sorciers, empoisonneurs de Saint-Domingue à Haiti* (Paris, 1987), pp. 259–60, 263–67; David P. Geggus, *Slavery, War and Revolution: The British Occupation of Saint Domingue 1793–1798* (Oxford, 1982), p. 27; and McClellan, *Colonialism,* p. 136.

that the disease seemed to select particular people and that it particularly decimated the slave population:

> There are perhaps no other countries where venereal disease is as common as it is in these islands. All the male and female slaves carry it from Guinea; the children who are born there are consequently infected, engendering others even more corrupted than themselves.
> There are very few Whites who would not have had commerce with these Negresses, and it would be a great miracle that they would not communicate their disease to them.[49]

Doctors didn't know what caused the disease. On the one hand, Jean-Damien Chevalier suggested that environmental considerations produced this brutal sickness. He believed that the 'tough' constitution of the skin, and the constant exposure to the sun and elements, caused pustules to erupt and cover the skin. The disease, transmitted by heredity, passed from generation to generation, and eventually degenerated into leprosy.[50] Building upon these insights, J.-B. Dazille, in his *Observations sur les maladies des nègres* (1776), insisted that slavery caused disease and depopulation amongst African slaves. He remarked: 'It is to be presumed that the venereal virus exercises its activity principally on poorly nourished, tired and nervous bodies, since then it produces accidents more serious, more murderous and less susceptible to being cured.'[51]

On the other hand, some physicians saw the disease as an inherent, pathological stigmata of the black. According to Antoine Bertin:

> Negroes [have] a particular, predisposing cause, one that is not found in Whites, or that is not found in the same proportion, since if pians is not an illness from which Whites are excluded, it is always very rare among them, while it is very common with the former. It is necessary, by consequence, that a humor exists that has a particular analogy with the nature of this virus.[52]

Such differences aside, physicians used these encounters to experiment with venereal cures. Of particular interest (due to their volatile and uncertain effectiveness) were mercury treatments. Historians have suggested that colonial doctors tested unorthodox or dubious cures upon helpless slaves (even judged by the standards of the day).[53] Eighteenth-century French physicians followed this tradition. Antoine Bertin argued that doctors should test healing techniques in the colonies before introducing them to the mainland. He did not object to physicians administering heavy mercury treatments to blacks who suffered from yaws and leprosy, although he warned that

---

49   Chevalier, *Lettres*, p. 84. Henri Grégoire referenced yaws in the colonies in his *Mémoire en faveur des gens de couleur ou sang-mêlées de St.-Domingue, et des autres îles françaises de l'Amérique* (Paris, 1789), p. 26.

50   Chevalier, *Lettres*, pp. 50, 53.

51   J.-B. Dazille, *Observations sur les maladies des nègres, leurs causes, leur traitements, et les moyens de les prévenir* (Paris, 1776), pp. 255–56.

52   Bertin, *La santé*, p. 90.

53   'Yaws', *The Cambridge World History of Human Disease*, ed. Kenneth Kiple (Cambridge, 1993), p. 1099.

slave owners expected a high success ratio.[54] Jean Damien Chevalier experimented with extensive purging and bathing regimes on yaws-infected patients, and he announced that his mercury treatments had an unusual record of success. He did not mention slaves who were not cured.[55] Not only was the African cadaver a source of knowledge; live, docile patients provided a new terrain for medical therapeutics.

Nevertheless, some physicians claimed that slavery itself caused so many slaves to fall sick and die. In defending this belief, these doctors drew upon long-standing claims in Western medicine. Originally, the Hippocratic *Corpus* suggested that oppressive government and climate had moulded the 'mental flabbiness', 'cowardice' and poor constitution of Asian peoples. Following these beliefs, eighteenth-century thinkers speculated that tyranny could deform a people's body and character.[56] Significantly, Georges-Louis Leclerc de Buffon had argued this in his influential 'De la dégénération des animaux' (1766) that made organisms deviate from a primordial or pristine form.[57] Nevertheless, most medical practitioners didn't believe that slavery and poverty alone caused disease. Rather, they thought that African sicknesses reflected some *a priori* degeneracy.

Physicians accentuated this relationship between sickness and slavery in the colonial literature about tetanus. Although tetanus appeared to afflict both settlers and slaves, physicians concerned themselves with the occurrence of lock jaw within the slave communities in general and the high disease frequency within the black infant population in particular. The eighteenth-century doctor knew that that cuts and abrasions had something to do with tetanus. Doctors attributed an attack of the disease to an exposure of the body (for example, through an open wound) to the exogenous, non-natural bad airs from without.[58] Observers thought that blacks were vulnerable to such occurrences, and that the conditions of slavery perpetuated the sources of infection.

In 1786, Félix Vicq d'Azyr approved a volume addressed to the Royal Society of Medicine in Paris that documented the prevalence of tetanus and neonatal tetanus within the Antilles colonies. The physicians concluded that both settlers and slaves suffered from the dreaded illness; nevertheless, tetanus seemed to afflict the black populations on a far heavier level. According to these doctors, the slave lifestyle caused the illness:

> In truth, the whites are infinitely less subject to this disease [tetanus] than are the blacks, although both are equally exposed to the impressions of the same air; but the particular reasons that could determine or encourage the invasion of these sicknesses are multiplied in the blacks. Their particular cares and their precautions are much less; their lifestyle [*manière de vivre*], exercises, and the means of both are vastly different: the blacks are

---

54 Bertin, *La santé*, pp. 89, 102–04.

55 Chevalier, *Lettres*, pp. 57, 79–82, 88–91.

56 'Airs, Waters, Places', in *Hippocratic Writings*, ed. G. E. R. Lloyd, trans. J. Chadwick and W. N. Monn (Harmondsworth, 1978), pp. 148–69 (at p. 160).

57 Buffon, *Œuvres*, vol. 14, pp. 3–114 (at p. 9). See also Manchuelle, 'Regeneration of Africa'.

58 On the causes of tetanus, and especially the incidence of exposure amongst children, see Joseph Raulin, *De la conservation des enfans* (2 vols, Paris, 1768), vol. 2, pp. 136–37; and Nicolas Chambon de Montaux, *Des maladies des enfans* (2 vols, Paris, Year VII).

more exposed to the intemperance and vicissitudes of the air; they are always exposed to it without precaution, whether for themselves or whether for the affairs of their masters; they are less covered, engaged in the longest, roughest, and most exhausting labour; the blacks go about with their legs and feet naked; though heated or in a sweat, they walk on cold objects, go into the water, cross through marshes, streams and rivers; they are exposed to the rain, evening dew and wind. Finally, blacks are more subject to wounds than are the whites; they go about with naked feet; they walk on hard, often sharp ground that injures them; and they often make use of their feet in their work and are more exposed to wounding them.[59]

However, the authors did not impugn the institution of slavery and instead blamed childbirth practices and midwifery within the slave population.[60] Often, black midwives cut the newborn's umbilical cord with sharpened sticks or rocks, and West African tradition encouraged birth attendants to pack the navel area with dirt, so to ward off evil spirits. European medical personnel, already hostile to continental midwifery and folk medicine, were less tolerant of African medicine. Colonial law kept slaves and free people of colour from practicing midwifery in Saint Domingue, and non-white administration of basic medical care, including first aid, was punishable by death.[61] Nevertheless, physicians' obsession over African childbirth suggests that traditional African practices persisted. Doctors complained that black midwives took few precautions in severing the umbilical cord and, in a further act of negligence, they failed to remove the residual blood and fluid within the exposed navel area. According to them, the congealed and putrefying blood caused humoral imbalances and, ultimately, tetanus in the newborn child. These physicians, their productive sensibilities sickened by this waste of human life, argued that authorities must teach colonial midwives more recent, continental forms of childbirth. Preferably, only qualified surgeons should supervise this critical procedure. As a consequence, in 1764 and 1773, colonial authorities brought licensed midwives from France into Saint Domingue, and then appointed a physician-obstetrician to regulate colonial midwifery.[62]

In this discussion, however, the physician focused upon the exogenous causes of disease. Not only did the tropical environment cause disease, perhaps the 'peculiar institution' of slavery was to blame. Everywhere, the black suffered under appalling conditions: immense physical labour in the hot and humid climate, poorly ventilated living quarters, newborn children exposed to foul airs and the burning rays of the sun, malnutrition and overcrowding on the slave galleys all contributed to disease. Whereas physicians such as Antoine Bertin thought that racial predisposition caused

---

59   *Projet d'instruction sur une maladie convulsive fréquente dans les colonies d'Amérique connue sous le nom de Tétanos* (Paris, 1786), pp. 29–30.

60   SEM, c. C, Amable Chèze, chirurgien, 'Mémoire sur le tétanos des îles et les moyens de le guérir', 10 Nov. 1808. On slave women and childbirth, see the excellent study by Arlette Gautier, *Les soeurs de solitude: la condition féminine dans l'esclavage aux Antilles du XVIIe au XIX siècles* (Paris, 1985).

61   Pluchon, *Vaudou*, p. 19; McClellan, *Colonialism*, pp. 134, 136.

62   McClellan, *Colonialism*, pp. 134–35; and Brau, *Trois siècles*, pp. 90, 92, 111.

blacks to get sick, other observers, such as J.-B. Dazille, suggested that slavery itself called disease. Slavery, perhaps, was hazardous to African health.

While some physicians may have expressed paternalistic concern for African health, they did not suggest that blacks could control their own bodies and enjoy good health. Quite the contrary: the plantation slave-owner must diligently regulate slave health – simply to promote his own economic interest. The physicians reporting to the Royal Society of Medicine warned:

> It is still easier to prevent than to stop [tetanus]; the precautions that will appear minute, subjugative and unpleasant, could be very important, and one could do irreparable harm in wanting to avoid them: the Owners of Negroes, interested in their conservation, ought to be the first to take the precautions that could be beneficial to them.[63]

These physicians, including Antoine Poissonnier-Desperrières, encouraged slave-holders to exercise diligent medical care over their property. In their view, the masters should 'entrust' their slaves to the 'methodical treatment' of *gens de l'art* in order to conserve 'a mass of individuals who are still more useful to them than the State'.[64] As J.-B. Dazille described it:

> the introduction of Negroes into a colony is the major and fundamental means of its prosperity, and the conservation of these unhappy beings is what renders this means efficient. Seeking the causes of [black] illnesses in their beginning, their progress, their termination and indicating the means of remedy, forming a result that tends to stop the ghastly depopulation of the species, is to occupy oneself with that which is useful to the Colonists in particular, to the Commerce of the Nation in general, and to the prosperity of the State.[65]

But policing black health care raised political problems – in terms of the types of medical services provided (and by whom) and whether medical intervention (either public or private) potentially interfered with the sacrosanct property relation between master and slave. In an immediate sense, physicians such as Antoine Poissonnier-Desperrières, Pierre Poissonnier and J. B. Dazille saw the centralization of colonial medicine as a means of increasing the naval health services' authority over the established (and fiercely independent) local medical communities. It was no accident that Dazille dedicated his *Les maladies des nègres* to the state minister of the navy, Sartine.[66] Yet there were broader ideological issues at stake, as well. As we have seen in Chapter 2 above, population thought during the Enlightenment, in form of either mercantilism or physiocratic doctrine, associated individual health with the physical well-being of the state. Both organisms needed self-regulating and disciplinary apparatuses to promote productivity, power and prestige. In old regime society, social commentators rejected the corporate model of society and thus turned individual health into a highly charged political idea.[67] In this manner, ideas about 'political economy' and the 'animal economy' of living beings converged, and

---

63 *Projet d'instruction*, p. 44.
64 Ibid., pp. 95–96.
65 Dazille, *Les maladies des nègres*, pp. 2–3.
66 McClellan, *Colonialism*, pp. 138–42.
67 See Chapter 4 below.

appear almost indistinguishable in the complex Enlightenment plays on notions of regeneration and therapeutics for the social body. If the state decided to assimilate the Caribbean slave into the restructured social body, it followed that blacks must adopt the same disciplinary mechanisms. At this point, medical questions over the health of the slave population began to dovetail with abolitionist concerns over slave conditions and morality – including health and hygiene.

Health and emancipation

Given debates over the 'right to health' throughout the French Revolution, it is not surprising that abolitionist writings on the so-called colonial question also explored slave morbidity and mortality. As David Geggus has brilliantly argued, the colonial question 'tested the universalistic claims of the French revolutionaries', raising powerful questions about autonomy, racial equality and the incongruence of slavery with bourgeois liberal society. But as historians have stressed, the French abolitionist movement suffered from many internal ambivalences and obstacles. Although antislavery opinion found an organizational base with the founding of the Société des Amis des Noirs by Jacques-Pierre Brissot in February 1788, it was an elite movement that, unlike its British or North American counterparts, failed to attract large-scale popular or grassroots support. Furthermore, powerful colonial lobbyists fiercely opposed abolitionism – notably the notorious Club Massaic – and the full-scale revolt in Saint Domingue in 1791 intensified political divisions within the Constituent Assembly.[68] Not surprisingly, the French revolutionaries could not obtain a consensus on legislation related to ethnicity and slavery. The piecemeal Jewish emancipation of 1791, decrees on colonial racial equality in 1792, and the full abolition of slavery in 1794 (reinstated by Napoleon Bonaparte in 1802) each encountered determined detractors and stringent qualifications.

More significantly, even ardent abolitionists, such as abbé Henri Grégoire, J.-P. Brissot and A.-N. de Condorcet, believed that the immediate abolition of slavery remained an unfavourable and pre-emptive event. According to them, any veritable change in the plantation system and slave society needed both international cooperation and the gradual assimilation of the black population.[69] For example, although Grégoire claimed that blacks did possess the 'capacity for improvement',

---

68   David P. Geggus, 'Racial Equality, Slavery and Colonial Secession during the Constituent Assembly', *American Historical Review* (1989): 1290–308 (at p. 1291). On the politics of abolition, see Drescher, 'Ending of the Slave Trade and Evolution of Scientific Racism'; Boulle, 'Defense of Slavery'; F. Thésée, 'Autour de la Société des Amis des Noirs', *Présence africaine* 125 (1983): 3–82; Serge Daget, 'Les mots esclave, nègre, noir et les jugements de valeur sur la traité négrière dans la littérature abolitionniste française de 1770 à 1845', *La Revue française d'histoire d'outre mer* 221 (1973): 511–48; and Edward D. Seeber, *Anti-Slavery Opinion in France during the Second Half of the Eighteenth Century* (New York, 1969).

69   See the comments in Grégoire, *Mémoire en faveur des gens de couleur*; Sébastien-André Sibire, *L'aristocratie négrière, ou refléxions philosophiques et historiques sur l'esclavage et l'affranchissement des Noirs* (Paris, 1789), p. 49. This subject is covered in

his efforts to have blacks 'become our equals' meant inculcating European ideas about Christianity, monogamous marriage, work ethic and personal hygiene.[70] 'If their physical and moral degradation is our work', the abbé S. A. Sibire noted, 'the less they reflect on it, the more it must interest us.'[71] Abolitionists must reform the vices created by slavery and encourage blacks to become good and virtuous citizens.[72]

These debates were by no means isolated to the issue of African slavery. Similar concerns appeared in Grégoire's widely circulated pro-emancipationist paper of 1788, *Essai sur la régénération physique, morale et politique des juifs*. Here, Grégoire used naturalist and medical ideas about degeneration to argue that European Jews had degenerated because of self-imposed archaic religious practices, the confinement of the ghetto and oppressive legal and religious institutions. Whereas Grégoire dismissed antisemitic prejudices, particularly blood libel and male menstruation, he nevertheless claimed that Jews, 'in carrying in the mass of humors numerous acrimonious particles', were predisposed to various pathologies, including melancholia, nymphomania and excessive masturbation. On one level, Grégoire's text encapsulates contemporaries' belief that the diseased somatic constitution of a state's citizenry reflected its 'degraded' social and political environment. By overturning tyrannical religious and social institutions, Jews could become healthy and moral people, and they would eventually convert to Christianity.[73] On another level, however, emancipationist and abolitionist discourse reflected the deep-seated eschatological, *secular* convictions of many contemporaries who believed that the French Revolution provided a *tabula rasa* for constructing both a new social order and a new type of 'man', one invariably based on the organicist precepts embedded in the doctrine of natural law. For these writers, 'regenerating' disenfranchised

---

great detail in Cohen, *French Encounter with Africans*, pp. 152–54 and Duchet, *Anthropologie au siècle des Lumières*, pp. 137–226.

70   Grégoire, *An Enquiry concerning the intellectual and moral facilities, and the literature of negroes*, trans. D. B. Warden (Brooklyn, 1810), p. 158. He later insisted that blacks were 'capable of great improvement' (p. 160). See also his *Mémoire en faveur des gens de couleur*, p. 28.

71   Sibire, *L'aristocratie*, p. 122.

72   'The blacks have the seed for all virtues', declared Henrion de Pansey; given the Revolutionary fascination with polarized discursive frameworks, such as vice/virtue, it is not surprising that many abolitionist writers adapted 'virtue' as means of rehabilitating the black; see Henrion de Pansey, *Mémoire pour un nègre qui réclame sa liberté* (Paris, 1770), pp. 13–14. On the eighteenth-century concept of virtue, see Carol Blum, *Rousseau and the Republic of Virtue: The Language of Politics in the French Revolution* (Ithaca, 1986).

73   Henri Grégoire, *Essai sur la régénération physique, morale et politique des juifs, ouvrage couronné par la Société royale des Sciences et des Arts de Metz, le 23 août 1788* (Mezt, 1789), pp. 34–35, 44–54 (at p. 35). For the general context of these remarks, see Richard Popkin, 'Medicine, Racism, Anti-Semitism: A Dimension of Enlightenment Culture', in G. S. Rousseau (ed.), *The Languages of Psyche: Mind and Body in Enlightenment Thought* (Berkeley, 1990), 405–42; Mitchell and Kottek, 'Diseases of the Jews'; and John M. Efron, 'Images of the Jewish Body: Three Medical Views from the Jewish Enlightenment', *Bulletin of the History of Medicine* 69 (1995): 349–66.

ethnic/social bodies would not only create virtuous, productive citizens; it would also play a centrifugal role in regenerating the entire nation of France.[74]

Whereas emancipationists alleged that traditional Jewish religion and culture caused Jews to get sick, antislavery activists looked elsewhere for the physical causes and possible cures for African degeneration. To be sure, much abolitionist discourse drew upon this same missionary zeal. Yet unlike Jewish emancipation, the regeneration of the African slave depended specifically on the eradication of the slave trade and, ultimately, slavery itself. One of the foremost concerns remained the devastating rates of morbidity and mortality in the slave population. In this manner, the persistence of earlier medical themes about the African body is striking. The reason for this wholesale slaughter, argued an anonymous author, were transportation conditions: 'It is certain that the mortality of the Negroes far exceeds their birth-rate by almost half. This is neither the fault of the *colons*, nor the rigorous discipline in their housing, but the result of the sufferance that the Negroes endured in the slave trade'.[75] Théophile Mandar expanded this critique, blaming the death rate on epidemics, seafaring accidents, the 'ferocity and intemperance of whites' and 'improper space and poor nutrition'.[76] Another writer insisted that, by abolishing slavery, the African death rate could only decrease.[77]

Often, abolitionists discussed economic productivity, prosperity and the eradication of 'depopulation' in the Antilles colonies or along the African coasts.[78] Although antislavery writers may have expressed a reserved outrage (so to speak) over the problem of slavery, the damage done to the colonial or African population did inflame their productive-minded sympathies. For example, Pruneau de Pommegorge, a former slave trader, argued in his *Description de la nigritie* (1789) that the slave trade significantly depleted the African coasts, marking the African population with a brutal and 'ferocious' character.[79] The demographic estimates of this devastation varied widely. J.-P. Brissot, Jérôme Pétion and Benjamin-Sigismond Frossmand figured the population loss anywhere between four, sixty or 300 million.[80] According to one

74 Sibire, *L'aristocratie*, pp. 10–12, 15; *Traité des nègres: à messieurs les députés à l'Assemblée nationale* (Paris, 1789), pp. 1–4; Bonnemain, *Régénération des colonies*, p. 84; Lecointe-Marsillac, *Le More-Lack, ou essai sur les moyens le plus doux et les plus équitables d'abolir la traite et l'esclavage des Nègres d'Afrique, en conservant aux Colonies tous les avantages d'une population agricole* (Paris and London, 1789), pp. 198–207; Pepin, *Adresse d'un patriote françois à l'Assemblée nationale sur la Traite des Noirs Avril 1791* (Paris, 1791), pp. 3–4.

75 *Du commerce des colonies, ses principes et ses lois: la paix est de temps de régler et d'agrandir le commerce* (n.p., 1785), p. 59.

76 Théophile Mandar, *Observations sur l'esclavage et le commerce des Nègres* (Paris, 1790), p. 23.

77 *L'esclavage des Nègres aboli, ou moyens d'améliorer leur sort* (Paris, 1789), p. 11.

78 See, for example, Mandar, *Observations sur l'esclavage et le commerce des Nègres*, pp. 24–25; *Discours sur la nécessité d'établir à Paris une Société pour concourir, avec celle de Londres, à l'abolition de la traite et de l'esclavage des Nègres* (Paris, 1788), p. 18.

79 On Pommegorge, see Cohen, *French Encounter with Africans*, pp. 148–49; and Manchuelle, 'Regeneration of Africa'.

80 Jérome Pétion, *Discours sur la traite des noirs* (April 1790), pp. 8–9; B.-J. Frossmand, *Observations sur l'abolition de la traite des nègres présentées à la Convention nationale*

anonymous writer, European colonists had created the African diaspora to supplement the slaughtered indigenous population of the Antilles, mistakenly believing that blacks were biologically adapted to the exigencies of the 'torrid' climates.[81] As the author put it, 'The suffering of the Negroes during the [Atlantic] crossing weakens their strengths and chafes their temperament; the grievous illness that they sustain in America and, usually, their short life-span, only demonstrate that they are imperfectly accustomed to this temperature.'[82] Therefore, the plantation owners' desire to fill the colonies with 'a generation of robust Blacks, attached to their masters by habit and by recognition' and capable of 'sustaining the hardest labours' proved an illusory hope. Quite simply, 'Without liberty, man is a degraded being in his moral and physical faculties'.[83] Antoine Bonnemain's later volume, *Régénération des colonies* (1792), argued that only the abolition of the slave trade and tempered care of the Caribbean slaves would encourage a burgeoning, healthy black population and thus facilitate full-scale abolition and assimilation.[84]

Within abolitionist circles, Daniel Lescallier was one of the first writers to discuss African health problems. Throughout his book, he focused upon slavery and France's economic productivity and he saw health problems as part of this relationship. Straight away, Lescallier acknowledged that the sugar and coffee trade were treated, with good reason, as though they were France's greatest political interest.[85] He nevertheless connected the slave trade to the morbidity and mortality, and he insisted that the state should take active interest in promoting the physical well-being of blacks. Lescallier quoted the 4 November 1788 decree adapted by the colonial assembly at Grenade and then argued:

> 'One should only attain a goal as desirable as fixing reasonable boundaries on the power of the Masters and the persons put in charge of supervising the slaves, whether in compelling them to provide for lodging, food and garments of an appropriate manner; whether in obtaining the knowledge of, and instruction in, the Christian Religion; occupying themselves essentially in the perfection of their morals; engaging them in the contraction of legitimate marriages, and protecting them, and respecting the rights of this State.'
>
> The legislation ... thus decreed and written, would be read and published amongst the workplaces and renewed from time to time. It would provide, with certainty, for nourishment for the Negroes ...; for their clothing and their lodging: one would assure the property of their gardens, poultry and barnyard; one would provide for their treatment in sickness, for the relief of the aged and disabled, for the care of pregnant women, wet nurses and children; and for the maintenance of good morals, instruction of youth and good order in the families, etc.[86]

(Paris, 1793), p. 20; Sibire, *L'aristocratie*, p. 4.

81 See J.-J. Virey, *Histoire naturelle du genre humain, ou recherches sur ses principaux fondemens physiques et moraux; précédées d'un discours sur la nature des êtres organiques, et sur l'ensemble de leur physiologie* (2 vols, Paris, Year IX), vol. 1, pp. 377–8.

82 *Réflexions sur l'abolition de la traite et la liberté des Noirs* (Orleans, 1789), p. 6.

83 Ibid., p. 7.

84 Bonnemain, *Régénération*, pp. 30–57.

85 Daniel Lescallier, *Réflexions sur le sort des Noirs dans nos colonies* (Paris, 1789), p. 3.

86 Ibid., pp. 47–49.

According to Lescallier, the French had to impart moral norms and values amongst the Caribbean slaves before they could emancipate them. A stable society demanded these actions. According to him, the slave trade caused the poor moral and physical quality of the black slaves. Like the abbé Grégoire, Lescallier did not want to immediately emancipate black slaves; legislators must first, in gradual terms, assimilate them into French society. Above all, legislators must always consider wealth and productivity when debating the different ways to emancipate the slaves. In the end, he promised that through the abolition of the slave trade, and careful attention to the living conditions of the Caribbean slaves, the subsequent release of human and economic vitality would prove far more profitable than the current situation.[87]

In powerful prose, Lecointe-Marsillac denounced the slave trade and how it affected African health. He divided his impassioned 1789 book into two parts. The first described the horrific middle passage between Africa and the New World (ostensibly based on the English memoirs of a former slave named More-Lack); and the second discussed the political and social consequences of abolition. Lecointe-Marsillac gave his readers heart-wrenching scenes of sickness and death – as illustrated by his provocative chapter titles, such as 'Treatment of sea-sick Negroes', 'Mortality of slaves at sea' and 'Causes of the depopulation and the mortality of Negroes'. In his twelve-point outline for the abolition of slavery, Lecointe-Marsillac put nutrition and untainted food supplies as the third step toward emancipation.[88]

According to Lecointe-Marsillac, both the slave trade and the plantation system bred African sicknesses. The galley ships, for example, were so unsanitary that even the surgeons dreaded to treat the diseased blacks, because 'they themselves fear breathing the pestilential air'. As a result, he estimated that almost a quarter of the slaves died before they reached the Caribbean. Their health deteriorated after arrival, as 'a quarter more slaves' succumbed to phthisis, putrid fevers or 'a sharp species of fever which indistinctly attacks all strangers'.[89] The attending physicians provided little help. Lecointe-Marsillac's narrator exclaimed:

> [The surgeons] remain with us for only a few instants, and prescribe to us haphazardly those remedies that, always poorly indicated and poorly administered, do us more harm than good ... .
>
> At the crack of a whip, they force us to swallow those poorly-made remedies that increase our grievous distress, and we are thus made to die. Finally, it is in these sepulchres of pestilential corruption that all the horrors of convulsions, putrefaction, despair and the most painful miseries of the end of the man seem to unite to offer sensible souls the most revolting spectacle of human sufferings; no, not even Hell would be so cruel.[90]

---

87 Ibid., pp. 6, 10, 57.
88 Lecointe-Marsillac, *Le More-Lack*, p. 279.
89 Ibid., pp. 61, 63.
90 Ibid., p. 61.

These surgeons served another agenda, for they assured that the slaves were healthy enough to fetch a good price on the open market. Lecointe-Marsillac further denounced the slave lodgings, working conditions and diet.[91]

Despite his outrage, Lecointe-Marsillac did not want to abolish slavery outright. For him, French society must first assimilate the Caribbean slave before they received freedom. Lecointe-Marsillac never placed this prerogative into the hands of the Caribbean slave; rather, French authorities (doctors included) must push good treatment, religious and civil values and even dietary controls from above. In this manner, when discussing sickness and death, abolitionists echoed the beliefs held by medical practitioners: they could not trust the Caribbean slaves to care for their own bodies. And while abolitionists vehemently opposed racist ideas, they still suggested that, given the social and political realities, black men and women could not regenerate themselves without European help and support.[92]

Conclusion

Like doctors concerned with degeneracy and depopulation in the mainland, colonial doctors and social commentators used medical science to advance specific political agendas. Originally, colonial medicine emphasized the critical interaction between the endogenous and exogenous causes of disease. By controlling bodily functions and lifestyle, the individual could avoid disease and prolong life. Within its continental eighteenth-century context, doctors used health and hygiene to change relations between sex and class. In the Antilles colonies, by contrast, Europeans used medicine to help reinforce powerful racial boundaries and defend the practice of slavery. In a sense, the diseased body signified not just the pathological milieu, but the total lack of self-control exercised by the individual.

With regard to the Caribbean slaves, physicians believed high levels of sickness and death meant Africans were racially predisposed to disease or that slavery itself made them sick. On the eve of the French Revolution, however, abolitionist writers insisted that both slavery and the slave trade caused black health problems and they hoped that abolishing both would eventually restore the African to his own political, physical and moral well-being. These writers believed that health regimen, along with the more obviously enunciated contingencies of Christianity, education, family life and respect for property, could assimilate the emancipated African slave. In this case, abolitionists must first regenerate the African slaves before they were included in the new revolutionary society. This belief played out, on an even broader scale, on the political stage of the French Revolution.

---

91   Ibid., p. 37; also, *Il est encore des Aristocrates, ou Réponse à l'infâme auteur d'un écrit intitulé: Découverte d'une conspiration contre les intérêts de la France* (Paris, 1790), p. 7.

92   Bonnemain, *Régénération*, pp. 19–21 n. 1; Grégoire, *Enquiry*, 28–29; also Ottobah Cugoano, *Réflexion sur la traite et l'esclavage des nègres, traduites de l'anglais d'Ottobah Cugoano, africain, esclave à la Grenade et libre en Angleterre*, trans. Antoine Diannyère (London and Paris, 1788), pp. ix, 51–56.

CHAPTER FOUR

Doctors, Regeneration and the Revolutionary Crucible, 1789–1804

On 10 August 1793, as the morning sun rose over Paris, the recently landscaped Place de la Bastille filled with the sound of F.-J. Gossec's *Hymn to Nature*, performed by a young girls' choir clad in virginal white. That daybreak, an enormous crowd had gathered upon the site of the demolished fortress to celebrate the republic's first anniversary with a festival of 'unity and indivisibility'. As Gossec's cantata, which adapted J.-J. Rousseau's pantheistic text, faded into silence, the president of the National Convention, M.-J. Hérault de Séchelles, climbed a flight of steps leading to an imposing 'fountain of regeneration'. Above the water basin towered a statue of the Egyptian goddess Isis, flanked by two seated lions; an allegory of nature and fertility, her folded arms cupped her marmoreal breasts, from which jetted streams of water. Slowly, Hérault de Séchelles filled a goblet with this fluid, first consecrating the ground with a few drops before pressing the cup to his own lips. In ritual synchronization, this act was repeated by the eighty-six elders who circled the fountain, each representing the eighty-six new departments of the French nation. As each elder stepped forward, Gossec's orchestra added brass fanfare; then the throng fell into silence as he clasped the chalice and drank the fluids. Finally, as the representatives descended, they were accompanied by an artillery salvo and greeted with the fraternal embrace.[1]

Choreographed by the revolutionary painter J.-L. David, this scene from the Festival of Unity and Indivisibility powerfully encapsulates one of the great dreams of the French Revolution: 'physical and moral regeneration'.[2] Revolutionaries hoped to create a 'new man' and a 'new society', both of which were generated from the decayed remnants of pre-1789 society. This dream is vividly illustrated by Isis's maternal body and fluids, revitalizing the atrophied males of the old regime. Given this rich symbolism – motherhood, fertility, growth, development, sickness, decay and rebirth – recent historians have found regeneration a key facet in political

---

1   I am following the synopsis in 'David, au nom du Comité d'Instruction publique présente à la Convention son rapport sur la fête de la Réunion républicaine du 10 août' (11 July 1793), AN C*172, fol. 4513; the text is reproduced in Daniel Wildenstein and Guy Wildenstein (eds), *Documents complémentaires au catalogue de l'oeuvre de Louis David* (Paris, 1973), no. 459 (pp. 53–54). Cf. the description in Jules Michelet, *Histoire de la Révolution française* (2 vols, Paris, 1961–62), vol. 2, p. 541.

2   See Lynn A. Hunt, *Politics, Culture, and Class in the French Revolution* (Berkeley, 1984); and Serge Bianchi, *La révolution culturelle de l'an II: élites et peuple (1789–1799)* (Paris, 1982).

rhetoric.[3] According to them, revolutionaries used the language of regeneration to capture 'linguistic authority' and thus seize a contested political terrain.[4] Though these historians have greatly enriched how we understand revolutionary discourse, they often emphasize the metaphoric aspects of regeneration, overlooking the fact that doctors and naturalists originally used this idea to describe real processes in living things and that revolutionaries had these specific processes in mind when they evoked ideas about social rebirth. In this manner, as Nina Gelbart Rattner and Emma C. Spary argue, contemporaries understood regeneration in very literal, not figurative, terms, and applied this idea in concrete efforts to improve public health, population, agriculture and animal husbandry.[5] Seen in this socio-scientific context, then, regeneration responded to powerful anxieties, dating from the 1750s, about nervous disease, luxury, libertinism and demographic decline.[6]

Whilst regeneration addressed pre-revolutionary concerns, it also extended beyond the Reign of Terror into the Thermidorean Convention, Directorial Republic and Napoleonic Consulate (1794–1804), a period that was utterly crucial for modern French education, family law, science and medical practice. But recent historians have largely overlooked this extensive post-Thermidorean debate about regeneration. This chapter shows that doctors affiliated with the new Paris hospitals, medical faculties and the Institut National hoped to use the human body to improve political morality and remake society along more moderate lines. These doctors rejected the utopian dreams of the radical revolutionaries and recycled regeneration into new private practices of self-control, rebirth and perfectibility. In this regard, I argue, practitioners participated in a broader public discussion – alongside legislators, jurists, lawyers, bureaucrats and educators – on how to stabilize chaotic sociopolitical conditions by using education, festivals and domestic law to mould personal behaviour.[7]

---

3   Mona Ozouf, 'La Révolution française et l'idée de l'homme nouveau', in *The Political Culture of the French Revolution*, vol. 2, *The French Revolution and The Creation of Modern Political Culture*, ed. Colin Lucas (Oxford, 1988), pp. 213–32; Antoine de Baecque, 'L'homme nouveau est arrivé: la "regeneration" du français en 1789', *Dix-huitième siècle*, no. 20 (1988): 193–208; and M. Peronnet, 'L'invention de l'ancien régime en France', *History of European Ideas* 14 (1992): 52.

4   See K. M. Baker, *Inventing the French Revolution: Essays on French Political Culture in the Eighteenth Century* (Cambridge and New York, 1990), pp. 4–5; also Hunt, *Politics*, pp. 10–16.

5   Nina Rattner Gelbart, 'The French Revolution as Medical Event: The Journalistic Gaze', *History of European Ideas* 10 (1989): 417–27; Emma C. Spary, *Utopia's Garden: French Natural History from Old Regime to Revolution* (Chicago, 2000), pp. 99–102.

6   Daniel Gordon, *Citizens Without Sovereignty: Equality and Sociability in French Thought, 1670–1789* (Princeton, 1994), p. 229; Julia V. Douthwaite, *The Wild Girl, Natural Man, and the Monster: Dangerous Experiments in the Age of Enlightenment* (Chicago, 2002), pp. 161–63; Anne C. Vila, *Enlightenment and Pathology: Sensibility in the Literature and Medicine of Eighteenth-Century France* (Baltimore, 1998), 296; Carol Blum, *Strength in Numbers: Population, Reproduction, and Power in Eighteenth-Century France* (Baltimore, 2002).

7   See the discussions in Martin S. Staum, *Minerva's Message: Stabilizing the French Revolution* (Montreal, 1996); and Carla Hesse, *The Other Enlightenment: How French Women Became Modern* (Princeton, 2001), pp. 104–29. On these developments, see especially Lynn

Doctors had their own ideas about regeneration. According to them, recent clinical and physiological discoveries proved that human nature was more rigid and unstable than earlier revolutionaries had believed. For these reasons, they doubted whether progressive law and education could extensively change human nature and society. Rather, as they thought, revolutionaries could only regenerate or heal civil society by using greater elements of emotional and physical self-control, values which were ideally taught by doctors and then adopted by the family. This new medical idea about regeneration radiated across three levels, moving from elite clinical practitioners to a kind of medical 'literary underground'. It involved, first, a health regimen to control limited amounts of vital energy; second, a physical and moral hygiene to keep women in the domestic sphere; and, finally, sexual strategies to breed a new generation of moderate republican citizens.

In this post-Thermidorean discourse on regeneration, doctors drew heavily upon a physiological idea that I call 'limited sensibility'. I mean two things here. As discussed in previous chapters, doctors habitually evoked sensibility when discussing the mind–body problem, seeing it as a fundamental element of human nature. For them, sensibility was a dynamic but unstable property that vivified all living things and determined moral faculties. After the Reign of Terror, however, doctors worried greatly about sensibility's unpredictable qualities, and feared that any display of excessive 'emotion' and 'imagination' could spark radical or reactionary upheaval.[8] As doctors saw it, recent clinical and physiological evidence suggested that individuals had a limited amount of sensibility in their bodies – a kind of precious but potentially explosive fuel – and that, without proper discipline and guidance, it could manifest itself in atrophic or convulsive display and thereby cause anarchy and violence. To truly regenerate society, then, citizens had to contain their precious sensibility through personal control or an imposed discipline. As the following analysis shows, this responsibility fractured overwhelmingly along sexual lines. Consequently, at the twilight of the revolutionary decade, doctors claimed that only the family could help individuals control their sensibility and thus regenerate their minds and bodies. In trying to heal a wounded society, then, doctors reaffirmed the family as a natural, hereditary institution and prefigured the conservative domestic law of the 1804 Civil Code.

A. Hunt, *The Family Romance of the French Revolution* (Berkeley, 1992), Ch. 5; Suzanne Desan, 'Reconstituting the Social after the Terror: Family, Property, and the Law in Popular Politics', *Past and Present*, no. 164 (August 1999): 81–121, and 'What's after Political Culture? Recent French Revolutionary Historiography', *French Historical Studies* 23 (2000): 163–96; Ewa Lajer-Burcharth, *Necklines: The Art of Jacques-Louis David After the Terror* (New Haven, 1999); and Sergio Moravia, *Il pensiero degli Idéologues: scienza e filosofia in Francia (1780–1815)* (Florence, 1974).

8   See W. M. Reddy, 'Sentimentalism and Its Erasure: The Role of the Emotions in the Era of the French Revolution', *Journal of Modern History* 72 (2000): 109–52; and B. H. Rosenwein, 'Worrying about Emotions in History', *American Historical Review* 107 (2002): 821–45. See also Jan Goldstein, 'Enthusiasm or Imagination? Eighteenth-century Smear Words in Comparative National Context', in Lawrence E. Klein and Anthony J. La Vopa (eds), *Enthusiasm and Enlightenment in Europe, 1650–1850* (San Marino, 1998), pp. 29–49.

In the post-Thermidorean period, regeneration raises important issues about medical power and authority. Indeed, modern medicine – the Paris clinic, pathological anatomy, experimental physiology, psychiatric care – was born during the French Revolution, an event that observers traditionally call the 'medical revolution'.[9] In the literature on this vast topic, historians often split between an 'Old Medical History' (focused upon 'internalist', cognitive aspects of medical practice) and a 'New Medical History' (centred upon 'history from below', sociological approaches).[10] The debate often hinges upon how historians interpret upper-class attitudes towards two things: the urban poor, who were the primary recipients of hospital care; and popular or 'folk' medicine, which was the therapeutic norm for the general population. At times, learned practitioners appear either as benevolent activists or nefarious agents of social control. Needless to say, both interpretations have found poignant critics. As L. J. Jordanova has argued, traditional historiography of the medical revolution often relies upon studies of '"great names", major institutions and professional organizations'; as she points out, we still know too little about the 'social and cultural features of science and medicine' during the French Revolution and should thus refrain from broad generalizations.[11] Fortunately, recent work on eighteenth-century medicine suggests new ways to explore social, political, cultural and corporal settings when reconstructing past medical practice, offering a wider, more nuanced 'range of contextualizations'.[12] By adopting this medico-historical 'thick description', historians can better understand the interactions between science and politics and move beyond the Foucauldian power/knowledge rubric. Consequently, they should look for ambivalence and contingency in medical thought and not dismiss doctors as simple handmaidens of social control.[13]

---

9   Michel Foucault, *Naissance de la clinique*, 4th edn (Paris, 1994); Erwin H. Ackerknecht, *Medicine at the Paris Hospital, 1794–1848* (Baltimore, 1967); David M. Vess, *Medical Revolution in France, 1789–1796* (Gainesville, 1975). For recent historiography on the 'medical revolution', see Caroline Hannaway and Ann La Berge (eds), *Constructing Paris Medicine* (Amsterdam, 1998).

10   See Colin Jones, '"New Medical History in France": The View from Britain', *French Historian* 2 (1987): 3–14; L. Brockliss and Colin Jones, *The Medical World of Early Modern France* (Oxford, 1997); Roy Porter and Andrew Wear (eds), *Problems and Methods in the History of Medicine* (London, 1987); and L. J. Jordanova, 'Has the Social History of Medicine Come of Age?', *Historical Journal* 36 (1993): 437–49.

11   L. J. Jordanova, 'Medical Mediations: Mind, Body and the Guillotine', *History Workshop*, no. 28 (1989), 39–52 (at pp. 40, 50), and her *Nature Displayed: Gender, Science, and Medicine, 1760–1820* (London, 1999).

12   Colin Jones, 'Pulling Teeth in Eighteenth-Century Paris', *Past and Present*, no. 166 (2000), 100–45, at 144, and 'The Great Chain of Buying: Medical Advertisement, the Bourgeois Public Sphere, and the Origins of the French Revolution', *American Historical Review* 101 (1996): 13–40.

13   See Karl Figlio, 'Sinister Medicine? A Critique of Left Approaches to Medicine', *Radical Science Journal* 9 (1979), 14–68; and Jan Goldstein (ed.), *Foucault and the Writing of History* (Oxford, 1994). The basic points of departure remain Michel Foucault, *Power/Knowledge: Selected Interviews and Other Writings, 1972–1977*, ed. Colin Gordon, trans. Colin Gordon, John Mepham and Kate Soper (New York, 1980); and Ivan Illich, *Medical Nemesis: The Expropriation of Health* (New York, 1982).

In this vein, this chapter underscores the contested boundaries of medical knowledge, those complex ways that doctors sought to explain their sociopolitical universe through medical language and ideas. Whilst doctors believed the new clinical science gave them powerful tools for deciphering human nature and prescribing social behaviour, it was an attitude characterized by uncertainty, confusion, negotiation and sometimes utter panic. During the 1790s, revolutionary agents – all across the political spectrum – worried about the raw mechanics of power: doctors, for their part, specifically struggled with concrete questions about human nature and how innate biological limits might keep legislators from improving society for the better. Unlike the natural philosophers of seventeenth-century England, who looked to the new mechanistic philosophy to reform Christian manners after the Civil War and Glorious Revolution, French medical practitioners wanted to find a more secular but vitalist model upon which to ground republican conservatism. Doctors asked: how could physical and moral hygiene help France 'get out' of the Revolution?[14]

The poetics of regeneration

What did regeneration mean for revolutionaries? At first glance, regeneration was one of those emotive words that appeared during the French Revolution – alongside 'nation', 'patrie', 'constitution', 'law', 'virtue', 'vigilance', 'republic', 'indivisibility', 'rights of man', 'equality', and so on – although historians have rarely placed its meanings in a broader cultural context.[15] However, as the following analysis suggests, regeneration had vast political meanings, carrying its particular languages and practices. It embodied, foremost, a desire to rehabilitate and to integrate all citizens (whether 'active' or 'passive') into the great body of the nation.[16] Consequently, revolutionaries introduced politics into all forms of everyday life, hoping to transform private life and behaviour and thus regenerate all of society. Unlike earlier medical crusaders, who had wanted to reform immorality and poverty, revolutionary regeneration sought to transform all social bonds and unite the body politic under new organic bonds.

---

14 On this point, see B. Baczko, *Ending the Terror: The French Revolution After Robespierre* (Cambridge and New York, 1994). On comparisons with the English revolutionary context, see J. R. Jacob, 'The Heavenly City of the Natural Philosophers: Boyle, Wilkins, and Locke as Social Engineers, c. 1649–89', unpublished ms.; and Simon Schaffer, 'Regeneration: The Body of Natural Philosophers in Restoration England', in Christopher Lawrence and Steven Shapin (eds), *Science Incarnate: Historical Embodiments of Natural Knowledge* (Chicago, 1998), pp. 83–120.

15 See Hunt, *Politics, Culture, and Class*, p. 21; and also François Furet and Mona Ozouf (eds), *A Critical Dictionary of the French Revolution*, trans. Arthur Goldhammer (Cambridge, MA, 1989), pt 3 ('Institutions and Creations') and pt 4 ('Ideas').

16 On these notions of citizenship, see especially William H. Sewell, Jr., 'Le citoyen/la citoyenne: Activity, Passivity, and the Revolutionary Concept of Citizenship', in Lucas (ed.), *Political Culture: The Political Culture of the French Revolution*, pp. 105–23.

Before the French Revolution, regeneration meant three things: religious, embryological and surgical. Originally, as Antoine de Baecque has shown, regeneration had a religious meaning. In works such as Furetière's *Dictionnaire universel* (1690), Trévoux's *Dictionnaire universel français et latin* (1704), and Richelet's *Dictionnaire de la langue française* (1732), regeneration meant the spiritual rebirth provided by baptism, or the incarnation of the word of God in Mary's womb, or the resurrection of the dead at the final judgment.[17] Over the course of the eighteenth century, however, regeneration also acquired a physiological meaning, one concerned with the generation of organic form. Between 1712 and 1741, René Réaumur's and Abraham Trembley's embryological experiments had demonstrated cases of regeneration in the crayfish and polyp (a hydra or fresh-water coelenterate).[18] The fact that an organism could regain its lost appendages (for instance, a hydra sliced in half 're-generated' into two separate hydras) forced contemporaries to debate what agency, if anything, governed reproduction and growth. Naturalists wondered whether organic form – 'the simple evolution of what was already engendered', as naturalist Charles Bonnet put it – was a stable essence, fixed at birth.[19]

By 1740, therefore, the *Dictionnaire de l'Académie* defined regeneration in both spiritual and biomedical terms; and Denis Diderot's and Jean de la Ronde d'Alembert's *Encyclopédie* also accepted this double meaning. Regeneration, the *Encyclopédie* said, 'is the act by which one is reborn into a new life'. Human beings experienced regeneration twice: 'Our first *regeneration* renders us children of God, accords us innocence, and gives us right to eternal life, which is the inheritance of the regenerated. But in the second *regeneration*, resurrection puts us in possession of this heritage.'[20] By contrast, regeneration's '*surgical sense*' (wrote Dr Antoine Louis) '[is] commonly used in treatises about wounds and ulcers, for explaining the restoration of lost substance'.[21] The *Encyclopédie* shows how medicine gradually eclipsed the sacred meaning; in fact, Louis emphasized the surgical over the theological. Further evidence appears in other entries: 'incarnation' dealt with the tissue regeneration;

---

17   See Antoine de Baecque, *The Body Politic: Corporeal Metaphor in Revolutionary France, 1770–1800*, trans. Charlotte Mandell (Stanford, 1993), pp. 132–33. Significantly, neither Bayle's nor Voltaire's respective dictionaries included the term.

18   See Charles W. Bodemer, 'Regeneration and the Decline of Preformationism in Eighteenth Century Embryology', *Bulletin of the History of Medicine* 38 (1964): 20–31; and Aram Vartanian, 'Trembley's Polyp, La Mettrie, and Eighteenth-Century French Materialism', *Journal of the History of Ideas* 11 (1950): 259–86.

19   Charles Bonnet, *Considérations sur les corps organisés* (2 vols, Neuchâtel, 1779), vol. 1, p. 120.

20   'Régénération', *Encyclopédie, ou dictionnaire raisonné des sciences, des arts, et des métiers*, ed. Denis Diderot (36 vols, Geneva, 1777–79), vol. 28, p. 566a–b.

21   Ibid., p. 567a. See also the later expositions in *Encyclopédie méthodique ou par ordre des matières: médecine*, ed. Félix Vicq d'Azyr (13 vols, Paris, 1782–1832), s.v. 'Régénération'; and the prestigious *Dictionnaire des sciences médicales*, ed. N. P. Adelon et al. (60 vols, Paris, 1812–22), vol. 40, pp. 341–46.

whilst 'resurrection' said it was unlikely that a person's decomposed body could rise from the grave at the end of days.[22]

After 1789, however, revolutionaries built upon earlier moral hygiene concerns and turned these scientific meanings of regeneration into more concrete plans for social improvement. In this sense, regeneration implied political reform; at least, it was defined this way in Boiste's *Dictionnaire universel de la langue française* and the *Dictionnaire de l'Académie* (both 1798). Reinhardt's *Le néologiste français, ou vocabulaire portatif des mots les plus nouveaux* (1796) was clear: it said that regeneration was '[a] term of theology and chemistry. Recently, it has been given a wider scope. Today it signifies the improved, perfected reproduction of a physical, moral, or political object.'[23] Throughout, this meaning shifted according to the political moment. Over the revolutionary decade, contemporaries spoke of 'a regenerating plan to liquidate State debts';[24] a 'moral revolution' that 'just regenerated the political order';[25] 'the numerous enemies who were opposed to the regeneration [of France]';[26] or 'that happy epoch of the regeneration of public instruction'.[27]

In the early phases of the Revolution, at least, regeneration expressed three agendas: revolutionaries could regenerate laws and institutions (such as seigniorial traditions or fiscal policy), specific social groups (such as the debauched aristocracy) or, finally, the whole social body (the nation-state itself, all its peoples and customs). In the first instance, regeneration implied legal-legislative improvement. In the National Assembly on 7 September 1789, the wives and daughters of several prominent artists, having donned vestal gowns and adorned their hair with cockades, presented the deputies with a casket full of their jewellery, a sacrifice meant to help liquidate the nation's public debt. This scene was inspired by Nicolas-Guy Brenet's 1785 salon exhibition: this painting had captured Plutarch's patriotic parable, in which the elite Roman women gave the Senate their gold to commemorate the victory over Veii.[28]

On one level, this stylized gesture shows how revolutionaries actively identified with neo-classical ideals and aesthetics in their public and private acts. And yet the women's words deserve further emphasis. Their speech to the deputies declared:

---

22   *Encyclopédie*, s.v. 'Incarnation' (vol. 18, pp. 521a–524a) and 'Résurrection' (vol. 28, pp. 970a–972b).

23   Quoted in de Baecque, *The Body Politic*, p. 134.

24   AN F^{17}1310, d. 6, *Adresse du conseil général de la commune de Soissons à l'Assemblée nationale, du 5 novembre 1790* (Soissons, n.d.), pp. 1–2.

25   AN F^{17}1002, d. 192 (Les Citoyens du district de Marcigny-sur-Loire), 'Citoyens législateurs', 25 Nov. 1792 [Year I].

26   AN F^{17}1144, d. 2, 'Aux citoyens représentants du peuple, membres du Comité d'instruction publique' (n.d.).

27   AN F^{17}1147, d. 20, Le Conseil de Commerce de la ville de Lyon au Ministre de l'Intérieur, letter of 8 Germinal, Year X.

28   Nicolas-Guy Brenet's painting was entitled *Piété et générosité des dames romaines*. Louis Gauffier returned to this scene in the piece he submitted for the Salon of 1791 (under the same title) and later in his *Cornélie, mère des Graecues, solicitée par les dames romaines de donner des bijoux à la patrie* (1792). See Robert Rosenblum, *Transformations in Late Eighteenth-Century Art* (Princeton, 1967), pp. 86–87.

> The regeneration of the state will be the work of the representatives of the Nation. The liberation of the state must be the work of all its citizens. When the Roman women presented their jewellery to the Senate, it gave the Senate the gold without which it could not carry out the vow made by Camillus to Apollo before the capture of Veii.[29]

The wording is significant. The 'regeneration of the state' was a specific legal moment; it was executed by male legislators and actualized through law. Reform, therefore, was a rational but circumscribed question of policy. By contrast, the allusive 'liberation of the state' (as these women called it) lurked elsewhere, entangled within the citizen's private life. If the women's gesture provides a clue, this liberation involved a domestic sensibility that had surmounted old regime decadence and debauchery. By changing their lifestyle, people could alleviate the current social crisis and solidify the political regime. When the women distinguished between the public and private reform, then, they used the language of regeneration in a formal sense; they echoed Louis XVI's words when he convened the Estates-General on 6 July 1788, heralding the 'great enterprise I have undertaken for the regeneration of the Kingdom and re-establishment of good order in all its parts'.[30]

For other revolutionaries, however, regeneration meant more than balancing the royal chequebook or overturning taxation without representation. In this case, private liberation converged with the 'regeneration of the state'. And this reveals the second meaning of regeneration: the desire to ameliorate civil status. Accordingly, regeneration could rehabilitate marginal social groups and thus encourage them to assimilate in order to receive civil status. Needless to say, revolutionaries couldn't agree whether they could – or even should – integrate these groups. A good example appears in the Metz academy's 1788 essay competition on regenerating Alsatian Jews. To make Jews happy and useful, the abbé Henri Grégoire said, Jews themselves should abandon traditional Judaism and embrace a French linguistic, religious and even corporal identity – essentially forgetting their former identity and converting to Christianity.[31] Indeed, revolutionaries expressed similar concerns about Protestants, actors and, as seen in Chapter 3 above, African slaves.[32] Since contemporaries believed these groups were degenerate in body and mind, they ought to cleanse themselves before they could feast at the banquet of civil society.[33]

---

29   *Procès-verbaux de la Convention nationale* (72 vols, Paris, 1792), 4, n. 69, pp. 1–5, quoted in Claudette Hould, *Images of the French Revolution* (Quebec, 1989), p. 187.

30   Quoted in Jean Egret, *La pré-Révolution française, 1787–1788* (Paris, 1962), p. 358.

31   See Arthur Hertzberg, *The French Enlightenment and the Jews* (New York, 1968); cf. Gary Kates, 'Jews Into Frenchmen: Nationality and Representation in Revolutionary France', in Ferenc Fehér (ed.), *The French Revolution and the Birth of Modernity* (Berkeley, 1990), pp. 103–16.

32   See, for example, the dramatist Jean-Louis Laya, *La régénération des comédiens en France, ou leurs droits à l'état civil* (Paris, 1789). Note that Laya's interests also ran into medicine; he reviewed Dr P.-J.-G. Cabanis's *Rapports du physique et du moral de l'homme* (Year X [1802]) for the *Magasin encyclopédique*, vol. 45 (Year XI [1802]), p. 153.

33   Cf. Lynn Hunt, 'The Origins of Human Rights in France', *Proceedings of the Western Society for French History* 24 (1997): 9–24, and 'Forgetting and Remembering: The French Revolution Then and Now', *American Historical Review* 100 (1995): 1119–35.

Beginning in 1788–89, some revolutionaries used this same rhetoric in the polemics of class struggle. In his renowned pamphlet, *Qu'est-ce que le Tiers État?*, abbé E.-J. Sieyès used the language of 'regeneration' to attack the aristocracy itself. In his work, a manifesto that inspired the Third Estate to create the National Assembly, Sieyès asked whether the Second Estate (the nobility) could 'regenerate itself' or whether it would expropriate the 'vaunted regeneration … for [itself] alone'. He feared that aristocrats could seize revolutionary energy and thereby rejuvenate their declining authority, transfusing this vivifying force into their blue-blooded veins. But Sieyès also directed these medical metaphors towards his bourgeois constituency, as he challenged his readers to overcome their sickly servitude and regenerate themselves for the national good. In his words: 'The health of the body and the free play of its organs must be restored so as to prevent the formation of one of these malignancies which infect and poison the very essence of life itself.'[34]

Nonetheless, these meanings of regeneration, whether expressed by Louis XVI, or by the women delegates, or by Grégoire or Sieyès, differed from the mass spectacles and pageantry found in the radical revolution – such as the meanings attached to David's imposing 'Fountain of Regeneration' at the Champ de Réunion in 1793. In broad fashion, this monument celebrated not particular interests, but rather the indivisible republic, that 'great body of the people'. Here, regeneration stretched across the individual life cycle and through all levels of society, regardless of rank or status. And this highlights the final meaning of regeneration: a collective baptism or rebirth. In this case, revolutionary activists dreamed of regenerating every citizen, from the vilest executioner to the working classes, marginalized Jews and slaves, women, the bourgeoisie, the aristocracy and the royal family itself. Even the sickly dauphin Louis-Charles must regenerate himself, a barrister from Dijon declared, should he one day lead the French race.[35] To achieve this goal, revolutionaries must rationalize all aspects of social life, believing that shared behaviour produced a common spirit and beauty. For these reasons, they abolished the old irregularities and asymmetries and standardized currency, tariffs, weights, measures and even time itself. The best-known examples are the metric system and the revolutionary calendar. As one legislator said, 'The Revolution has renewed the souls of Frenchmen; it educates them each day in republican virtues. Time opens a new book in history; and in its new march, as majestic and simple as equality, it must engrave with a new and vigorous instrument the annals of regenerated France.'[36]

As these examples demonstrate, revolutionaries applied regeneration to anything and anybody, making it synonymous with the Revolution itself. It is difficult to impart the sense of urgency that infused this language and practices. According to

---

34   Emmanuel-Joseph Sieyès, *What is the Third Estate?* ed. S. E. Finer, trans. M. Blondel, intro. by Peter Campbell (New York, 1963), pp. 92, 140–41, 174.

35   AN F^{17}1309, d. 4, Delmosse, homme de loi à Dijon, 'Système de l'éducation physique, morale, civique et politique, qui doit être suivie, à l'égard de Louis-Charles, prince-royal' (n.d.); two other such extraordinary projects, albeit not as detailed, can also be found in AN F^{17}1310, d. 8.

36   Romme, 'Report on the Republican Era' (20 September 1793), in *The Old Regime and the French Revolution*, ed. Keith Michael Baker (Chicago, 1986), p. 363.

François Furet and Lynn Hunt, revolutionaries wanted to make a transparent society in which virtue, not interest, held people together – but, at the same time, many feared that they couldn't attain these goals and would therefore fail to achieve a genuine social rebirth.[37] Indeed, the rhetoric of regeneration intensified as political consensus crumbled, suggesting that these ideas plastered over deep ideological cracks in the social body. In a telling passage, Grégoire wrote: 'The French people have gone beyond all other peoples; however, the detestable regime whose remnants we are shaking off keeps us still a great distance from nature; there is still an enormous gap between what we are and what we could be. Let us hurry to fill this gap; let us reconstitute human nature by giving it a new stamp.'[38]

Historians have made much, quite correctly, of the Reign of Terror as a force of regeneration. During the radical revolution, regeneration assumed its most disturbing guises, drawing upon images of heroic sublimation, self-sacrifice, redemption through violence and purification by blood. These ideas appear, for instance, in J.-L. David's violent tableau, *The Triumph of the French People* (1793–94) and J.-L. Pérée's image of masculine rebirth, *L'homme régénéré* (1795). But lest historians simply characterize regeneration as totalitarian indoctrination – one scholar has called it 'Mao-think' – the archival evidence suggests that revolutionaries experienced physical and moral rebirth as profoundly authentic and associated it with individual emancipation.[39] It is crucial to consider what these historical actors originally hoped and desired. As one provincial activist put it in a letter to the committee on public instruction in 1792, France must do more than reclaim her liberty; rather, she 'must conserve it and assure it for our future races'. Liberty cannot exist without virtue, but without regeneration virtue could not last.[40] And here the emphasis on 'liberty' is decisive, making it difficult to accept that revolutionaries understood regeneration as a false consciousness or 'cynical reason', in which disbelieving agents accepted ideological mandates out of calculated interest. Records indicate that contemporaries, from a variety of social backgrounds, believed that regeneration was a hallmark of self-emancipation. These writers and activists believed that revolution was good for a person's health, and that individual health was good for the revolution. This radical coupling of ideas about political and physical well-being underscores that individuals saw revolution as a positive force in transforming personal identity.

---

37 François Furet, *Interpreting the French Revolution*, trans. Elborg Forster (New York, 1981), pp. 1–79; and Hunt, *Politics*, pp. 49, 56.

38 *Rapport sur l'ouverture d'un concours pour les livres élémenatires de la première éducation, par Grégoire* (séance du 3 pluviôse an II), quoted in Hunt, *Politics*, p. 2.

39 J. A. Leith, *Media and Revolution: Moulding a New Citizenry in France During the Terror* (Toronto, 1968), p. 10; he describes the revolutionary government as 'a prototype of the modern totalitarian state' (p. 5). For Ozouf, regeneration connects the great society of the revolutionaries to the gulag and the concentration camp of the twentieth century; see her 'L'homme nouveau'. Cf. Hunt, *Politics*, p. 72 n. 50.

40 AN F[17]1309, d. 1, *Arrête du Directoire de l'administration du département du Lot, rélatif à l'instruction publique, du 17 octobre 1792, l'an Ier de la République* (Cahors, n.d.), p. 1.

Doctors and limited regeneration

The Thermidorean and Directorial regimes, which followed the fall of the Robespierrists, changed these radical meanings of regeneration. The propertied classes, traumatized by terror and civil war, insisted that the government must re-establish the rule of law. Specifically, they wanted to dismantle radical family legislation, which they thought had caused anarchy and terror because it allowed divorce, egalitarian inheritance and civil rights for children. In terms of political health, revolutionaries sought to balance individual emancipation and social stability. Consequently, they wanted the family, not the state, to help regenerate society. Legislators should limit reform and use paternal authority to control personal change and snuff out potential radicalism.[41]

In all this, post-Thermidorean legislators insisted that earlier revolutionaries had miscalculated how popular ignorance and domestic disorder had undermined regenerative efforts. Given revolutionary radicalism, these authorities increasingly distrusted human nature, and they hoped to discover a moral or biological instinct that made people act responsibly in civil society. Once they discovered it, they could nurture it in a more favourable social and political climate. At the vanguard of this search were the so-called Idéologue thinkers of the Institut National: the grammarian A.-L.-C. Destutt de Tracy, the geographer C.-F. Volney, and doctor and anthropologist Pierre Cabanis. These intellectuals blended Lockean sensationalism, sceptical empiricism and conservative republicanism, and developed their own philosophic system – *idéologie* (the 'science of ideas'). Throughout, they maintained that authorities had to cultivate any innate human qualities leading to sociability and consensual politics. Moral values were not simply 'out there', as *a priori* imperatives, as the more conservative Kantian intellectuals would have it; rather, they were like pale and exquisite flowers that had to be potted in favourable soil and tended with firm but loving care so the roots would take hold and the pedals would bloom. In important ways, the Idéologues influenced the Directory's ambitious educational reforms, whose impact upon France cannot be exaggerated. The École Normale, Institut National, École Polytechnique, École des Langues Orientales and the central schools became the institutions to shape citizens who were both moderate *and* republican.[42]

The health blueprint was provided by Constatin Volney's *La loi naturelle, ou catéchisme du citoyen française*. This book appeared in September 1793 after the Convention proscribed the Girondin faction and the Reign of Terror began to get underway.[43] In this chaotic setting, Volney informed readers that the 'law of nature'

---

41   On family law, see M. Garaud and R. Szramkiewicz, *La Révolution française et la famille: histoire générale du droit privé française (de 1789 à 1804)*, ed. Jean Carbonnier (Paris, 1978); James Traer, *Marriage and the Family in Eighteenth-Century France* (Ithaca, 1980); and Desan, 'Reconstituting the Social'.

42   B. Baczko, 'La Constitution de l'an III et la promotion culturelle du citoyen', in François Azouvi (ed.), *L'institution de la raison: la révolution culturelle des Idéologues* (Paris, 1992), pp. 21–37.

43   See Sergio Moravia, *Il tramato dell'illuminismo: filosofia e politica nella società francese (1770–1810)* (Bari, 1970), pp. 196–97. On this text, see L. J. Jordanova, 'Guarding

was still 'inherent in the existence of things'. Its core principle was simple: people had an innate faculty of 'self-conservation' and this faculty ultimately influenced how people understood good and evil, vice and virtue, justice and injustice, truth and error. The greatest threats, he cautioned, were ignorance and passion (a quality apparently found in Jacobin radicals and popular activists), so it was important that people learned to control their bodies through a kind of stoic virtue. For Volney, this involved scientific knowledge, temperance, strength, labour and cleanliness, all of which enhanced the 'physical attributes inherent in man's organization' – namely, 'equality, liberty and property'. So long as citizens learned self-control, they could use their own bodies as they saw fit, just like they used any other property: '[e]very one is the absolute master, the entire proprietor of his body'. For him, individual morality ultimately promoted collective well-being. In his words: '[A]ll individual virtues have, for their more or less direct and proximate end, the conservation of the man who practices them; and by the conservation of each man, they tend toward that of the family and of society, which is composed of the united sum of those individuals'.[44]

After the Terror, politically conscious doctors hoped to apply Volney's insights to mould a moderate citizenry, especially those who were associated (or sympathetic) with the Idéologue circle and the martyred Girondins. Now, a number of doctors had been pressing their own political agendas – both for radical change and health reform – since the first days of the French Revolution. Given that medical crusaders originally blamed physical degeneracy and depopulation upon old regime immorality and administrative incompetence, some hoped that political revolution might vastly improve personal health for all French people.[45] Like other revolutionary actors, then, they too picked up the banner of regeneration. For them, though, this idea meant something more specific: regeneration could potentially change popular health habits and learned medical skills. These beliefs emerge in a number of letters and manuscripts. For example, as Dr C.-L. Dufour put it, political revolution bade well for an analogous revolution in personal health, and he awaited immanent change in national health and morality – almost as though the Revolution could spontaneously generate a new and healthy society. Like Dufour, Dr Linacier of Chinon said that political change could heal people just by itself, noting that nervous disease had declined after Louis XVI had called the Estates-General. According to the records of the Royal Society of Medicine, even the climatic timing seemed opportune for good health: the time was ripe for substantial change. Of course, not all doctors were convinced. Sceptical observers noted that the popular outbursts surrounding the storming of the Bastille had caused neuroses amongst women and the common sort. In Paris, Dr Geoffroy encountered 'nervous maladies' such as jaundice, diarrhoea

---

the Body Politic: Volney's Catechism of 1793', in Francis Barker (ed.), *1789: Reading, Writing, Revolution* (Colchester, 1982), pp. 12–21.

44 C.-F. Volney, *La loi naturelle, ou catéchisme du citoyen français*, ed. Gaston-Martin (1793 [Year II]; Paris: Armand Colin, 1934), 108, 113, 138–39, 148.

45 AP 564 Foss 14, *Voeux d'un patriote sur la médecine en France, où l'on expose les moyens de fournir d'habiles médecins au royaume, de perfectionner la médecine et de faire l'histoire naturelle de la France* (Paris, n.d.), vi–vii.

and false labour; and fifty-five people, he said, had 'lost their heads' to madness on July 14 (presumably, this did not include Delaunay, the governor of the Bastille, who was decapitated on the steps of the Hôtel de ville in Paris).[46]

These examples were not anomalous. For doctors, political change raised questions about the relation between the animal economy of the individual and the larger political economy of the nation-state itself. Equating personal and political health meant that one reflected the well-being or pathology of the other. A sick polity created sick citizens and vice versa. These ideas emerged, for example, in the writings of the republican, Dr F.-X. Lanthenas, who agitated for a variety of radical causes and was a member of the reforming group called the Cercle Social. In a fascinating pamphlet, Lanthenas claimed that the government must concern itself with the health of its citizens. Tyranny, he said, made people sick. Absolutism blinded men to nature, making them forget the values that made them healthy and happy.[47] Fortunately, however, the Revolution would waken the hearts of men, leading them back to the kinds of health practices and policies that would raise them up in body and spirit.

Crucially, Lanthenas transposed his complaints from old regime debates: luxury, consumption, squalor and hereditary degeneration ending in sterility. Some doctors went farther, writing that the very act of revolution had regenerated the body politic – especially after the monarchy was overthrown. In 1792, medical popularizer Joseph-Marie Audin-Rouvière claimed that a republican government encouraged population growth. He wrote, 'Our new morals [*moeurs*], republican virtues, and the benefits of peace and constitution will support the necessary equilibrium and will provide all parts of the republic with that equal and uniform movement that tends to vivify everything'. Before the Revolution, Paris was filled with feminine spectacle and debauchery; but now, the sea change of revolution had swept away the infection. Following J.-J. Rousseau, Audin-Rouvière insisted that urban living caused disease, so the habitant must keep up good personal hygiene, or the government would have to intervene. He said, 'Often, men are only what the government makes them to be'.[48]

But after the Terror, politically engaged doctors feared radicalism. Now they wanted stability, not change. These doctors claimed that they could intervene in political events and regenerate society for the better – by controlling extremism and forming more moderate and self-controlled citizens. To prove these beliefs, they cited their special understanding of how the human organism reacted to environmental

---

46 SRM 177, d. 1, C.-L. Dufour, 'Topographie médicale de la ville de St Fargeau et du pays de Puisaye, suivie de quelques observations de médecine et de chirurgie, et des réflexions sur les changements que l'état actuel de la médecine et l'administration laissent à désirer' (n.d.); SRM 165, d. 10, no. 45–46, Linacier, letters of 8 Feb. and 23 Apr. 1791; Geoffroy, 'Constitution de l'année 1789, avec le détail des maladies qui ont régné pendant les différentes saisons de cette année', *Histoire de la Société Royale de Médecine* (10 vols, Paris, 1779–98), vol. 10, pp. 9–10, 16–17. See also Gelbart, 'Revolution as Medical Event'.

47 F.-X. Lanthenas, *De l'influence de la liberté sur la santé, la morale et le bonheur* (Paris, 1792), pp. 4–5.

48 J.-M. Audin-Rouvière, *Essai sur la topographie physique et médicale de Paris* (Paris, Year II), pp. 7, 8, 46–47.

determinants, especially politics.[49] They asked themselves whether political change was good for a person's health and whether medicine could intervene constructively in this process.

First, doctors said, true regeneration needed a biomedical study of human nature – something they called the 'science of man' – and then derive concrete policies from this knowledge.[50] This post-Terror science of man rejected the Cartesian mind–body divide and focused instead upon the physiological sources of human identity ('the physical and the moral'). In this project, doctors returned to earlier ideas about sensibility, especially the pre-revolutionary Montpellier vitalism, which medical reforms had put at the centre of the new biomedical curriculum.[51] But this discourse on sensibility began to change in new and marked ways. At this stage, doctors began questioning established images of the sensible man and woman of feeling found in pre-1789 literature. Undoubtedly thinking of Jacobin excess, doctors now diagnosed the man of feeling as a person suffering from a nervous disorder (particularly melancholia). Admittedly, Enlightenment literati had found sensibility's various expressions unsettling, ranging between true illumination and convulsive display, 'enlightenment and pathology'.[52] Yet revolutionary radicalism brought earlier anxieties about sensibility into political relief, foregrounding self-control and the limits of personal transformation. Post-Thermidoreans hoped that doctors might solve these pressing problems. In Idéologue circles, the 'attack on sensibility' – so closely associated with Mary Wollstonecraft's literary anti-sentimentalism in England – unfolded as a medical question following the Reign of Terror.

In his inaugural lectures at the Institut National in March 1796, Dr Pierre Cabanis first took up these concerns about sensibility and perfection, and later expanded them in his renowned book, *Rapports du physique et du moral de l'homme* (1802). As a prominent Idéologue and Directorial insider, Cabanis conspired with Napoleon Bonaparte to overthrow the republic – he was rewarded with a Senate post but later purged – and his remains are now resting at the Panthéon.[53] Cabanis was clearly concerned with political stability and he wanted to use medical anthropology to stabilize civil society. As he told sympathetic listeners: 'Under this point of view, the physical study of man is particularly interesting. It is here that the philosophe, the moralist, and the legislator ought to fix their gaze, so they can simultaneously

---

49   A remarkable instance of this kind of thinking can be found in a Lyonais manuscript (a city that had suffered some of the worst horrors of the Revolution); see FMP, ms. 5212, fol. 68, M.-A. Petit, chirurgien-en-chef de l'hôtel-Dieu de Lyon, 'Discours sur l'influence de la Révolution française sur la santé publique (prononcé à l'ouverture des cours d'anatomie et de chirurgie de l'hôtel-Dieu de Lyon)', 30 Sept. 1796. See also J.-L. Alibert, 'De l'influence des causes politiques sur les maladies et la constitution physique de l'homme', *Magasin encyclopédique, ou Journal des sciences, des lettres et des arts* 5 (1795): 298–305.

50   C.-L. Dumas, *Discours sur les progrès futurs de la science de l'homme, prononcé dans l'École de médecine de Montpellier, le 20 germinal an XII* (Montpellier, n.d.), pp. 74, 76–77.

51   On 'anthropological medicine', see the comments in the introduction to this volume.

52   Vila, *Enlightenment and Pathology.*

53   The authoritative biography remains Martin S. Staum, *Cabanis: Enlightenment and Medical Philosophy in the French Revolution* (Princeton, 1980).

discover new understandings about human nature and fundamental insights on its perfectibility.'[54] The physician not only advised the legislator, but he could help create moderate republican citizens. Cabanis thus argued thought that physical and moral hygiene could perfect society.

Like Cabanis, many revolutionary doctors had high hopes for health science. Indeed, Cabanis's desire 'to perfect human nature in general' dovetailed nicely with ideas about the regenerative benefits of personal hygiene.[55] In 1791, Antoine Fourcroy's journal *La médecine éclairée par les sciences physiques* issued a veritable manifesto on the subject, and the future chair of hygiene at the Paris health school, Jean-Noël Hallé, established the epistemological contours for this new science. For the first time in medical history, Hallé distinguished between public and private health care, claiming that '[i]n public hygiene, the Enlightened physician [*le médecin philosophe*] becomes the counsellor and spirit of the legislator'.[56] Subsequently, in his 1792 project for medical reform, the comparative anatomist Félix Vicq d'Azyr ranked hygiene alongside clinical practice and the science of man in terms of curricular importance. In 1794, after legislators had reopened the medical schools, Hallé and Philippe Pinel taught classes on hygiene and health care at the École de Santé de Paris. At the Lycée Républicain, Dr J.-L. Moreau de la Sarthe – whose views on women we will examine shortly – claimed that hygiene could control the 'cruel passions' that were as dangerous as contagious diseases. Hygiene and morality, he suggested, reinforced one another.[57]

For his part, Cabanis believed that hygiene could regenerate individual temperament. In this discussion, he was original because he emphasized that living organisms potentially could improve or degrade their internal functions, though nature always put limits on potential change. Nevertheless, there always remained some opportunity for progressive change. Since a physical sensibility determined consciousness, the physician could alter ideas, moral qualities and reason itself by modifying a person's body. The means were through directed regimen, whether internalized by the individual citizen or imposed by public health agencies. Broadening earlier medical teaching about moral hygiene, Cabanis understood regimen as a sweeping range of human habits that impacted not just particular

---

54 P.-J.-G. Cabanis, 'Considérations générales sur l'étude de l'homme et sur les rapports de son organisation physique avec ses facultés intellectuelles et morales', *Mémoires de l'Institut national des sciences et arts*, 2e classe, *Sciences morales et politiques* 1 (Year VI): 64.

55 Cabanis, *Rapports*, vol. 1, pp. viii, 69–70, 79, 82–83, 480.

56 'Introduction', in Antoine Fourcroy (ed.), *La médecine éclairée par les sciences physiques* (4 vols, Paris, 1791–92), vol. 1, pp. 13–14, 26–27; 'Exposition du plan dun traité complet d'hygiène, communiqué par J.-N. Hallé à A. F. Fourcroy', ibid., vol. 4, pp. 225–26; J.-N. Hallé, 'Hygiène', in *Encyclopédie méthodique: médecine*, vol. 7, p. 432.

57 AN F^{17}1310, d. 6, [Félix Vicq d'Azyr] 'Nouveau plan de constitution pour la médecine en France' (n.d.); and BN 8°Z Le Senne 12.075, *Plan général de l'enseignement dans l'école de santé de Paris, imprimé par ordre du Comité d'instruction publique de la Convention nationale* (Paris, Year III), pp. 23, 24, 25; J.-L. Moreau de la Sarthe, *Esquisse d'un cours d'hygiène, ou de médecine appliquée à l'art d'user de la vie et de conserver la santé* (Paris, n.d.), pp. 27, 51–56.

organs, but rather the systemic determinants that maintained health and therefore encouraged improvement.[58]

But in this analysis, Cabanis shifted the long-standing Enlightenment debate over human education and experience. Balancing views about innatism and environmentalism (associated with Shaftesbury and John Locke), he believed that organisms had inherent mimetic faculties, faculties which allowed them to acquire new behaviour and thus adapt to a changing environment. Like Jean-Baptiste Lamarck, he thought that received impressions could change organic form and function, and, in some instances, individuals could inherit these adaptations, 'propagating themselves from race to race'. Although these observations suggested that nature tended towards perfection, Cabanis concluded that the acquired 'force of habit' had its boundaries. The mind was not a tabula rasa; rather, the 'cerebral pulp' was constrained by its sensibility and instinctual drives. Here the doctor encountered limits to regeneration. As Cabanis suggested, doctors could not entirely change human nature.[59]

Cabanis's hesitant views on regeneration were developed by Xavier Bichat, the celebrated pathologist and creator of the Société d'Émulation Médicale. Best remembered today for introducing the tissue concept, the young Bichat was one of the leading doctors and teachers in late revolutionary Paris. By 1800, he attracted a dedicated coterie of young students and the Paris faculty readily incorporated his works into clinical instruction (indeed, his friends, pupils, and colleagues viewed his premature death in 1802 as utterly calamitous). His ambitious masterpiece, *Recherches physiologiques sur la vie et la mort* (1800), moved physiology towards a specialization based upon vivisection and had an enormous influence on the medical and intellectual establishment.[60] However, underneath Bichat's rigorous levels of experimentation and elemental analysis was a withering rumination on human nature.

---

58   Cabanis, *Rapports*, vol. 1, pp. 76, 215, vol. 2, pp. 6–7, 8, 89–90, 210–11. For a similar view on temperament, see C.-L. Dumas, *Principes de physiologie, ou introduction à la science expérimentale, philosophique et médicale de l'homme vivant* (4 vols, Paris, 1800–03), vol. 1, pp. 9–10, 458, vol. 2, pp. 73, 77–78.

59   Cabanis, *Rapports*, vol. 1, p. 287, vol. 2, pp. 79–80, 81–82, 250–51, 253–54. Although it is impossible to explore here in any depth the connection between Lamarck's ideas of transformism and medical regeneration, suffice to say that Lamarck rejected a simplistic model of direct environmental influence of the organism. For him, species change originated from a shift in the exterior milieu that engendered new needs within in the internal economy of the organism. On the possible affinities between Lamarck and Cabanis, see Staum, *Cabanis*, pp. 182–89; Moravia, *Il pensiero degli Idéologues*, pp. 75–86.

60   On Bichat's contributions to histology and vitalistic thought, see Elizabeth L. Haigh, *Xavier Bichat and the Medical Theory of the Eighteenth Century* (London, 1984); John V. Pickstone, 'Bureaucracy, Liberalism and the Body in Post-Revolutionary France: Bichat's Physiology and the Paris School of Medicine', *History of Science* 19 (1981): 115–42; Geoffrey Sutton, 'The Physical and Chemical Path to Vitalism: Xavier Bichat's *Physiological Researches on Life and Death*', *Bulletin of the History of Medicine* 58 (1984): 53–71; and Sean M. Quinlan, 'Apparent Death in Eighteenth-Century France and England', *French History* 9 (1995): 27–47.

Going further than Cabanis, Bichat argued that unstable vital phenomena threatened the body's sensibility, causing people to 'soar to the highest pinnacle of excellence, or fall to the lowest abyss of wretchedness'. In this discussion, Bichat introduced an important idea that every organism possessed a degree of 'limited sensibility' (or what Elizabeth A. Williams has called 'limited energy'). As Bichat explained, 'The perfection of animals is in proportion to [the dose of sensibility] which has been given to them'. He thus rejected Enlightenment philosophers who believed that people could improve their intelligence and moral sense by improving education and environment. Since sensation in one body part necessitated decrease elsewhere, the organism maintained a 'determinate *sum*' of vital powers that should remain constant throughout its life cycle. If people could not maintain this judicious equilibrium, he said, the body drained its animating agent – sensibility – and it consequently suffered from disease and disorder.[61]

Of course, pre-revolutionary doctors had worried that organisms could quite literally 'run out of matter'. Enlightenment doctors long maintained that the body could exhaust its vital spirits and cause atrophic nervous disease. The best example is the novelist Samuel Richardson, who had notoriously suffered from hypochondria ('spleen'), an eighteenth-century form of depression. Consequently, his physician, George Cheyne, built for him a 'chamber horse' – a prototype, one might suspect, for modern home exercise equipment – and this contraption allowed Richardson to regenerate his nerves with 'all the good and beneficial Effects of a hard Trotting Horse except the fresh air'.[62]

Although this whimsical, Shandean image of the rotund Richardson, riding his own hobby-horse to good health, reveals a mid-century optimism that nervous disease could be cured, the grim Bichat, at the dawn of the Napoleonic era, would have none of it. In his *Recherches physiologiques*, Bichat argued that the organism struggled against the omnipresent forces of death, balancing its fragile will against dangerous vital drives. Though other clinicians had described vital functions in similar terms, Bichat underscored the political import of limited sensibility.[63] Society, argued Bichat, ought to prescribe status and limits, so it could better manage human sensibility. To do so, he proposed a tripartite division of society, based upon unequal levels of vital energy distributed amongst artists, scientists and labourers – a division that inspired later social thinkers such as the Utopian socialist Henri de

---

61   FMP, ms. 5144, Xavier Bichat, 'Notes de physiologie: (4°) sympathies', p. 17; and his *Physiological Researches Upon Life and Death*, trans. Tobias Watkins (Philadelphia, 1809), pp. 5, 6–7, 9, 27–28, 43–44, 46, 52, 56, 6–2, 67. On 'limited energy' and Paris medicine, see Williams, *The Physical and the Moral: Anthroplogy, Physiology, and Philosophical Medicine in France, 1750–1850* (New York, 1994), pp. 99–101.

62   Charles F. Mullet (ed.), *The Letters of Doctor George Cheyne to Samuel Richardson (1733–43)* (Columbia, Mo., 1943), 26–27, quoted in Carol Houlihan Flynn, 'Running Out of Matter: The Body Exercised in Eighteenth-Century Fiction', in G. S. Rousseau (ed.), *The Languages of Psyche: Mind and Body in Enlightenment Thought* (Berkeley, 1990), pp. 147–48.

63   Bichat, *Physiological Researches*, pp. 63, 70, 75–77, 109–10, 112. See also B.-A. Richerand, *Nouveaux élemens de physiologie*, 2d edn (2 vols, Paris, 1802); and Dumas, *Principes de physiologie*, vol. 1, passim.

Saint-Simon and the sociologist Auguste Comte, even earning him a special place on the 'positivist calendar'.[64]

Although Bichat was pessimistic about improving people and society, he acknowledged that civilization could sometimes 'invert the natural order' of 'animal life' for the better. With this rather backhanded statement, he did recognize a degree of social mobility. Yet he was unimpressed with human nature, and doubted that individuals could exercise sufficient 'will' over their vital functions. As he concluded, inequality was 'one of the grand laws of the animal economy, and will remain as immutable as the base upon which it rests'.[65] Limited sensibility, and thus limited ability, formed a natural law that wise legislators should follow. Following these insights, ambitious practitioners sought to develop hygienic habits to conserve this precious sensibility. In their view, the family could equalize this precious property and rejuvenate self-control – a need evidenced by Jacobin excess and popular upheaval. This was true for that group whose sensibility always threatened the social body: women. As a consequence, doctors often returned to earlier ideas about women and moral hygiene that had first appeared in the 1760s and 1770s, but now hoped the changed political landscape would allow them to implement this programme of regeneration.

The natural history of women

Pierre Cabanis and Xavier Bichat were clear: medicine should help control human feeling, not engage in reckless social engineering. Yet doctors still hoped to regenerate society by transforming bodily practices; after all, France still needed to re-establish civil and civic harmony. However, clinical science suggested that some groups simply lacked the moral and physical strength to control their own bodies. Legislators constantly returned to this question when they debated citizenship for minority groups such as slaves, Jews and women. These concerns had first been raised, in inadvertent fashion, by the philosopher A.-N. de Condorcet. When debating women's rights, he declared that legislators first must show that women were physically unfit for citizenship. In other words, science must first demonstrate biological inequalities before lawmakers deprived people of their civil rights.[66] Presumably, Condorcet believed that these natural facts did not exist and that men of science could not invent them with a clear conscience.

This debate about biological inequalities took an acrimonious turn when discussing women's rights. When revolutionaries moved the locus of regeneration back into the

---

64   Barbara Haines, 'The Inter-Relations Between Social, Biological and Medical Thought, 1750–1850: Saint-Simon and Comte', *British Journal for the History of Science* 11 (1978): 19–35.

65   FMP, ms. 46, n. 9, Xavier Bichat, 'De la volonté et de son influence, considérées relativement aux deux vies de l'animal'; and his *Physiological Researches*, pp. 34, 107–09, 112–13, 115.

66   A.-N. de Condorcet, 'Sur l'admission des femmes au droit de cité', in *Oeuvres* (Stuttgart, 1968), vol. 10, p. 129, cited in Londa Schiebinger, *Nature's Body: Gender in the Making of Modern Science* (Boston, 1993), pp. 143–44.

family, they made women into an integral agent of social change. For this reason, physicians carefully studied women's physical and moral qualities, asking what social and political roles they could play in the new polity – and they concluded that women must stay under paternal authority because of their convulsive sensibility. But legislators did not wait for doctors to approve. In 1792, the National Convention expanded male suffrage but then denied citizenship to all women (including women of property). That same year, the Jacobins suppressed female clubs and associations because they feared popular violence. From now on, they said, women must discuss political news in their proper place: the hearth. During the Reign of Terror, Marie Antoinette, Mme Roland, Charlotte Corday and Olympe de Gouges were guillotined after they had been systemically defamed. In 1794, public authorities imprisoned former club leaders such as Claire Lacombe and Pauline Léon. In May 1795, after the Parisian risings of Germinal, Floréal and Prairial, the Directory banned women from its galleries and put all Parisian women under house arrest. Those who appeared in the streets in groups of five or more were dispersed by force.[67]

The republic's antifeminist violence emanated from two things: the revolutionary experience itself (legislators believed that lower-class women had been powerful agitators in the revolutionary crowd) and long-standing anxieties about gender transgression within the elite household. The pre-1789 biomedical image of the 'disorderly woman' in the public sphere returned in post-Thermidorean politics.[68] Under the old regime, doctors said, women had participated too much in public culture; they neglected family values and made themselves physically and morally sick. As a consequence, women had caused physical degeneracy, depopulation and political instability. To regenerate these denatured women, doctors believed they must reform domestic behaviour. As we have seen in Chapter 1 above, these concerns ran like an *idée fixe* through medical texts and appeared in Pierre Roussel's notorious text, *Système physique et morale de la femme* (1775). This was not the same 'gender panic' that Dror Wahrman has distinguished in Britain after the American Revolution.[69] In France, the sexual backlash began in the turbulent 1750s. Rousseau was perhaps the most notable Enlightenment celebrity suffering from this malady, but it seemed contagious amongst medical men, especially those concerned with the 'vapours' diagnosis. In the campaign against degeneracy, doctors returned to the public presence of women and the disorder they caused.

However, when medicine and post-Thermidorean politics collided, some doctors moved from 'gender trouble' to outright hostility.[70] In medical writings, doctors

---

67   Dorinda Outram, *The Body and the French Revolution: Sex, Class, and Political Culture* (New Haven, 1989); Joan Landes, *Women and the Public Sphere in the Age of the Frrench Revolution* (Ithaca, 1988); Hunt, *Family Romance*, pp. 153–55; Madelyn Gutwirth, *The Twilight of the Goddesses: Women and Representation in the French Revolutionary Era* (New Brunswick, 1992).

68   The idea of female 'disorderliness' follows Natalie Z. Davis's classic 'Women on Top', in *Society and Culture in Early Modern France* (Stanford, 1975), pp. 124–51.

69   Dror Wahrman, '*Percy*'s Prologue: From Gender Play to Gender Panic in Eighteenth-Century England', *Past and Present*, no. 159 (1998): 113–60.

70   The expression is from Judith Butler, *Gender Trouble: Feminism and the Subversion of Identity* (London, 1990).

argued that there were simply innate differences between men and women. Like their Enlightenment predecessors, post-Thermidoreans insisted that women's true destiny was motherhood – but they now added that this duty, for better or for worse, filled their lives with sickness and pain. Nature mandated that all living beings must die and return to their primordial state, but she still wanted to preserve the species. For this reason, she had invented sexual dimorphism. Consequently, as Dr J.-M.-J. Vigarous explained, '[m]en and women are utterly distinct beings, each with their own passions, morals, customs, temperaments and diseases'.[71]

In explicit and implicit ways, these comments contained a political agenda. Since a woman was destined for motherhood, nature made her body weak and fleshy, so she could endure pregnancy and nourish the foetus; and her innate mental inferiority meant that she couldn't realistically participate in public exchange. In some senses, then, women's hypersensibility was a survival strategy; but this sensibility soon caused disease if women had abandoned nature's duties. Under Napoleon's Consulate – which became increasingly authoritarian and centred upon male display – major physicians such as Pierre Cabanis and C.-L. Dumas privileged what they called the genital system in human temperament, showing that sexuality obliterated choice, judgment and reason. At the same time, other doctors reintroduced the uterus, once again, as a nosological principle when discussing female disease.[72]

Although doctors transposed many ancien régime obsessions, they were specifically responding to the changed status of women in Directorial society. Following the Reign of Terror, French society saw an outpouring of hedonistic fashions. At the centre of this perceived Directorial decadence were the so-called new women of affluence and fashion, who were epitomized by Parisian socialites such as Mme Tallien and Juliette Récamier. During this period of profound cultural transgressiveness, both men and women appropriated earlier Jacobin thinking about the body. Through style, post-Thermidoreans used the body for self-fashioning rather than collective indoctrination. These techniques included shocking modes that aped the look of guillotined victims (the *coiffure à la victime* or the *croisures à la victime*), the alleged victim's balls attended only by people whose relatives had died on the guillotine, flamboyant youth gangs and reactionary male fashions.

---

71   J.-M.-J. Vigarous, *Cours élémentaire de maladies des femmes, ou essai sur un nouvelle méthode pour étudier et pour classer les maladies de ce sexe* (Paris, Year X [1801]), vol. 1, p. 6; see also Joseph Capuren, *Traité des maladies des femmes, depuis la puberté jusqu'à l'âge critique inclusivement* (Paris, 1812), pp. 1, 38–51; and Richerand, *Nouveaux élemens de physiologie*, vol. 1, pp. xxiv, xxvii–xxviii. On mid-century views on female sickness, see François Azouvi, 'Woman as a Model of Pathology in the Eighteenth Century', trans. Michael Crawcour, *Diogenes*, no. 115 (1981): 22–36.

72   See Capuren, *Maladies des femmes*, p. 3; and Vigarous, *Cours élémentaire*, vol. 1, pp. xvii, 50–52, 63, 71. Indeed, the 'convulsive woman' of high and low society remained a pervasive concern for medical practitioners, even past the revolutionary decade. See SEM, c. D, Desjardins, officier de santé, 'Observations sur les convulsions des femmes en couches (sept exemples dans un millier d'accouchements)', 21 Aug. 1818; and SEM, c. D, Delaporte, 'Hystérie reconnaissant pour cause une vive frayeur, et guérie par une autre frayeur', 29 Feb. 1818. However, these later manuscripts suggest a medical command over nervous disorder; this constitutes a contrast to the panicked writings of the later eighteenth century.

Yet these decadent practices ran afoul of Directorial moral authorities (like the Idéologues), who wished to consolidate political stability through family controls. These tensions emerge in the anonymous print *La mère à la mode* (which dates from the later 1790s). The engraving contrasted the fashionable woman of elite culture, who abandoned her children to an abusive wet-nurse, to the doting mother ('la mère telle que toutes devraient être'), who dedicated herself to moral rectitude and the tender education of her children. As these images implied, Jacobinism had not cured maternal degeneracy.[73]

In the post-Terror period, doctors wanted to use family values to regenerate society. Since women were the rock that grounded the holy family, doctors must cure them first. For some observers, women should become active agents in their own regeneration and learn moral hygiene. In a petition to create a vocational school for women, a woman identifying herself as 'citizeness Acrin of Paris' insisted that public authorities had 'not sufficiently meditated on [the condition of] the timid sex, who, because of her weakness and the dangers which she is constantly surrounded, seems to call for a more pronounced protection'.[74] For others, women must learn domestic hygiene or society would fail to regenerate itself: '[O]ne must transform the physical education of women to assure the success of their moral instruction and we believe that by fortifying their bodies we can fortify their souls'.[75] According to the maverick popularizer Pierre Boyveau-Laffecteur, who had gained notoriety in the 1780s for his syphilis remedies, moral hygiene could regenerate that 'lovable sex' who was often 'disturbe[d]' by the 'contagion of bad example'. By learning domestic duties, libertine women would again submit to the 'social order'.[76]

However, the Idéologue books on the 'natural history of women' best exemplify post-Terror efforts to regenerate women. These titles included J.-F. Saint-Lambert's *Analyse de l'homme et de la femme* (1798–1801), A.-L. Thomas's *Essai sur le caractère, les moeurs et l'esprit naturel de la femme* (2d edn, 1803), J.-L. Moreau de la Sarthe's *Histoire naturelle de la femme* (1803), and Gabriel Jouard's *Nouvel essai sur la femme considérée comparativement à l'homme* (1804).[77] Indeed, these works formed a unique genre in French science and letters. Although rooted within

---

73   See Jacques Godechot, *La vie quotidienne en France sous le Directoire* (Paris, 1977); and Lajer-Burcharth, *Necklines*, pp. 181–204, 242–47.

74   AN F[17]1144 (dos. Secrétariat [an VIII–1811]), 'Projet d'établissement d'écoles de métiers pour les filles, présenté par la citoyenne Acrin', Paris, Year VIII. The legislative report derided Acrin's project, arguing that institutions that purported to foster virtue and skills amongst young women invariably facilitated moral corruption and sexual commerce. 'Les filles ne peuvent, comme les garçons, être élevées en commun', they wrote.

75   AN F[17]1310, d. 2, [Chaudan?] 'Sur l'éducation des femmes' (n.d.).

76   Pierre Boyveau-Laffecteur, *Traité des maladies physiques et morales des femmes*, 4th edn (1798; Paris, 1812), vi, 4.

77   These natural histories, whilst frequently cited, have yet to receive systematic study. See the provisional albeit suggestive comments in Yvonne Knibiehler, 'Les médecins et la "nature féminine" au temps du code civil', *Annales: E.S.C.* 31 (1976): 824–45; Paul Hoffmann, *La femme dans la pensée des Lumières*, 2d edn (Geneva, 1995), pp. 157–71; and Geneviève Fraisse, *Reason's Muse: Sexual Difference and the Birth of Democracy*, trans. Jane Marie Todd (Chicago, 1994), pp. 72–102.

the science of man, the very moniker – 'the natural history of women' – indicated a different agenda. These doctors and moralists did not analyse human identity (as did the science of man); rather, they made naturalist observations, describing women's true character and what civilization had since made of it. Like race theorists working on natural history, these doctors wanted to prove that 'independently of all political institutions, nature herself has formed the human species into castes and ranks'.[78] Throughout, these doctors insisted, women were *terra incognita*, as though they had been built from some dense substance that wouldn't yield under the male gaze. They wanted to emphasize one particular point: biological sex determined a woman's social destiny. In this manner, the natural history of women was timely because it combined cutting-edge science with a significant political agenda.[79] These medical practitioners often identified with the moderate, pro-republican and monist philosophy associated with the Idéologues, and at least one – Moreau de la Sarthe – moved within high-ranking medical and philosophic coteries, despite his reputation as a consummate vulgarizer.

The books had a standard structure. Each doctor described basic anatomy and physiology, female temperament, and the social aspects of womanhood; each doctor claimed to observe female nature without 'prejudice' or 'superstition'. In his *Nouvel essai sur la femme*, Dr Jouard said that moralists must consider human biology when discussing women, since their minds were constrained by a small cranial cavity, a sensible uterus and the mammary systems. But Jouard insisted that sex went beyond reproductive anatomy: 'In every age, from their birth to extreme old age, we find again in a woman general characteristics that distinguish her from a man of the same age.' People could improve their temperament, like Condorcet and Cabanis had promised, but they certainly could not change their sex. Although Jouard didn't believe the uterus totally controlled a woman's nerves and muscles, he still insisted they suffered from a chronic neurasthenia which kept them from participating in civic life.[80]

Dr Moreau de la Sarthe, the chief librarian at the Paris medical faculty and former instructor at the Lycée Républicain, provided the most obdurate generalizations about female nature in his voluminous *Histoire naturelle de la femme*, a book that was clearly intended to complement Cabanis's *Rapports du physique et moral de l'homme* (Moreau de la Sarthe benefited from Cabanis's patronage). He divided his work into two sections: the first detailed the physiology and natural history of women (including novel sections on female racial characteristics); and the second examined women's health and addressed a broader readership (including women).

---

78   William Smellie, *The Philosophy of Natural History* (Edinburgh, 1790), vol. 1, pp. 521–22, quoted in Schiebinger, *Nature's Body*, p. 145.

79   As indicated by the classroom notes of a Parisian medical student, Jules Cloquet, the views of Roussel, Cabanis, Moreau de la Sarthe and Vigarous persisted in the educational curriculum during the Restoration (their potential materialism and ideological scepticism notwithstanding). See ANM, ms. 1062, v. 11, Desmormaux, 'Cours de maladies des femmes et des enfants', 11 Apr. 1820.

80   Gabriel Jouard, *Nouvel essai sur la femme, considérée comparativement à l'homme, principalement sous les rapports moral, physique, philosophique, et avec les applications nouvelles à sa pathologie* (Paris, Year XII [1804]), pp. 11, 17, 42–50, 66–67, 80, 89, 107, 124.

Like Jouard, he emphasized a basic female inferiority, claiming that every detail of her body, from her skin to her bones, offered a 'series of oppositions and contrasts' that were manifest in 'all parts of [her] organization'. In particular, he relied upon recent naturalist descriptions of the female skeleton (he especially praised Thomas von Soemmering's controversial images), and he even included an engraving that emphasized that the female pelvic bones were bigger than her skull. Like Capuren and Vigarous, Moreau de la Sarthe also claimed that a 'uterine temperament' commanded the female psyche. Little wonder, he implied, the young republic had filled its new insane asylums with deranged women.[81]

In a unique way, Moreau de la Sarthe justified his claims about female inferiority by using embryological science. He followed Italian naturalist Lazzaro Spallanzani's work on amphibious development, which had galvanized Parisian medical circles by shifting embryological sentiments in the 1790s towards a theory of ovist pre-existence (that is, a belief that the embryo existed beforehand in the womb). Following this research, Moreau de la Sarthe insisted that microscopy showed sexual traits appeared in the female egg before fertilization. Moreover, these embryos were lodged within the ovaries, and were thus an integral part of the female body. In procreation, the male simply contributed an animating seminal fluid. As Moreau de la Sarthe concluded, embryology thus showed the mother alone was responsible for her child. For these reasons, female self-pollution caused the species to degenerate.[82]

In this discussion, Moreau de la Sarthe had a political agenda, since his embryological evidence supported Directorial and Consulate attitudes towards family law. At this time, jurists were busy finishing a unified Civil Code (adopted in 1804). As historians have made clear, this central document in French law reconstituted society upon 'property, the certainty of the law and the authority of fathers and husbands'.[83] For French women, the Code was a juridical debacle. According to law, women had no legal status beyond their husbands, and men controlled all property, including dowries and earnings. The code also instituted the sexual double-standard (men could imprison women for adultery) and curtailed divorce. As under the old regime, fathers could imprison their children and they could not marry without consent before age of twenty-five. Moreover, the law disinherited illegitimate children and prohibited paternity searches. Using embryological data, Moreau de la Sarthe established that the pre-existing embryo was simply a maternal charge.

---

81   J.-L. Moreau de la Sarthe, *Histoire naturelle de la femme, suivie d'un traité d'hygiène appliquée à son régime physique et moral aux différentes époques de la vie* (2 vols, Paris, 1803), vol. 1, 15, 62, 102–03, 120–23, 695, 700. On the female skeleton, see Londa Schiebinger, 'Skeletons in the Closet: The First Illustrations of the Female Skeleton in Eighteenth-Century Anatomy', in Catherine Gallagher and Thomas Laqueur (eds), *The Making of the Modern Body: Sexuality and Society in the Nineteenth Century* (Berkeley, 1987), pp. 42–82.

82   Moreau de la Sarthe, *Histoire naturelle de la femme*, vol. 2, pp. 23–31, 211, 221; see also Jouard, *Nouvel essai sur la femme*, p. 11 (who did not mention Spallanzani's experiments); and Richerand, *Nouveaux élemens*, vol. 2, pp. 373ff. On eighteenth-century ovism, see John Farley, *Gametes and Spores: Ideas About Sexual Reproduction, 1750–1914* (Baltimore, 1982), pp. 25–29; and Walter Bernardi, *Le metafisiche dell'embrione: scienze della vita e filosofia da Malpighi a Spallanzani (1672–1793)* (Florence, 1986), pp. 309–486.

83   Desan, 'Reconstituting the Social', pp. 119–20.

By contrast, the father thought of it only in terms of descent and inheritance, and had no other responsibility for it – other than what he decided to bestow upon his offspring.[84]

Above all, Moreau de la Sarthe wanted to derive practical health practices from this mass of biological detail. According to him, hygiene was a patriotic duty, because it could make women what they ought to be: dutiful wives, mothers and daughters. In terms of advice, however, Moreau de la Sarthe didn't offer many new insights. Predictably, he denounced wet nursing, conspicuous consumption, bookishness, libertinism and fashion. He loathed current styles such as corsets and petticoats, although he found the neo-Athenian Directorial styles more natural, so long as the gowns weren't too revealing. He even advertised a republican corset designed by the citizen La Croix, which accentuated the breasts without crushing the rib cage. Moreau de la Sarthe then moralized about unauthorized sexuality, especially female masturbation and lesbianism. Whenever in doubt, good hygiene boiled down to 'father knows best'. Moreau de la Sarthe seemed unclear whether women existed for anything more than male pleasure, procreation and primary child care.[85]

The natural history of women changed how many doctors thought about sex and gender. Over the course of the Enlightenment, doctors had discussed women's health and the social causes of female disease. Yet consistently, medical crusaders ignored dangers associated with pregnancy and childbirth, preferring to write about an imaginary world of upper-class indulgence and abuse. In this discussion, doctors used biomedical science to reinforce domestic roles, claiming that men and women complemented each other in their rights as well as their inequalities. In this manner, doctors refused to separate the natural world of sexuality and the cultural world of gender: gender and sex were one and the same thing. There could be no interplay, no acknowledgment, between these categories.[86] In a revealing passage, Moreau de la Sarthe discussed hermaphrodism, concluding that it was so monstrous that science could not comprehend it. One can hardly glance at his illustrations of hermaphrodism without feeling queasy from their pornographic violence, or embarrassed by his desire to maintain sexual difference. Paternalistic law and science would make the female body clean and healthy and thus regenerate society. But women must first accept their place and embrace their new domestic roles, for they too must become active agents in regeneration. The home was their own private republic.

---

84   On the Civil Code, see Jean-Louis Halpérin, *L'impossible code civil*, foreword by Pierre Chaunu (Paris, 1992), and *Histoire du droit privé français depuis 1804* (Paris, 1996). See also André-Jean Arnaud, *Essai d'analyse structurale du code civil français: la règle du jeu dans la paix bourgeoise* (Paris, 1973).

85   Moreau de la Sarthe, *Histoire naturelle de la femme*, vol. 2, pp. 2–6, 223–25, 267–74.

86   On the distinction between sex and gender in English dramatic literature, see Wahrman, '*Percy*'s Prologue', passim; for the social construction of catergories of sex and gender, see Butler, *Gender Trouble*, pp. 6–7.

Sexual healing

A year after Bichat's *Recherches physiologiques* and two years after Napoleon's coup d'état of 18 Brumaire (1799), there appeared a little volume, bearing the odd title of *Essai sur la mégalanthropogénésie*. Penned by the young Dr L.-J.-M. Robert, the text constituted a systematic exposition, dedicated to the Institut National, instructing administrators how to increase the nation's demographic reserves and regenerate the citizenry's physical constitution. In short, Robert promised to breed so-called 'great men' [*grands-hommes*], worthy of the Panthéon, in the neo-classical style.

Robert focused upon two things. On the one hand, he was impressed by naturalist G.-L. Leclerc de Buffon's claim that ill-advised marriages produced sickly offspring; but he was equally dismayed, on the other, by moralist C.-A. Helvétius's assertion that education alone made 'great men of genius'. Incensed by Helvétius's biological naiveté, Robert insisted that sexual hygiene and instruction could tame reproductive chance, and thus breed republican citizens along quantifiable lines of beauty developed by physiognomists such as Peter Camper and J. K. Lavater.[87] These reproductive objectives were so important, Robert thought, because the state must balance an inequitable division of corporeal faculties – almost as though citizens had the right to have a good body.

In Robert's view, government needed to regulate sexual hygiene in a process he called 'mega-anthropogenesis'. The urgency was clear. He warned, 'The daily history of societies teaches us that vices are transmitted within families'; unfortunately, these precious embryos, containing the seeds of future generations, pre-existed within the wombs of uneducated women.[88] Robert thus wanted to change family life and snatch the malleable child from its well-intentioned but simple-minded parents. The government should establish two primary schools, or Athenaeums, to regenerate citizens: one at the Paris military school for men, the other at the château de Versailles for women. Using basic physiognomic knowledge, the Ministry of the Interior would identify promising children and put them in special schools, and there they should remain until a national jury declared their education complete. The young women should learn science, literature, home economics and good mothering; after graduation, they would marry their male schoolmates and receive a state pension proportionate to their merit. Adolescent males would learn the arts and sciences, too, but with greater emphasis on classics and natural philosophy; their education should inculcate a patriotic and militaristic attitude. In particular, Robert concerned himself with the space of learning, dividing the males' education between a hall of Mars and a hall of Minerva, whose walls were adorned with marble tiles and edifying neo-classical works, so to control the pubescent boy's sensible nerves and perhaps discourage libertine thoughts and acts.

Finally, at the annual Festival of the Republic, the First Consul (Napoleon) would confer a national award upon the six most distinguished male and female students of the Athenaeum; and the youngsters would then celebrate their 'mega-

---

87   L.-J.-M. Robert, *Essai sur la mégalanthropogénésie, ou l'art de faire des enfans d'esprit, qui deviennent des grands-hommes* (Paris, Year X [1801]), pp. 14–15, 17, 19–20.

88   Ibid., p. 16.

anthropogenetic' marriages with all the dignity that good republican citizens deserved. Robert concluded: 'Oh, government of France! It is you who must calculate the happy influence of mega-anthropogenesis and its effect upon the Republic and the well-being of nations.'[89]

Robert's plans, as bizarre as they might appear, underscore the continuing concerns about regeneration in the post-Thermidorean period. His book provoked a storm of discussion in the literary and popular press and it immediately went into a second edition (it even inspired satirical vaudeville plays in Paris and in northern Italy). Following clinical ideas about limited sensibility, Robert's mega-anthropogenesis signals how contemporaries conceived regeneration in terms of heredity and domestic hygiene. These concerns unfolded along two alternating levels: the first related to bodily self-fashioning, the second to sexual hygiene. Throughout, gender politics dominated both.

As part of this shift, regeneration made the individual body into a medium of self-expression. The marked resurgence of physiognomy, as seen in Robert's text, constitutes a revealing symptom. Physiognomists wanted to create an objective science to read facial features and decipher the psyche lurking behind them. One striking example, albeit non-medical, was the dramatic interest in portraiture in Directorial society. In contrast to the pantomime eloquence found in neo-classical paintings, Directorial artists returned to Baroque physiognomy, centring upon the intimate attributes of facial expression. Although aesthetic critics found this physiognomic taste decadent (associating it with the so-called new women of high society), the genre points to a compelling need, within elite culture, to assert individuality through the most material means possible. For these reasons, fashionable elites were fascinated by mirrors and specular images, and they purchased personal objects such as so-called psyché mirrors (free-standing mirrors) and viewing fans (fans that had mirrors on the blades).[90] In this manner, bodily self-fashioning, as found in portraiture and sartorial fashion, allowed people to assert their own sense of individual self and personal agency.

Alongside these transformations, physiognomy helped spread the belief, espoused by doctors such as Cabanis and Bichat, that biology shaped intelligence and ability. In his renowned *Traité médico-physique sur l'aliénation mentale* (1800), the psychiatrist Philippe Pinel argued that physiognomy showed a 'connection between an imperfect structure of the cranium and an imperfect operation of the intellectual faculties'.[91] In a similar vein, J.-M. Plane, a disciple of Lavater, used physiognomic insights to label political types. He used profile portraits of radical Jacobins such as Georges Danton, J.P. Marat and Maximilien Robespierre to demonstrate their 'sanguinary' temperament.[92] In this taxonomy of images, Plane implied that physicians could literally read signs of political pathology on the body itself.

---

89   Ibid., pp. 33–34, 47–49, 60, 230–31.

90   Lajer-Burcharth, *Necklines*, pp. 239–41.

91   Philippe Pinel, *A Treatise on Insanity*, trans. D. D. David, with an intro. by Paul F. Cranefield (1800; New York, 1962), pp. 114–33 (at p. 121).

92   J.-M. Plane, *Physiologie ou l'art de connaître les hommes sur leur physionomie* (2 vols, Meudon, 1797).

By introducing physiognomy into discussions about regeneration, doctors linked family hygiene to aesthetic concerns over 'beautiful bodies' and 'ideal values'.[93] Before the Revolution, aesthetic authorities, following the famed art historian J. J. Winckelmann, generally agreed that Graeco-Roman sculpture, what they considered to be the pinnacle of Western art, expressed ideal human forms and thus incarnated society's highest desires and imagination. But by the late 1790s, debates over ancient anatomical knowledge associated with the prominent art critic T.-B. Émeric-David and the physician and amateur artist J.-G. Salvage suggested that Graeco-Roman art did not simply project ideal values, but instead faithfully transcribed a past corporeal reality, one that had since been lost in the modern decadent age.[94] As they thought, people in Antiquity actually looked like the figures found in their sculptures and images. Following this belief, aesthetes and doctors suggested that men and women could regain these sensuous, historical bodies in the revolutionary present.

To achieve these aesthetic goals, contemporaries hoped that doctors could cure ('regenerate') the physical defects that detracted from their sense of personal worth. Orthopaedic surgeons, for instance, promised great results during this period.[95] But given the evidence of limited sensibility, several doctors argued, people had to start cultivating their bodies at the earliest possible age. In their youth, Dr Étienne Tourtelle explained, people acquired the temperament that followed them throughout their lives. When parents raised their children in a lackadaisical or slothful way, they caused bodily alienation and self-misery for their adult selves. Like Robert, Tourtelle blamed mothers for these physical faults, and said that women must become first the object and later the conduit of medical discipline. 'Only through their faithful observation', he said, 'can we hope for a regeneration of the human species'.[96] Following these insights, several physicians insisted that all citizens should have access to health knowledge. These convictions emerge in the transcripts of the Paris medical faculty, where elite practitioners such as Philippe Pinel and J.-L. Baudelocque drafted ornate broadsides apparently to advise poor parents about

---

93   Alex Potts, 'Beautiful Bodies and Dying Heroes: Images of Ideal Manhood in the French Revolution', *History Workshop*, no. 30 (Autmn 1990): 10.

94   Dorothy Johnson, *Jacques-Louis David: Art in Metamorphis* (Princeton, 1993), pp. 156–66.

95   P.-F.-F. Desbordeaux, *Nouvelle orthopédie, ou précis sur les difformités que l'on peut prévenir our corriger dans les enfans* (Paris, Year XIII [1805]), pp. xvi, xx, 71, 76–77.

96   Étienne Tourtelle, *Élémens d'hygiène, ou de l'influence des choses physiques et morales sur l'homme, et des moyens de conserver la santé*, 3d edn (2 vols, Paris, 1815), vol. 2, pp. 341–42, 378.

child-rearing techniques.[97] Similar printed works addressed a more sophisticated, but not too cultivated, lay audience.[98]

Still other practitioners, following Robert's mega-anthropogenesis, eagerly connected sexual hygiene and regeneration. These doctors wanted to limit the more subversive possibilities offered by hygienic self-fashioning. This desire characterizes the works of naturalist J.-J. Virey. He distinguished between public and private physical education, saying that the former promoted social utility whilst the latter perpetuated 'particular interests'. Hence, physical instruction imparted civic values to all citizens, treating them 'as integral members of a fractional family of the nation'. Parents must do more than enlighten their children; rather, they must 'purify their hearts, inspire respect for proper morals, a love of virtue, country, and humanity and instil fear of dishonour, contempt, and the infamy of vices. Virtue must arise before science.'[99]

In his later L'art de perfectionner l'homme (1808), Virey pushed this argument even further by arguing that public education must promote physical education and sexual hygiene. In approaching this problem, the doctor and legislator must use medical anthropology – pioneered by Cabanis and Bichat, amongst others – to explain proper civil and civic behaviour. But throughout, Virey worried about nervous degeneracy amongst elites and was alarmed by reports of idiocy and cretinism in the countryside, all of which he suspected were hereditary in nature. As a result, he doubted that doctors could treat 'monstrosities' acquired at birth and he asked whether society needed government-sponsored breeding programmes.[100]

In 1801, surgeon J.-A. Millot proposed a similar system of physical rehabilitation. In the previous year, the aging Millot (who had delivered Marie Antoinette's children) entered Directorial debates over reproduction and domestic hygiene with his successful manual on procreating male offspring; these were techniques imminently useful, he boasted, for providing both heirs and conscripts.[101] Millot believed that paternal authority and family life preserved social cohesion; and it was upon these

---

97 AN AJ[16]931 (dos. 'Tableaux des soins à donner dans certains états physiologiques et dans quelques accidents ou maladies contagieuses'): [Jean-Louis] Baudelocque, 'Avis aux femmes enceintes' (ventôse, Year VII), and 'L'éducation physique et médicale des enfans, depuis le moment de la naissance, jusqu'au temps du sevrage' (ventôse, Year VII); [Philippe] Pinel, 'Principes de l'éducation physique et médicale des enfans depuis le sévrage jusqu'à la 5e ou 6e année' (ventôse, Year VII), and 'Tables des moyens propres à conserver la santé des enfans' (n.d.).

98 L.-C.-H. Macquart, Dictionnaire de la conservation de l'homme, ou d'hygiène et d'éducation physique et morale, ouvrage élémentaire et à la portée de tous les citoyens (2 vols, Paris, Year VII), vol. 1, p. i.

99 J.-J. Virey, De l'éducation publique et privée des français (Paris, Year X [1802]), pp. v–vii, xiii, xvii, 1, 71–72, 81.

100 J.-J. Virey, L'art de perfectionner l'homme, ou de la médecine spirituelle et morale (2 vols, Paris, 1808), vol. 1, pp. vii–viii, 240, vol. 2, pp. 26065, 271–72, 298–99.

101 J.-A. Millot, L'art de procréer les sexes à volonté, ou système complet de génération, 4th edn (Year IX [1800]; Paris, n.d.).

tenets that he based his reproductive science.[102] Significantly, his books addressed women readers. Having first taught them about procreation, Millot claimed, he would now teach them how to care for their children's bodies (his text even deployed catechist devices, in form of a paternalistic dialogue between physician and naive mother). After all, in his eyes, the well-being of the *patrie* was in question, but he was confident that women would submit to 'everything that depended' on them – such as breast-feeding.[103]

Millot denounced the Jacobin and Directorial republics and hoped that the authoritarian Consulate would create a more thoroughgoing programme of physical education. Following Bichat and Cabanis, Millot said doctors and legislators must transform the body before they could regenerate moral and intellectual qualities. Through physical education, practitioners could preserve individual and national health, transmitting force, beauty and intelligence through racial bloodlines. Millot wrote, '[E]ducation shall correct, improve and perfect the French nation, since that is what made the *grands hommes* of Greece and Rome'.[104] By refining the body, young children learned to control their passions (an essential quality in post-Thermidorean society) and promoted the requisite moral attributes for every citizen. These included parental obedience, duty, respect, patriotism and moral virtue.

Nevertheless, Millot emphasized that regeneration had limits. Every individual had a 'genius proper to him' or a specific 'manner of sensation' that provided a 'particular disposition', 'aptitude' or 'degree of attention' for the 'acquisition of science, spirit and genius'. Education might refine biological characteristics, but in the end it created nothing truly new: '*Memory, imagination, attention, reflection* and *genius* depend upon a certain nature of the fibres, a certain disposition of the brain'.[105] Whereas maternal neglect created sickly bodies, he also believed that pathological causes were 'inherent in our primordial constitution' or stemmed from 'a fault in the abundance of our vital fluids', assuring that 'the nation has degenerated and is continuing to degenerate'.[106] Like Bichat, Millot claimed that humans were born with an 'individual and particular organization' that determined social status. Given this power of heredity, Millot concluded: 'I desire that physical education might correct a part of the hereditary vices of children who are born feeble, by procuring for them a temperament fashioned for anything … . With health of such calibre, one would be sure to be happy and attain an old age without infirmity.'[107]

Following Cabanis, Bichat, and Moreau de la Sarthe, doctors such as Robert, Virey and Millot understood that human nature had a biological underpinning and that this underpinning limited regeneration. In many ways, these popular writers ultimately saw regeneration as a problem of race. This was clearly true

---

102 J.-A. Millot, *L'art d'améliorer et perfectionner les hommes au moral comme au physique* (2 vols, Paris, Year X [1801]), vol. 2, pp. 162–66.

103 Ibid., vol. 1, pp. v, vol. 2, p. 27, and id., *Médecine perfective, ou code des bonnes mères* (2 vols, Paris, 1809), vol. 2, pp. 1–22.

104 Millot, *L'art d'améliorer*, vol. 1, pp. 11, 14–15, 19, 81.

105 Ibid., vol. 1, pp. 27, 28, 29.

106 Millot, *Médecine perfective*, vol. 1, pp. 144–45, vol. 2, 23–24.

107 Millot, *L'art d'améliorer*, vol. 1, pp. 22–24, 27–29, 32–33, 95, vol. 2, 74–75.

for Millot and Virey, who stated that racial interbreeding caused degeneration. For these reasons, Virey said, the government must improve the nation's racial stock. For Millot, French degeneracy came into sharper relief when doctors compared their compatriots to the well-formed German and Swiss physiques; however, physical education could make French citizens into a new race of poet-warriors, reminiscent of the Greeks and Romans of old. In a flight of fancy, Millot even wanted to create public bath houses alongside the Seine, so young children could bath in the river's healthful waters. Following Rousseau's *Émile*, Millot believed that the cool water toughened the young child's fibres, rendering him strong and healthy; and he predicted that in fifteen years, contemporaries could observe a marked change in their offspring.[108] In truth, however, doctors offered many ideas already advanced by old regime moral crusaders such as Antoine Le Camus, N. Brouzet de Béziers and C.-A. Vandermonde. To control physical sensibility, physicians reverted to traditional domestic hygiene: temperance, propriety, diet, exercise, clean air, light sleep, emotional self-control, moderate sexuality, regularity, paternal authority, female obedience and breast feeding. These practices, doctors said, would finally regenerate the social body and make it what it ought to be.

In the end, given the burdens of regeneration, post-Thermidoreans said that what society really needed was love. For them, *l'amour* constituted the most troubling aspect of human experience and as such it had to be subjected to scientific study and control. According to Virey, citizens must rethink moral values so they could accommodate the drives and desires caused by sensibility (particularly passion and desire); only in this way could society avoid the sexual degeneracy that had contributed to the French Revolution in the first place. In his manuscript on political economy, A.-L.-C. Destutt de Tracy conceded that, given the failure of republican institutions, only the family could regenerate society. Family values allowed the nation to achieve political harmony and helped the population grow. As he concluded, 'the transformation that I would desire in society remains, in its substance, a complete regeneration ... affectionate sentiments and charitable passions shall re-establish their powers, and we will see born a national character that is entirely new'.[109]

Conclusion: medicine and polity – the revolutionary years

In French political life following the Reign of Terror, biomedical science transformed how revolutionaries thought about the social world. Doctors applied physiological models to pressing social concerns about sensibility, gender destabilization and

---

108 Virey, *De l'éducation*, vol. 1, pp. 142–43; Millot, *Médecine perfective*, vol. 1, pp. 142–43 and *L'art d'améliorer*, vol. 1, pp. 92–93.

109 Millot, *L'art d'améliorer*, vol. 1, p. 281, vol. 2, pp. 149–52; Ambroise Ganne, *L'homme physique et moral, ou recherches sur les moyens de rendre l'homme plus sage, et de le garantir les diverses maladies qui l'affligent dans ses différens âges* (Strasbourg, 1791), pp. 88–90, 94–95; J.-J. Virey, *Histoire naturelle du genre humain, ou recherches sur ses principaux fondemens physiques et moraux* (2 vols, Paris, Year IX), vol. 1, pp. 62–63, 74–75, 112, 286, 303, 313, vol. 2, pp. 32, 246; A.-L.-C. Destutt de Tracy, *De l'amour*, ed. Gilbert Chinard (Paris, 1926), p. 36.

domestic authority, and they thus made medical science into a major ideological force in shaping the social and political configurations of post-Thermidorean France. In this period of profound social upheaval, doctors provided a common vocabulary for talking about dramatic sociopolitical changes and prescribing therapeutic responses. In their eyes, political radicalism, war and terror had destroyed the nation's physical and moral health, causing both physical degeneracy and social disaggregation. But doctors promised that public authorities could use medical knowledge to restructure domestic life and thus cure the morbid social body. Medical science could thus regenerate French society. In this manner, doctors helped define pressing concerns about the sensibility, sexuality and domesticity in a rapidly changing France.

Historians have traditionally identified the French Revolution as a period of momentous medical change. But as this chapter has shown, doctors were not solely concerned with promoting biomedical science in its own right. Rather, they wanted to use their specialized knowledge to improve the nation's physical and political health. In this case, doctors moved from specific concerns over patient care and hoped to build a more perfect society. Physiological knowledge of human sensibility, doctors such as Cabanis and Bichat argued, could improve the citizenry and make a more harmonious social order. Through physical and moral hygiene, policy-makers could regenerate society by instilling morality, self-control and paternal restraints. For Jouard and Moreau de la Sarthe, medical science could transform domestic relations by establishing natural parameters between men and women, and by emphasizing women's roles as wives and mothers within the domestic sphere. Finally, through sexual hygiene, doctors such as Robert, Virey and Millot hoped to breed a new generation of moderate republican citizens to perpetuate this regenerated polity.

This multilayered medical discussion about regeneration sheds new light upon the interplay between science and society during the 'Age of Revolution'. In terms of eighteenth-century France, the debate has traditionally split in two ways. In his classic analysis, Charles C. Gillispie argued that the relationship between science and polity in the old regime was one of mutual, if not harmonious, scientific and political tradeoffs. The government supported scientific institutions and research in return for applied scientific knowledge and technological expertise. In response, scientists created an autonomous sphere for scientific inquiry and were unconcerned with the political dimensions of their research, except that it contributed to public utility and progressive works. This model, Gillispie suggests, continued into the French Revolution, when scientists entered public service in staggering numbers irrespective of their political or ideological convictions.[110] By contrast, historians

---

110 C. C. Gillispie, *Science and Polity in France at the End of the Old Regime* (Princeton, 1980), 549–50: '[This] behavior, I have come to think, was characteristic of the general relation between science and the state, which has been one of partnership rather than one of partisanship, whatever the strife of factions within the political process ... Science was not the source of a reform movement or of liberalism' (p. 550). On science and the Revolution, see his 'Science in the French Revolution', *Behaviorial Science* 4 (1959): 67–73, and 'The *Encyclopédie* and the Jacobin philosophy of science: a study in ideas and consequences', in M. Clagett (ed.), *Critical Problems in the History of Science* (Madison, 1969), pp. 255–89. He has fully developed these themes in his recent *Science and Polity in France: The Revolutionary and Napoleonic Years* (Princeton, 2004). Cf. especially Terry Shinn, 'Science,

such as Keith M. Baker and Harvey Mitchell have identified a stronger pull of politics and ideology in scientific practice. Pre-revolutionary authorities were frustrated by corporate privilege, particular interests and local tradition, and they appealed to scientific authority in order to provide an objective, rational and, above all, disinterested basis for public policy. Public figures thus turned divisive political issues into scientific or technical equations to be solved by a specialized technocratic elite ('politics in the service of knowledge', as Mitchell has put it). Though these historians deny a social constructionist or relativist perspective, they highlight that scientists work under specific sociopolitical constraints and claim that these constraints can sometimes frame the questions that scientists ask and ultimately try to answer. Accordingly, Gillispie's harmonious interchange between science and polity gives way to one framed more by issues of political power and interest.[111] In this case, Enlightenment science in France reveals long-term continuities in the social uses of natural philosophy, which had been evolving since the Scientific Revolution of the seventeenth century.[112]

The shift from Jacobin democracy to Thermidorean republic throws the relationship between science and polity into dramatic relief. After 1794, republican legislators clearly hoped that science could stabilize the Revolution (unlike Napoleon Bonaparte, who eventually turned to religious coercion).[113] In the Thermidorean period, as François Furet suggested, civil society triumphed over popular sovereignty, as legislators saw that political authority lay in political 'special interests' rather than ideological abstractions of the 'general will'. 'Henceforth', Furet writes, 'ideological notions were subordinated to pragmatic action ... . Men began to use those values to justify themselves, now that values had ceased to identify them.'[114] But the cacophony of special interest voices – Jacobin, Idéologue, sentimentalist, neo-Kantian, Brumairian, revivalist, royalist – overwhelmed post-Terrorist efforts to reconstruct civil society. So like pre-revolutionary thinkers, post-Thermidoreans

---

Tocqueville, and the State: The Organization of Knowledge in Modern France', in Margaret C. Jacob (ed.), *The Politics of Western Science, 1640–1990* (Atlantic Highlands, 1994), pp. 47–80.

111 Keith M. Baker, 'Scientism at the End of the Old Regime: Reflections on a Theme of Professor Charles Gillispie', *Minerva* 25 (1987): 21–34; and Harvey Mitchell, 'Politics in the Service of Knowledge: The Debate Over the Administration of Medicine and Welfare in Late Eighteenth-Century France', *Social History* 6 (1981): 185–207.

112 See especially James R. Jacob and Margaret C. Jacob, 'The Anglican Origins of Modern Science: The Metaphysical Foundations of the Whig Constitution', *Isis* 70 (1980): 251–67; Steven Shapin, 'Social Uses of Science, 1660–1800', in Roy S. Porter and G. S. Rousseau (eds), *The Ferment of Knowledge* (Cambridge, 1980), pp. 93–139; James R. Jacob, 'The Political Economy of Science in Seventeenth-Century England', in Margaret C. Jacob (ed.), *Politcs of Western Science, 1640–1990*, pp. 19–46; and Margaret C. Jacob, *Scientific Culture and the Making of the Industrial West* (Oxford, 1997).

113 Staum, *Minverva's Message*; for this context, see C. Langlois, 'Le renouveau religieux au lendemain de la Révolution', in J. Le Goff and R. Rémond (eds), *Histoire de la France religieuse*, vol. 3, *Du roi Très Chrétien à la laïcité républicaine (XVIIIe–XIXe siècle)* (Paris, 1991), pp. 415–23.

114 Furet, *Interpreting*, pp. 58, 72, 74–78.

hoped to solve divisive problems by using the objective and disinterested world of science. After the Terror, however, medicine assumed a far more conspicuous role in this process, eclipsing the physical, chemical and mathematical sciences as a source of advanced social thought.[115] For social and moral authorities, medicine provided the therapeutic and diagnostic tools to help diffuse sociopolitical chaos and create a more harmonious social order. In turn, revolutionary doctors self-consciously directed their work towards a broad lay audience and proposed utilitarian solutions in a language that the elite classes found appealing and convincing. They claimed that mechanical and mathematical models were unable to explain human complexity, and they emphasized the limits of human nature and social improvement. In this case, then, the political and social concerns determined how doctors approached with their research, writings and patients. If we define 'pure science' as science's 'insulation from external pressures', then post-Thermidorean medicine constitutes what Steven Epstein has called 'impure science'.[116] Nowhere is this more striking than in the medical discussions about gender and sexuality, in which political and biomedical concerns proved mutually reinforcing. But politics did not seep as much into the cognitive realm of science as medical men stepped forward to engage the big political issues of the day.

Nevertheless, a major conclusion of this chapter is that the medical debate over physical and moral regeneration did not represent a disciplinary 'will to power', a political ruse that practitioners used to advance professional or institutional interests. Nor were medical views completely 'hegemonic', in that they formed a unified ideological front. In terms of regeneration, French practitioners expressed a plurality of ideological and political interests: Cabanis's moral anthropology, Bichat's experimental physiology, Moreau de la Sarthe's natural history of women and Robert's mega-anthropogenesis all reveal social and ideological concerns that transcended any single disciplinary or ideological agenda. Overall, however, these doctors – whether consciously or not – veered towards authoritarian political solutions. Post-Thermidorean practitioners rejected Jacobin civic virtue and sought to combine regeneration with an emerging model of family politics, all which assumed an increasingly paternalistic and authoritarian tone. By emphasizing limited sensibility and sexual self-control – particularly on the part of women – these doctors reified ideas of domesticity and biological difference, whilst at times opening up space for corrosive self-fashioning practices. Above all, they wanted to regenerate compromised social hierarchies within the context of post-Thermidorean conservatism. In this manner, medical regenerative projects were a heavy stone

---

115 A similar trend already appears in natural history during the early and radical phases of the Revolution; see the excellent analysis in Spary, *Utopia's Garden*, pp. 99–239; and also R. W. Burkhardt, Jr., *The Spirit of System: Lamarck and Evolutionary Biology* (1977; Cambridge, MA, 1995). For developments in politics and the general sciences, see Roger Hahn, *The Anatomy of a Scientific Institution: The Paris Academy of Sciences, 1666–1803* (Berkeley, 1971), pp. 252–312.

116 Steven Epstein, *Impure Science: AIDS, Activism, and the Politics of Knowledge* (Berkeley, 1996), p. 8. Cf. the classic statement in Robert K. Merton, 'Science and the Social Order' (1938), in *The Sociology of Science: Theoretical and Empirical Investigations* (Chicago, 1973).

of reactionary republicanism that stirred the political waters for Brumaire and the Civil Code. Part of this sociopolitical transformation was a new medical image of the regenerated self, one cast in a biological mould and emblazoned with all the inequities that human sensibility would allow.

CHAPTER FIVE

Uncertain Territory and Fragmented Agendas, 1804–1830

During the French Revolution, health crusaders had hoped that applied medical science could transform human nature and create a new, regenerated society. By using physical and moral hygiene, doctors and public officials could mould a moderate citizenry – not too radical, not too reactionary – that respected the so-called 'principles of 1789' and accepted law-and-order political solutions. But this vision did not survive the conservative backlash of the early 1800s. Under the Napoleonic Empire and the Restoration monarchy (1804–30), doctors revised their views on the self and social melioration, diverging in their attitudes towards health activism in form, function and intent. From here, doctors rejected their original quest for physical and moral regeneration, and began to fear a new kind of degeneration brewing within French society – this time, among the urban labouring classes. Simultaneously, they pushed government and scientific authorities to support greater intervention into society's health. In so doing, they shifted from the earlier ideas about moral hygiene and established social medicine as an accepted academic and public policy pursuit.

Generally, medical historians have approached post-1800 health activism in terms of the aetiological debate over contagion and infection: conservatives believed in disease contagion and supported quarantine policies, while liberals believed in atmospheric infection and rejected government regulations, preferring instead environmental sanitation. In this chapter, however, I move away from this debate by looking at health activism in terms of the continuing medical discussion about human nature and society. In these years, contemporaries developed new ideas about social hygiene as medical consensus about human nature and perfection began to unravel. Doctors posed three interrelated questions: first, they wanted to know whether hygiene could improve ordinary citizens (and whether or not this was a worthwhile endeavour); second, whether the nation even needed healthy individuals (and whether the government should subsidize health care); and third, whether or not population growth mattered for national power, productivity and prestige. Doctors thus used new ideas about political economy to study public hygiene, asking about the quality and quantity of the population and whether the government could improve individuals and society for the better. In so doing, hygienists raised new questions about the health and morals of labouring classes and framed them in socio-statistical terms.

Following the Napoleonic regime, there appeared three major approaches towards social medicine. First, there were the pragmatic hygienists and forensic specialists such as Paul Mahon and F.-E. Fodéré, who wanted to create a so-called political medicine [*médecine politique*] that reflected the legal, administrative and political realities of the Napoleonic and Restoration period. Second, there were the philosophic and idealistic reformers associated with the Idéologues, Eclectics and social Christians, notably J.-J. Virey and P.-J.-B. Buchez. These doctors wanted to create a new moral society, one characterized by social harmony and mutual interdependence. Finally, there were the sanitarians who led the new public health movement of the 1820s, such as Louis-René Villermé and Alexandre Parent-Duchâtelet. These doctors embraced socio-statistical methods and Malthusian sensibilities, and focused upon the moral condition of the labouring classes. These new sanitarians doubted that public authorities could improve the physical and moral health of the citizens, and they raised new anxieties about the increasingly dire social conditions in early industrial France.

Pragmatic constables: medicine for a well-ordered society

Between 1794 and 1803, doctors and public officials reorganized medical faculties, hospitals, certification criteria and charities and thus created the basis of modern medical practice in France. These reforms also generated unprecedented interest in public hygiene. In the new health schools in Paris, Montpellier and Strasbourg, prominent doctors offered pioneering courses on hygiene and forensic medicine, and used their faculty positions to push health-reform agendas within professional and administrative circles. A number of these outstanding faculty doctors, notably Antoine Fourcroy, François Chaussier, Étienne Pariset, J.-N. Hallé, Paul Mahon, F.-E. Fodéré and Étienne Tourtelle, turned hygiene into an important branch of medical science, and they raised government support for public health measures following the Reign of Terror.[1]

During this period, as William Coleman writes, these early hygienists borrowed important methodological approaches from colleagues who were pioneering the study of clinical medicine. In the hospitals, pathologists such as Xavier Bichat and Jean-Nicolas Corvissart were 'no longer content' to describe morbid appearances; rather, they 'sought out a more secure basis for diagnosis in pathological changes in the human body itself'. In short, they wanted to explain 'the underlying relations or supposed causes' behind disease.[2] These clinical ideas, which did so much to explain pathological phenomena, also inspired health activists in important ways. Like hospital doctors, hygienists wanted to discover the systemic causes of disease, but they concluded that the primary place for studying pathology was not the hospital or clinic, but rather society itself. Consequently, doctors had to put public health problems in a broader social and economic framework. To do so, they looked to the new science of political economy to study – as they described it – 'the different parts

---

1   See Dora B. Weiner, *The Citizen-Patient in Revolutionary and Imperial Paris* (Baltimore, 1993).

2   William Coleman, *Death is a Social Disease: Public Health and Political Economy in Early Industrial France* (Madison, 1982), pp. 21–22.

of the social body' and how these 'different parts' influenced sickness.[3] By using socioeconomic insights developed by Adam Smith and J.-B. Say, hygienists hoped to discover the natural laws that linked the so-called 'animal economy' and the 'social economy' of the body politic – laws that ultimately governed individual and collective health. In this manner, doctors connected corporeal and socioeconomic phenomena.[4]

Though health activists wanted to expand public health services, their political sensibilities were often cautious and conservative. This attitude was shaped by several complex factors. The first was the doctor's class status and his place in the social order. Often, doctors were members of the urban bourgeoisie and they understandably shared the upper-class belief that the world was well enough and it didn't need a terrible amount of change. Health activists thus rejected radical political solutions as either hopelessly idealistic or downright dangerous. Second, the doctor was decidedly indebted to government officials. During the Napoleonic regime, legal and bureaucratic reforms transformed the relation between doctors and the state.[5] In this time, public officials overhauled medical institutions, putting medical professors on public payrolls and guaranteeing medical training and licensing. In material terms, these reforms made physicians, more than ever, into handmaidens of the state, since they relied upon the government to keep their status and livelihood. These class and government loyalties caused many doctors to be more moderate and circumspect in their health plans.[6]

Nevertheless, post-revolutionary doctors cannot be dismissed as simple agents of bourgeois hegemony. Although they were obvious components of the new social order, medical practitioners apparently had mixed feelings about the authoritarian and reactionary governments that ruled France between 1799 and 1830. In general fashion, while physicians expressed a plurality of sociopolitical beliefs – ranging from radical republicanism to religious conservatism – it can be said that many consciously defined themselves as moderate reformers on the side of science and social progress, and even, at times, as agents of social and moral improvement. Like the Idéologues, they accepted the 'principles of 1789' so long as these principles were

---

3   J.-B. Say, *Cours complet d'économie politique pratique*, 2d edn (2 vols, Paris, 1840), vol. 1, p. 1, vol. 2, p. 237, quoted in Coleman, ibid., p. 275.

4   F.-E. Fodéré, *Essai historique et moral sur la pauvreté des nations, la population, la mendicité, les hôpitaux et les enfans trouvés* (Paris, 1825), pp. 45–46. On notions of the animal economy at the turn of the century, see Stephen J. Cross, 'John Hunter, the Animal Oeconomy, and Late Eighteenth-Century Physiological Discourse', *Studies in the History of Biology* 5 (1981): 1–110.

5   See Elizabeth A. Williams, *The Physical and the Moral: Anthroplogy, Physiology, and Philosophical Medicine in France, 1750–1850* (Cambridge and New York, 1994), pp. 115–22; and Jacques Léonard, *Les médecins de l'ouest au XIXe siècle* (3 vols, Lille, 1978), vol. 3, pp. 1207–18.

6   On this background, see Jan Goldstein, *Console and Classify: The French Psychiatric Profession in the Nineteenth Century* (Cambridge and New York, 1987), pp. 20–28, 35–40; Matthew Ramsey, *Professional and Popular Medicine in France: The Social World of Medical Practice* (Cambridge and New York, 1987), 71–125; and Léonard, *Les médecins de l'ouest*, vol. 1, pp. 197–302.

checked by the rule of law. In many ways, this progressive political attitude stemmed from the fact that the medical profession had inherited the empirical, rationalist mantle of the Scientific Revolution and the Enlightenment, and they clung to these ideas even in the reactionary and obscurantist atmosphere of the Restoration. These intellectual movements had given them the tools and methods that enabled them to transform medicine from a guild craft into a bona fide science. Doctors knew all these facts. They also knew that the French Revolution had allowed doctors to overhaul and reform medical schools and hospitals, thereby revolutionizing their professional and institutional practices for the better. For them, it was clear that revolutionary politics – despite all the memories of radicalism and violence – had moulded the profession and assured its status and power in French society, and they really couldn't say that the French Revolution had been bad for their professional as a whole. For all these reasons, doctors maintained an important but ambivalent debt to Enlightenment philosophy and revolutionary politics, even after these ideas had become unfashionable and seditious in post-revolutionary society.

Given these conflicting ideological and philosophic loyalties – moderate but potentially progressive – both the Napoleonic and Restoration governments mistrusted members of the medical profession because they feared doctors had seditious philosophic and political agendas. The Paris medical faculty, in particular, were well known for advocating sceptical empiricism, philosophic materialism and republican sentiments. Though these doctors defended moderate values against Jacobinism and reactionary royalism, Napoleon disliked independent thought and action, and thus preferred to use religious coercion, rather than scientific expertise, to control the masses.[7] Little changed after the Restoration. Under Louis XVIII and Charles X, reactionary officials were so threatened by the medical tradition of intellectual independence that they even tried to dismantle the entire post-revolutionary medical system, a project that liberal doctors managed to stonewall.[8] At the same time, medical students were also earning a reputation for their radical and materialistic spirit, and these attitudes sometimes exploded in public disturbances.[9] In 1820, for example, medical students rioted after the duc de Berry was assassinated, and the ultramontane Denis-Luc Frayssinous punished them by closing down the Paris medical school and purging eleven faculty members, several of whom were cherished pioneers in the medical revolution.[10] In all these respects, political realities shaped health activism, as public officials either censored progressive doctors or rewarded those who accepted official political values.

In response to these sociopolitical realities, doctors interested in social medicine developed a new model of health activism, something that I call 'pragmatic

---

7   Martin S. Staum, *Minerva's Message: Stabilizing the French Revolution* (Montreal, 1996), pp. 213–15.

8   AP 564 Foss 21, *Rapport de la commission nommée par l'ordonnance du roi du 9 novembre 1815, à l'effet de lui rendre compte de l'état actuel de l'enseignement de la médecine et de la chirurgie en France, et de proposer à sa majesté les modifications dont pourroient être susceptibles ces établissements* (Paris, 1816).

9   Francis Schiller, *Paul Broca: Founder of French Anthropology, Explorer of the Brain* (Berkeley, 1979), pp. 16–58.

10   Léonard, *Les médecins de l'ouest*, vol. 3, pp. 1214–16.

scientism'. Here, doctors self-consciously avoided political or theological debate. Rather, they claimed to serve the government – no matter the political form – in order to keep the social peace and make the nation healthy and strong. In so doing, doctors shifted from ideas about physical and moral regeneration to something they called 'legal medicine and medical police'. They revamped forensic medicine and combined it with the new juridical and administrative realities of post-revolutionary society, and championed this new science in medical and official circles.[11] Pierre Sue, for example, told his colleagues that legal medicine was a civic duty; and N.-P. Gilbert promised that it would assure the 'happiness of humanity, the assurance and security of peoples'.[12]

The most important medico-legal systems were developed by Paul Mahon in Paris and F.-E. Fodéré in Strasbourg. Both doctors combined forensic medicine with new European ideas about medical police pioneered by Johann Peter Frank and Andrew Duncan; in particular, Fodéré launched an ambitious project to reconcile traditional medical jurisprudence with all the exigencies of the new Civil Code and Penal Code of 1804.[13] For Fodéré and Mahon, medico-legal practice involved two levels: forensic medicine and medical police. The former dealt with juridical issues while the latter dealt with public health, broadly construed. In their books, Fodéré and Mahon painted with broad brushstrokes, starting with theories about natural law and the social contract. Both doctors approached traditional law and custom in rationalist terms, hoping to promote a 'vast medical enlightenment' amongst the population.[14] To meet these extensive needs, medico-legal practice combined a variety of fields: medicine, anatomy, physiology, botany, zoology, geography, anthropology, history

---

11   See, for example, AN AD XI, 21 ('Edits, arrêts, lettres-patentes, etc. [médecines, chirurgiens]'), no. 2 (1666). At present, we lack a monographic study of legal medicine in modern France; however, see the introductory comments in Jean Lecuir, 'La médicalisation de la société française dans la deuxième moitié du XVIIIIe siècle en France: aux origines des premiers traités de médecine légale', *Annales de Bretagne* 86 (1979): 231–50; as well as Lindsay Wilson, *Women and Medicine in the French Enlightenment: The Debate Over 'Maladies Des Femmes'* (Baltimore, 1993), passim. For a comparative study, see Catherine Crawford, 'Legalizing Medicine: Early Modern Legal Systems and the Growth of Medico-Legal Knowledge', in Michael Clark and Catherine Crawford (eds), *Legal Medicine in History* (Cambridge and New York, 1994), pp. 89–116.

12   Pierre Sue, *Aperçu générale, appuyé de quelques faits, sur l'origine de la médecine légale* (Paris, Year VIII); N.-P. Gilbert, *Quelques réflexions sur la médecine légale et son état actuel en France* (Paris, Year IX), p. 6. See also J.-J. Belloc, *Cours de médecine légale, théorique et pratique*, 2d edn (Year IX; Paris, 1811); and Jean-Baptiste Vigné, *De la médecine légale* (Rouen, 1805).

13   AN F¹⁷2165, Fodéré au Citoyen François [Neufchâteau], Ministre de l'Intérieur, Nice, 1 Frimaire Year VII; see also F.-E. Fodéré, *Les lois éclairées par les sciences physiques, ou Traité de médecine-légale et d'hygiène publique* (3 vols, Paris, Year VI), vol. 1, 'Advertissement'. See also 'Notices historiques sur le Professeur Mahon', *Journal de Médecine* (Germinal, Year IX): 91ff, reprinted in P.-A.-O. Mahon, *Médecine légale et police médicale*, ed. M. Fautrel (3 vols, Rouen, 1801).

14   Fodéré, *Les lois éclairées*, vol. 1, passim, and his *Traité de médecine légale et d'hygiène publique ou de police de santé, adapté aux codes de l'Empire français et aux connaissances actuelles* (6 vols, Paris, 1813), vol. 1, 'Introduction'.

and law. As they cautioned, however, medico-legal theories should never be seen in the abstract because they dealt with real-life concerns. Unlike utopian plans for social engineering, their science remained eminently practical.[15]

Significantly, medico-legal practice served class-conscious agendas. In terms of forensic medicine, doctors dealt with upper-class and bourgeois problems.[16] The main issues involved property and sexual propriety and the topics ranged from impotence to virginity, rape, sodomy, late birth, illegitimacy, abortion, insanity, suspicious death, and so on. In these cases, doctors were expected to evaluate claims over heritage, patrimony, sexuality and the family – especially when these claims concerned inheritance and titles. Here, Fodéré and Mahon saw the doctor as an objective and moral figure in bourgeois society, a self-possessed professional thrust into the seedy underworld of provincial family politics by judges and barristers. This persona marks an important development, as it reflects a new image of the doctor as a paragon of middle-class values, something seen (in different ways) in literary works such as Honoré de Balzac's *Le médecin de campagne* or Gustave Flaubert's *Madame Bovary*. According to Mahon and Fodéré, doctors must help jurists evaluate the intimate lives of the bourgeoisie and returning *émigrés* in order to clarify domestic disputes. Wealthy patrons asked: How could they determine whether a young bride had lost her virginity? If a husband had died, how many months after could the spouse give birth without casting doubt upon paternity and inheritance? At what stage in a mental illness were people unable to dispose of their property as they pleased? Given the embryological evidence, could doctors verify paternity searches in a reliable, scientific manner?

On the level of 'medical police', medical practitioners dealt explicitly with the health of the poor and labouring classes. According to Mahon, public hygiene was 'one of the most important aspects of that science we call police', because it assured the 'interior security' and 'happiness' of the 'body politic'. In this sense, physicians advised jurists and legislators about 'the sure methods of conserving the health of men united in a society'. By these means, the government could encourage population growth by ameliorating the pathologies caused by civilization itself. Mahon asked, 'Wouldn't it also be that the diminution and, above all, the degradation of the human species has finally forced them to encourage the study of the proper measures of remedying such a terrible affliction?'[17]

In all this, Mahon and Fodéré emphasized that medico-legal practice constituted a conservative force in society. Though they may have drawn precedents from the radical health activism associated with the French Revolution, they cautioned that they wanted to use health science to defend the status quo. In revealing ways, Mahon and Fodéré defined society just like pathologists defined life itself, believing that 'life is the totality of those functions which resist death'.[18] Following this insight, they

---

15 Fautrel, 'Préface de l'éditeur', in Mahon, *Médecine légale*, vol. 1, pp. xix–xxi.

16 Mahon, *Médecine légale*, vol. 1, p. 3.

17 Ibid., vol. 3, pt 2, pp. 3–4; see also F.-E. Fodéré, 'Police médicale', *Dictionnaire des sciences médicales*, ed. Adelon et al. (60 vols, Paris, 1812–22), vol. 44, pp. 42–91.

18 Xavier Bichat, *Physiological Researches Upon Life and Death*, trans. Tobias Watkins (Philadelphia, 1809), p. 1.

stressed that anarchic and corrupting forces threatened the social order. By whatever means, the doctor must improve personal health and hygiene, because physical well-being promoted morality and a happy civil society.[19] These goals, Mahon believed, had been made more attainable by recent medical progress. Botanical knowledge and veterinary medicine had improved rural health. Midwives were officially licensed and now learned improved obstetrical skills. Public officials had closed urban cemeteries and prohibited burial within church walls. The Revolution had revamped the old hospitals and promoted clinical training, and learned societies allowed doctors to exchange biomedical knowledge. The government even regulated the remedy trade.[20]

That said, further reforms were needed in the urban and rural environment. Medical practitioners and public officials needed to clean up urban centres. In towns and cities, the air was corrupted by human, animal and plant decompositions. Hospitals and manufacturers produced revolting human effluvia. Bodily wastes were indiscriminately spread around by the poor and labouring classes. The countryside had its own problems. Recurring epidemics were caused by stagnant waters and swamps. Everywhere there were quacks and empirics. Betwixt and between, society was still threatened by the twin scourges of luxury and libertinism. Echoing the moral hygienists of the old regime and revolutionary eras, Mahon wrote: 'The luxury which renders men effeminate, and by this alone, more susceptible to a great number of illnesses, merits as well, under several circumstances, the greatest impediments and should be discouraged by all manners'.[21] Despite all the medical advances wrought by the Revolution, therefore, the body politic was still menaced by degeneracy and decline.

In this regard, medical reform had failed to solve the gravest problem of all: depopulation. Fodéré and Mahon firmly embraced pro-natalist policies. As Mahon wrote, 'The power and wealth of an empire depends on its more or less large population. This truth needs no demonstration. The government must therefore direct all its attention to favour everything that can encourage it and to remove the obstacles that are dangerous for it.'[22] The primary causes of depopulation were epidemic and endemic disease, 'celibacy' among priests and soldiers, prostitution and concubinage, and hereditary diseases. To these factors, Mahon added bad physical education, smallpox, gastroenteritis and convulsions. Nevertheless, the government could possibly limit child mortality by inoculating children and regulating the wet-nursing industry.

Finally, Mahon and Fodéré wanted to regulate all the practices and rituals surrounding death itself. In his pro-natalist campaign, Mahon wanted a medically trained 'cemetery police' to administer last rites. These practitioners would verify death, record its causes and report suspicious cases. If the person had died from an epidemic disease, the physician would oversee the disposal of the body and they would examine cadavers for cases of apparent death. Doctors should search for

---

19   Fodéré, *Traité de médecine légale*, vol. 5, pp. 23–24.
20   Mahon, *Médecine légale*, vol. 3, pt 2, pp. 8–10.
21   Ibid., vol. 3, pt 2, pp. 2, 23.
22   Ibid., vol. 3, pt 2, pp. 32–33.

signs of pregnancy; in doubtful cases, the attendants should cut open the woman's body and 'extract the foetus that can still be living and conserved for society'. Crucially, mortality bills should be overseen by physicians, who would thus keep the all vital statistics and monitor mortality rates. Doctors should register the name of the deceased, age and sex, possible causes of death, the attending physician (to trace charlatans and fraudulent practitioners), and the place, hour, day and year of death. As Mahon concluded, '[t]his is the only method of evaluating the progress or diminution of the population, by comparing death registers with those of the sepulchres'.[23]

Mahon and Fodéré envisaged a large-scale medical system that could cover the citizen from conception to final decay, promising that medico-legal science could improve society and assure productivity and social tranquillity. But they wanted to protect and conserve the social body, not transform it. For some critics, however, Mahon's and Fodéré's plans still echoed more radical health plans to regenerate the nation, and so they wanted to limit health activism to strict legal or forensic questions. For example, Gibert said that 'medical police' applied strictly to medical licensing and regulation, and he urged that medico-legal practice should avoid social or political agendas.[24] However, as the next section shows, a number of physicians during the Empire and Restoration sympathized with Mahon and Fodéré and believed that that medicine could simultaneously improve society whilst guarding the status quo. As they saw it, doctors protected the social order and thus acted as a judicious and moderate force to maintain morals and manners. C.-L. Cadet de Gassicourt called this agenda '*médecine politique*', whereby medical practitioners joined the government in 'the interest of the governed'. In his words: 'Politics considers man in society under two respects, the physical and the moral. Medicine, which strives to understand the first, is not a stranger to the second, and pertains to their reciprocal influence. Under this point of view, medicine is an instrument of politics.' The question was how to implement this vision.[25]

Guarding society: public health, medical topography and yellow fever

Mahon and Fodéré's ideas complemented new legal and bureaucratic realities that were emerging in the post-revolutionary environment. Though public authorities wanted to avoid radical reforms, they managed to consolidate institutional changes made during the 1790s and continued to expand some health-care services. As a consequence, there emerged a fragmentary health system, an administrative mosaic that comprised the medical schools and networks, hospitals, the interior ministry, departmental prefects and municipal authorities. After the Reign of Terror, these bureaucratic and institutional structures complemented the creation of numerous

---

23 Ibid., vol. 3, pt 2, pp. 39, 41.

24 Gibert, 'Police médicale (Méd. lég. hyg. pub.)' [1827], *Encyclopédie méthodique ou par ordre des matières: médecine*, ed. Félix Vicq d'Azyr (13 vols, Paris, 1782–1832), vol. 12, pp. 205–11.

25 C.-L. Cadet de Cassicourt, 'Médecine politique', *Dictionnaire des sciences médicales*, vol. 31, pp. 535–46 (quote at pp. 534–35).

medical associations. Between 1794 and 1820, doctors formed prominent academies to pursue public health agendas, notably the Société de l'École de Médecine, Xavier Bichat's Société Médicale d'Émulation, Joseph Guillotin's Académie de Médecine (later called the Société Académique and the Cercle Médical) and, finally, the Académie Royale de Médecine. At the same time, the Paris Athénée taught public courses on hygiene in 1813 and the Institute of France also interested itself in physical education. Prominent thinkers such as Georges Cuvier and Joseph-Marie Degérando also published important works that increased public and intellectual interest in health and medical reform.[26]

In addition to these medical activities, the government also created new bureaucratic agencies. After revolutionary and Napoleonic reforms overhauled central and local government, departmental prefects asked the Ministry of Interior to take a lead in urban sanitation, infectious disease and rural health conditions.[27] In response, in 1802, C.-L. Cadet de Gassicourt helped create the Paris health council. This new body advised city authorities on unsanitary habitations, distributing mineral waters and first-aid techniques. In 1807, the health council became a permanent institution and it expanded its activities to include epidemics, the grain trade, cemeteries, factories, sewers, cesspools, public baths and so on.[28]

Public authorities also wanted to improve rural health. In 1805–06, the Ministry of the Interior inaugurated a departmental system of *médecins des épidémies*, and in 1813, it tried to create a nation-wide system for reporting endemic and epidemic diseases.[29] At the same time, Napoleon also sponsored national competitions on health issues.[30] Somewhat encouraged, in 1815, the Paris health council asked the ministry to establish a national organization of health committees modelled on the Paris example. Although public officials rejected the measure, local municipalities later took their own initiative and established similar councils in Nantes in 1817, Lyon in 1822, Marseilles in 1825, Lille in 1828 and Strasbourg in 1829 – a trend that intensified before the cholera epidemic of 1832.[31] By the early nineteenth century, public authorities had created, in embryonic form, a national system of medical police.

To coordinate health reform in the urban and rural areas, doctors and public authorities wanted to create a coherent epistemological and practical approach to

---

26 For background, see John E. Lesch, *Science and Medicine in France: The Emergence of Experimental Physiology, 1790–1855* (Cambridge, MA, 1984), 30–79; and George Weisz, *The Medical Mandarins: The French Academy of Medicine in the Nineteenth and Early Twentieth Centuries* (Oxford, 1995),pp. 3–20.

27 See, for example, AN F^{8}18, fol. I et seq.

28 On apparent death and resuscitation, see AN F^{8}3, dos. 1 (boîtes fumigatoires); on cemeteries, see AN F^{8}90, d. 1–2 and F^{8}91, d. 1, 6, 11, 13, 22, 24–26, 28, 30–31, 41–42; on slaughterhouses, see F^{8}96, d. 1–2; AN F^{8}93, d. 1–2; and on factories F^{8}94, dos. 2, 8–9; F^{8}95, d. 1, 4, 6.

29 AN F^{8}15 and F^{8}16, 'Régistre des épidémies qui ont régné dans les divers départements de l'Empire en 1813'.

30 AN F^{8}4^b, dos. 1 and 4, esp. 'Rapport présenté au Ministre de l'Intérieur', Paris, 9 Feb. 1808.

31 Anne La Berge, *Mission and Method: The Early Nineteenth-Century French Public Health Movement* (Cambridge and New York, 1992), pp. 113–47.

health policy. To do so, they returned to the pre-revolutionary project to create a national medical topography – a project, as seen in Chapter 2 above, famously associated with the Royal Society of Medicine. Although the Royal Society had been dissolved, doctors continued to make topographic surveys, remitting them to existing medical societies and sometimes even publishing them as full-length book studies.[32] In June–July 1800, the Minister of the Interior asked the Paris medical school to complete the Royal Society of Medicine's original national topography. Though doctors supported the idea, they cautioned that a new national topography needed large-scale funding and support in order to accommodate recent scientific innovations and bureaucratic and territorial changes. In particular, they emphasized that medical personnel needed new and sophisticated studies that assessed local climate, geography, disease and demography. Consequently, the Faculty asked public authorities to create a medical commission consisting of fifteen Paris-based physicians, even petitioning the Ministry of the Interior to create a new faculty chair of medical topography at the Paris medical school.[33] Throughout, doctors employed the long-standing rhetoric about family values and pro-natalism to justify this post.[34] But the government did not respond, and the project was only taken up twelve years later by the new Académie Royale de Médecine in 1820.[35]

However, public authorities often requested doctors to compile medical topographies as a kind of diagnostic tool to help them make health policies. Officials became concerned when they observed high mortality and morbidity in particular localities, and they asked doctors to investigate the problems and propose possible solutions. To answer these demands, doctors often crafted medical topographies as they had under the old regime, but now they now changed the scope and content by adding substantial data culled from local health councils, welfare bureaus and new government agencies for vital statistics. Consequently, medical topographies increasingly correlated vital statistics and environmental approaches to disease in striking ways. For example, this new emphasis appears in the writings of Dr Buquet, a physician who practiced in Laval. In 1807, the Ministry of Interior asked him to correspond with the Paris Medical School Society, hoping to explain the

---

32 See, for example, SEM, c. B (d. Boismare, no. 4), Boismare, 'Mémoire sur la topographie médicale de la ville de Quilleboeuf et de ses environs', Rouen, 12 Mar. 1812; SEM, c. T ('Topographie'), Roger (chirurgien-en-chef), 'Topographie de Thionville et des environs', 28 brumaire, Year V; and SME, c. 4, n. 1, H. L. D. (at Parthenay), 'Essai sur la topographie médicale du Mont Saint-Michel, aperçu sur la Maison centrale de cette ville' (1829). For published works, see especially J.-C. Lebrun, *Essai de topographie médicale de la ville du Mans et de ses environs* (Mans, 1812); and Claude Lachaise, *Topographie médicale de Paris* (Paris, 1820).

33 AAFM, c. 1, 'Rapport de la commission nommée d'après la lettre du Ministre de l'Intérieur, en date du 26 prairial, portant invitation à l'École de s'occuper de la topographie médicale de France', séance du 19 messidor an VIII.

34 AN F¹⁷2107, d. 1, [Antoine] Dubois, docteur en médecine de l'École de Paris ... à Monsieur le Conseiller d'État, directeur général de l'instruction publique, Comte d'Empire (n.d.).

35 Antoine Portal et al., 'Rapport de la commission chargée de rédiger un report d'instruction relativement aux épidémies', *Mémoires de l'Académie royale de médecine* 1 (1828): 245–79 (at p. 249).

high death rates in the cantons of Mayenne, Laval and Château. To do so, Buquet carefully researched two extensive local topographies which are notable largely for combining both clinical and statistical methods (he relied heavily upon conscription data provided by local authorities). He saw local health in grim terms, commenting on excessive poverty, bad physique and low fertility, and he particularly emphasized the role of child morbidity and mortality in affecting local demographic patters.[36] As he confirmed, a third of all children died before age ten, long before adolescence – and yet another third died before age twenty. Outraged, Buquet wrote, 'a little less than half reaches thirty years of age, so that there only remains, to produce a new generation, less than half of that which had preceded it, without including celibacy'.[37]

In 1807–08, a more extensive example of this kind of topographic inquiry appears in Paris. In the tenth arrondissement (the present-day sixth), public authorities were alarmed by high rates of sickness and child death, and the neighbourhood mayor turned to the Ministry of the Interior to study the problem and solve it.[38] In response, municipal authorities coordinated a thorough-going medical inquest that used local charity bureaus and the newly created Paris health council to generate raw demographic data. Directed by Dr Chappon, the inquest stretched across the better part of a year: it involved a series of official reports and meetings, and even attracted high-profile medical figures, such as the Montpellier-trained J.-J. Ménuret de Chambaud, who had previously written a medical topography of Paris in the 1780s (as discussed in Chapter 2 above).[39]

In this new Paris topography, doctors incorporated aetiological theory into new institutional and policy practices. Bureaucratic agencies gave doctors access to all existing vital records through which they figured the statistical incidence of sickness and death; institutional authorities gave doctors the wide authority to go into buildings, inspect homes, observe private behaviour and to directly question working-class families – powers not available to doctors writing topographies for the Royal Society of Medicine during the 1770s and 1780s.[40] In all these activities, these officials and physicians were still motivated by depopulationist fears, as they connected poverty, sickness and demographic loss – especially amongst the very young and the aged.

In different ways, medical practitioners heavily emphasized the unsanitary conditions in towns and cities, moving from the earlier worries about the urban corruption associated with libertinism and luxury. Rather, doctors now complained about poorly built housing, filthy bodies and immoral lifestyles, and identified dangerous and unhealthy occupations in the neighbourhoods. In this sense, doctors

---

36   SEM, c. B (d. Buquet), n. 14, Dr Boquet, 'Rapport sur la mortalité des années X, XI, XII et XIII d'après la demande du Ministre de l'Intérieur', Laval, 30 Nov. 1807 and, n. 16, 'Topographie médicale de la ville de Laval et de son territoire' (1808).

37   Buquet, 'Topographie médicale de la ville de Laval'.

38   AP 124 Foss 1, Chappon, letter of 19 Oct. 1807.

39   AP 124 Foss 1, Ménuret de Chambaud, 'Extrait de l'aperçu médico-statistique du 10e arrondissement' (n.d.).

40   AP 124 Foss 1, Gaultier, report of 13 July 1807; Brillouette, letter of 11 June 1807.

described urban conditions much like their predecessors had described rural health in the pre-revolutionary years, but now they apparently believe that urban health problems overshadowed the kinds of issues previously documented amongst rural inhabitants. According to them, towns had become the new health blight, the potential cause of degeneracy and depopulation.

On a second level, these medical practitioners also implied that the poor were largely responsible for their own sicknesses and death. Whereas the peasantry suffered because of ignorance and superstition, urban dwellers made themselves sick because of their wilful immorality and slovenly lifestyle. Doctors were repelled by public drunkenness, duelling, suicides, promiscuous and rakish behaviour – especially adolescent masturbation – and they believed these habits contributed to high levels of syphilis and tuberculosis amongst the urban poor.[41]

Throughout, medical practitioners tailored medical methods and approach to appeal to the authorities who staffed the post-revolutionary health and welfare institutions. As they saw it, doctors and officials had to understand disease aetiology before they could craft effective public policy, and so they used charity bureaucracies to track welfare recipients from public offices back to the home and streets in order to study disease and death more effectively. The government had to make public welfare as cheap and effective as possible, and medical knowledge could help contain the costs of poor relief.[42]

In more dramatic ways, pragmatic scientism and topographic medicine converged in the administrative response to a new epidemic threat: yellow fever ('la peste d'Amérique', as one administrator described it).[43] In 1804, the disease appeared in Cádiz, Spain and sparked an international crisis; four years later, it infected the Spanish towns of Córdoba, Grenada, Valencia and Catalonia. The most terrifying manifestations occurred in Barcelona and Gibraltar in 1819–21 and 1828: in Barcelona, almost 20 per cent of the population died; and in Gibraltar, doctors and public authorities watched 1,183 persons die.[44] Afterwards, any alleged sighting of this epidemic – whether in the Mediterranean or in the Americas – caused immediate panic.[45]

As historians of medicine have argued, yellow fever constituted a socio-medical watershed. Across Europe and the Americas, it caused doctors to re-examine

---

41 AP 124 Foss 1, Séance du conseil (n.d.).

42 AP 124 Foss 1, Chappon, 'Des vieillards de 70 à 80 ans la plus secourus par le Bureau de Bienfaisance de la division de l'ouest faisant partie du Xe arrondissement municipal de Paris', Conseil de salubrité, 2 Aug. 1807.

43 AN F^{8}9, fol. II, d. 2, letter of 24 May 1817.

44 See William Coleman, *Yellow Fever of the North: The Methods of Early Epidemiology* (Madison, 1987), pp. 18–19, 25–26.

45 Given the ravages wrought upon English and French troops in the Caribbean during the French revolutionary wars, statesmen were sensitive to the global implications of this disease. See especially AN F^{8}2, d. 1–2; F^{8}5, d. 4–5; F^{8}11, d. 1; and F^{8}19, d. 1, for good examples of the international apprehensions concerning yellow fever, which linked American outposts, Caribbean colonies and southern European trading ports as crucial disease contact zones.

traditional ideas about debate aetiology and health policies; in France, panic over the disease even forced the government to create a short-lined national agency for public health.[46] Oftentimes, historians have studied yellow fever in terms of the anticontagionist movement spearheaded by Dr Nicolas Chervin, which opposed the quarantine system established by the landmark 1822 sanitary code, alleging that the code cut off the 'principle sources of prosperity by prohibiting more and more [of our] commerce'.[47] However, the analysis here does not revisit the anticontagionist–contagionist debate but rather examines how ideas about health activism helped shape official responses towards yellow fever outbreaks. When seen in this light, yellow fever shows how doctors and public officials adapted aetiological theories and diagnostic tools to fit the 'law-and-order' bureaucratic, institutional and ideological sensibilities of post-revolutionary France.

In the early 1800s, public officials responded to yellow fever much like they responded to recent epidemics of prison fever and typhus. Using bureaucratic channels and medical networks, public officials sent doctors to observe the outbreak and then file an official report with the Paris medical school. In theory, any policy action would follow the diagnosis provided by the medical faculty.[48] So when the yellow fever kept appearing in Spain, Napoleon himself demanded that the Ministry of the Interior take immediate steps, since officials worried that yellow fever was contagious and could infect French territories. At this time, Spain and France still enjoyed an uneasy diplomatic alliance, but the Iberian peninsula was of extraordinary tactical importance in Napoleon's war against England. For these reasons, the Ministry contacted the Paris health school, which then sent an investigative team to Spain. The doctors included N.-R. Dufriche Desgenettes, Victor Bailly and Pierre Nysten. The doctors never saw yellow fever, but they spent their travel allowance and withheld their final report for nearly fifteen months – much to the ministry's disgust.[49]

In fact, the reason for the delay was that the commission was deeply divided in its aetiological beliefs. According to these practitioners, yellow fever was extraordinarily lethal – in Cádiz, for example, the disease killed 9,977 people out of a population of 71,499 – but they didn't know what caused it or where it came from. The evidence seemed inconclusive. When yellow fever first appeared in 1800, it seemed like a seasonal bilious fever, so local doctors failed to recognize its epidemic character. Allegedly, it came from Charleston or Havana on the ship *Delfin* and spread from Cádiz to Seville. Between 1801 and 1803, yellow fever returned again (possibly from Paraguay), but the biggest outbreak happened in 1804, when the disease infected several regions, including Málaga, Carthagine, Alicante, Cádiz,

---

46   The most important study remains George D. Sussman, 'From Yellow Fever to Cholera: A Study of French Government Policy, Medical Professionalism, and Popular Movements in the Epidemic Crises of the Restoration and the July Monarchy' (PhD thesis, Yale University, 1971). See also the recent appraisal in Sheldon Watts, *Epidemics and History: Disease, Power and Imperialism* (New Haven, 1997), pp. 213–68.

47   Nicolas Chervin, *Pétition contre la formation des lazarets projetés depuis 1822 dans la vue de mettre la France à l'abri de la fièvre jaune* (Paris, 1828), pp. 9–10.

48   SEM EFG, n. 2 (c), 'Rapport de M. Hallé à l'Institut', 6 frimaire, Year IX.

49   AN F⁸4ª, fol. II, d. 2, Le Ministre à M. Thouret, Directeur de l'École de Médecine de Paris, letter of 8 May 1807.

Cordone and Grenada. In Carthagine, local doctors said that a woman infected her neighbourhood after she purchased contraband goods. In a further twist, however, the epidemic spared the public hospitals, suggesting that it was not contagious.

When addressing public authorities, the Paris doctors first adapted a consensual and cautious tone. In their opinion, Spanish epidemics were likely the same yellow fever that had appeared in the Americas. Nevertheless, the epidemic seemed contained to the coastlines and the doctors believed the outbreak might have previously appeared in Spain (they identified similar epidemics in the eighteenth century). Consequently, they couldn't prove that the disease travelled from the New World into the Old (although Spanish doctors believed this was true). For them, environmental factors probably caused the disease and it became contagious only in particular instances. They thus urged pragmatic measures: the police should make sure the air circulated, keep clean water and remove urban filth. In the final analysis, public officials could institute quarantines, but they must do so at an early stage.[50]

One commission member, Victor Bailly, broke with his colleagues and rejected the joint report. The reason was that Bailly had been a doctor in Saint Domingue during the 1790s and he had observed yellow fever first-hand in the colonial wars against the English and Haitian revolutionaries. For this reason, he was troubled by the Spanish case. He firmly believed that yellow fever was contagious, arguing that it had travelled from the Caribbean to the Mediterranean; now it had apparently penetrated the Spanish mainland, away from the sultry coasts. According to him, yellow fever could not have crossed the Atlantic if it was strictly endemic or caused by environmental determinants (as Philadelphia physician Benjamin Rush argued). At the same time, Bailly conceded that the disease was not always contagious. Once introduced into a hospitable environment, however, this *endemic* disease could become *epidemic* and produce a 'morbid germ' or 'contagious miasma'. Given these observations, he argued that quarantines could stop yellow fever[51] – and prominent doctors such as Philippe Pinel endorsed his memoir.[52]

In response to Bailly's split, his disaffected colleague, Dr Pierre Nysten, wrote a lengthy report to public authorities which countered Bailly with an environmental argument. In his view, yellow fever was endemic to tropical climates and he blamed indigenous Spanish factors for the epidemic outbreaks. In particular, he said that the distance between Cádiz and Seville suggested that the disease hadn't journeyed from the coast to the mainland. But Nysten admitted yellow fever could become contagious under favourable conditions, just like doctors had seen with recent epidemics of prison fevers. Yellow fever was thus endemic in the New World but epidemic in the Old, but its exotic aetiology should keep this colonial disease from entering France. That

---

50   AN F⁸4ᵃ, fol. II, d. 2, 'Extrait du rapport sur la fièvre jaune qui a régné en Espagne dans les années 1800, 1801, 1803 et 1804, par la commission des médecins envoyée par le gouvernement français en 1805 pour étudier cette maladie' [1807].

51   AN, F⁸4ᵃ fol. II, d. 2, [Victor] Bailly ['l'un des commissaires envoyés en 1804'], 'Sur la contagion de la fièvre jaune d'Espagne' (n.d.).

52   AN F⁸4ᵃ, fol. II, d. 3, Le Secrétaire de la Société de Médecine, 'Rapport fait à la Société de la Faculté de Médecine sur un ouvrage de Monsieur le docteur Bailly intitulé "De la fièvre jaune"', Paris, 7 July 1814.

said, Nysten provided a similar approach to policy, recommending that public officials use quarantines to prevent it from infecting France's southern borders and ports.[53]

Given these aetiological uncertainties, the Ministry of the Interior carefully watched yellow fever in the New World. Public officials anxiously alerted the central government for all alleged sightings and they immediately set up quarantines in trading ports.[54] But merchants and manufacturers disliked government interference and drew upon aetiological debates to criticize quarantine policies. By this time, several physicians were forcefully suggesting that local factors caused yellow fever and even blamed the poor for intensifying unsanitary conditions.[55] The anticontagionist movement benefited when they were endorsed by the prominent hygienist, Jean-Noël Hallé. In 1817, the Ministry of the Interior tried to settle this aetiological and policy dispute by convening a new medical commission to study yellow fever and quarantine policies. Public officials asked doctors to decide whether yellow fever was contagious, whether it could it infect French territory, whether it was imported from the colonial Americas, whether it could contaminate people and goods, and whether they should institute quarantines and suspend trade.

Despite aetiological disputes, the medical commission balanced scientific controversy and the perceived need for public order. In the end, they advocated the same cautious policies that Bailly and Nysten had urged twelve years previously. As they said, doctors couldn't easily distinguish between epidemic and contagious diseases. People didn't necessarily get sick when they were exposed to a contagious disease, suggesting that hygiene, lifestyle and environment mattered. In other instances, local conditions altered disease patterns, making them either endemic, epidemic or contagious. After the commission qualified aetiological theories, they cautioned that yellow fever might be contagious and that public authorities should take moderate steps but keep quarantines in port cities. Clearly, these physicians understood that they had to balance aetiological beliefs, commercial interests and the demands of public order.[56]

In the case of yellow fever, these approaches to medical topography neatly dovetailed with pragmatic scientism. In this case, doctors simply wanted to maintain existing health standards and they rejected aetiological ideas and policies that might cast medical and social authority in any doubt. When dealing with authorities, they tried to move medicine into a consensual or even apolitical realm to support the demands of public health and public order. However, not all practitioners accepted this pragmatic and utilitarian approach to public health. Radical doctors still wanted to change human nature and create a more just society; liberal and conservative

---

53   AN F^{8}4^a, fol. II, d. 4, Nysten to the Ministry of Interior, Paris, letter of 6 Feb. 1806.

54   AN F^{8}9, fol. II, d. 2, 'Rapport présenté à son Excellence le Ministre Secrétaire d'État au département de l'intérieur', Paris, 4 Aug. 1817.

55   AN F^{8}10, fol. X, Mimant [Consultant de Carthagène], 'Aperçus et recherches sur la nature des maladies qui ont régné à Carthagène, et particulièrement sur celle de la fièvre jaune' (1819).

56   AN F^{8}9, fol. II, d. 2, *Rapport ... relativement à la nécessité de prévenir l'introduction de la fièvre jaune par la voie des communications commerciales* (Paris, 1817).

doctors rejected old pro-natalist policies and claimed that population growth caused poverty, sickness and social disorder. The analysis explores these contrary views next.

The contested Idéologue tradition: from moral hygiene to social-Christian medicine

Doctors still interested in 'physical and moral hygiene' reforms had to navigate an ideological minefield. Though Fodéré and Mahon offered a pragmatic approach to hygiene that couched medical activism in consensual terms, conservative doctors and intellectuals often attacked medical crusaders for their perceived materialism and republican sympathies. These were not just cranky ultramontanes like Louis de Bonald and Joseph de Maistre; even former sensationalists and neo-Kantians, so indebted to Enlightenment epistemology, joined this critique. The main targets were the Idéologue doctors associated with Pierre Cabanis. A number of factors were at work. For Restoration intellectuals, atheism and materialism had became, if not anathema, or at least terribly unfashionable. At the same time, diverging physiological models, coming from biomedical circles, undercut more holistic approaches to the mind-body problem and made general thinking about human nature and society more difficult.[57] These tensions appear in Charles-Louis Dumas's massive *Principes de physiologie* (1800), a text that attempted to combine materialist sensationalism and more metaphysical ideas about the self or soul.[58] But not all doctors accepted this conservative approach and some flamboyant personalities even pushed materialist philosophy in medical circles. For example, Franz-Joseph Gall, J.-C. Spurzheim and especially François-Joseph-Victor Broussais tried to localize discreet mental faculties in the brain and sparked great philosophic controversy about the physiological forces that caused sensation and will.[59]

The most damaging assault on medical thinking about human nature and society came from academic philosophers such as Pierre-Paul Royer-Collard, Victor Cousin and Théodore Jouffroy. These philosophers formed a philosophic school called Eclecticism, spiritualism or psychology – intellectuals who Karl Marx famously dismissed as the 'true interpreters' of 'bourgeois society in its sober reality'.[60] The Eclectics attacked science and Lockean sensationalism, and combined the Scottish commonsense psychology of Thomas Reid and neo-Kantian innatism. Throughout, they proclaimed the autonomy of 'the moi' or the soul's 'voluntary and free

---

57   See Williams, *Physical and the Moral*, pp. 176–243; and François Azouvi, *Maine de Biran: la science de l'homme* (Paris, 1995), pp. 13–34.

58   C.-L. Dumas, *Principes de physiologie, ou introduction à la science expérimental, philosophique, et médicale de l'homme vivant* (4 vols, Paris, 1800–03).

59   Edwin Clarke and L. S. Jacyna, *Nineteenth-Century Origins of Neuroscientific Concepts* (Berkeley, 1987); and Robert Young, *Mind, Brain, and Adaptation in the Nineteenth Century* (Oxford: Clarendon, 1970), 24–27. See also Goldstein, *Console and Classify*, pp. 245–57; and Williams, *Physical and the Moral*, pp. 105–14, 166–75, 182–88.

60   Karl Marx, 'The Eighteenth Brumaire of Louis Bonaparte' [1852], in *The Marx–Engels Reader*, ed. Robert C. Tucker (New York, 1972), pp. 436–525 (at p. 437).

activity'.[61] The word they used to describe this study – 'psychology' – was rife with political undertones. A.-L.-C. Destutt de Tracy rejected the word for its metaphysical connotations ('the science of the soul') and substituted his laicized neologism *idéologie* ('the science of ideas'). But at times, even Eclectic philosophy seemed too liberal and 'philosophical' for Restoration tastes. Hard-core ultramontanes such as Félicité de Lamennais said that only theologians should study human nature and thus rejected philosophical inquiry about the self. In the 1820s, even Cousin ran into political trouble and lost his faculty position at the Sorbonne.[62]

In terms of social medical thought, the most important Eclectic philosopher was François-Pierre Maine de Biran (1766–1824). Once a royalist legislator and sensationist philosopher, Maine de Biran totally refashioned Enlightenment psychology and conservative intellectuals praised him as the French version of Immanuel Kant. In 1797, he was purged from the Directory government on account of his conservative beliefs and he then returned to his native Bergerac (Dordogne), where he spent his remaining days writing about the science of man.[63] Though he first associated with Idéologue philosophers such as Cabanis and Destutt de Tracy, his philosophic thought became increasingly metaphysical. In his *Mémoire sur la décomposition de la pensée* (1804), for example, Maine de Biran began to criticize the materialist ideas advocated by the Second Class of Moral and Political Sciences in the Institute of France, and insisted that an independent and autonomous ego alone produced will and movement.[64] Like ultramontanes, then, he believed that an immaterial soul commanded the 'hyperorganic forces' associated with the brain and nervous system, and thus countered monism with metaphysics.[65]

Under the late Empire, Maine de Biran moved further towards spiritualism. In his Copenhagen memoir of 1811, he fully rejected the materialistic physiology associated with his former mentor Cabanis and now espoused an absolute Cartesian divide between soul and body. As he described it, 'it is only in the *sentiment intime* of its proper acts that the soul finds its ideas of substance, of force, of cause, of identity'.[66] Consequently, he rejected materialist doctors such as Gall and Spurzheim because they wanted to localize a non-material faculty in the brain and nervous tissue. After corresponding with psychiatrist Antoine-Athanase Royer-Collard (brother of Pierre-

---

61 Victor Cousin, *Introduction to the History of Philosophy*, trans. H. G. Linberg (Boston, 1832), pp. 414–15.

62 For discussion, see George Boas, *French Philosophies of the Romantic Period* (New York, 1964); and Jan Goldstein, *The Post-Revolutionary Self: Politics and Psyche in France, 1750–1850* (Cambridge, MA, 2005).

63 See Azouvi, *Maine de Biran*; and F. C. T. Moore, *The Psychology of Maine de Biran* (Oxford, 1970). For brief synopses, see Martin S. Staum, *Cabanis: Enlightenment and Medical Philosophy in the French Revolution* (Princeton, 1980), pp. 259–65; Goldstein, *Console and Classify*, pp. 258–62, and *Post-Revolutionary Self*, pp. 129–41.

64 F.-P. Maine de Biran, *Mémoire sur la décomposition de la pensée*, vol. 3, *Oeuvres*, ed. François Azouvi (Paris, 1984–).

65 Sergio Moravia, *Il pensiero degli Idéologues: scienza e filosofia in Francia (1780–1815)* (Florence, 1974), pp. 457–529.

66 F.-P. Maine de Biran, *Rapports du physique et du moral de l'homme*, vol. 6, *Oeuvres*, pp. 51, 71–72, 83–86.

Paul Royer-Collard, the Eclectic philosopher and politician), Maine de Biran further revised these manuscripts and completed a more complex work, called *Nouvelles considérations sur les rapports du physique et du moral de l'homme* (1820–22). In this new work, he insisted that philosophers and physiologists could not reduce the complex interactions between mind and body to simple material phenomena. Although the nervous system was a kind of organic envelope that surrounded the soul, physiological models could not 'imitate, figure, reproduce, nor by such explicate the effects or attributes proper even to the soul's will or motor force'. As a result, materialist physiology was unable to explain 'the fact of the *sens intime*, that of free activity, and even [that of] the existence of the *moi*'.[67]

Because of this sophisticated and nuanced reasoning, which combined both psychological and physiological approaches, Eclectic philosophers like Maine de Biran were able to challenge medical materialism with its own methods and tools and conservative doctors took this intellectual lashing to heart. The best example is J.-L. Alibert (1768–1837), who was a major figure in the Paris medical establishment. Born in Aveyron, he became the medical consultant to Louis XVIII, *médecin-en-chef* at the hospital Saint-Louis and a professor at the Paris Faculté de Médecine.[68] Like Maine de Biran, he initially sympathized with Idéologue philosophy but his politics and beliefs became increasingly conservative following the post-revolutionary backlash. In one of his first publications, for example, Alibert stated that the government should promote moral duty instead of democratic rights and freedom.[69] Under the Restoration, Alibert rejected both C.-A. Helvétius's environmentalism and Pierre Cabanis's biological materialism.[70] His most popular book, *Physiologie des passions* (1825), claimed that doctors could not understand man simply through physiological models. Following Kant, Alibert believed that all ethics came preformed in the soul.[71] From a public policy perspective, then, social and moral reform became difficult and even impossible, since mind and body formed an unchangeable, essential whole. In some ways, though, Alibert presents an unusual paradox. Although he believed in an immaterial soul, he still located the passions in the body and thus, in some ways, reflected a deeper biological innatism than colleagues such as Bichat, Maine de Biran and even Cabanis. For example, Bichat had argued that sensibility limited human aptitude and ability – education could only do so much – but he did not believe that all intellectual faculties were innate or preformed in the mind. By contrast, Alibert suggested all morals and human emotion – a kind of offshoot of

---

67   F.-P. Maine de Biran, *Nouvelles considérations sur les rapports du physique et du moral de l'homme*, vol. 9, *Oeuvres*, pp. 43, 53.

68   L. Brodier, *J.-L. Alibert, médecin de l'Hôpital Saint-Louis (1768–1837)* (Paris, 1923), cited in Williams, *Physical and the Moral*, pp. 122–34.

69   J.-L. Alibert, 'De l'influence des causes politiques sur les maladies et la constitution physique de l'homme', *Magasin encyclopédique, ou Journal des sciences, des lettres et des arts* 5 (1795): 298–305.

70   J.-L. Alibert, 'Du pouvoir de l'habitude dans l'état de santé et de maladie', *Mémoires de la Société médicale d'émulation* 1 (Year IV [1798]): 396–415.

71   J.-L. Alibert, *Physiologie des passions, ou nouvelle doctrine des sentimens moraux* (Paris, 1825), p. i, quoted in Staum, *Cabanis*, p. 250; see also Williams, *Physical and the Moral*, p. 124.

Kant's famous categorical imperative – were biologically hardwired in the physical passions. Alibert offered a contrast to the Eclectic belief in an autonomous *moi*, because they still put the soul at the doorstep of medical authority, and suggested that mental faculties might be biologically predetermined.[72]

Not all medical practitioners followed Alibert and saw human nature in such innatist terms. The most interesting combination of Idéologue and Eclectic beliefs was developed by Dr J.-J. Virey, who was a naturalist and consummate popularizer and whose prolific career spanned from the French Revolution to the July monarchy.[73] Steeped in Rousseauian primitivism (associated with writers such as Bernardin de St Pierre and L. S. Mercier), Virey wanted to promote moral virtue and civic harmony and he firmly believed that biomedical science could regenerate the moral and physical dimensions of man.[74] Throughout, Virey expressed the relation between body and society through the metaphor of the nervous system. Combining Cabanis and Condorcet, he equated the major periods of human sensibility – youth, virility (adulthood) and decline (old age) – with the historical stages of human progress – primitive, conquering and 'industrious' societies. Each socio-biological level required what he called a particular 'macrobiotic' response: a 'physical hygiene' for the young and primitive societies, a 'political hygiene' for conquering societies and a 'moral hygiene' for advanced or aging cultures.[75] The highest civilized stage – a stage exemplified by manufacturing and consumption – was 'a neurotic condition', literally a 'pathological prodrome of the nervous apparatus'.[76] In this 'extreme civilization, considered physiologically', men and women needed an extensive programme of self-hygiene to restore balance between the body and the outside corrupting forces associated with modernity. In this regard, then, Virey returned to the kind of physical and moral hygiene associated with pastoralists such as Samuel Tissot, who had believed that consumption and secular free-living had caused moral and physical decline.[77] In contrast to these pre-revolutionary doctors, however, Virey claimed his work addressed less high-risk groups (intellectuals, people of fashion, women, children, artisans) than the whole of the body politic itself.[78]

---

72 Williams, ibid., pp. 130–31.

73 For biographical details, see Claude Bénichou and Claude Blanckaert (eds), *Julien-Joseph Virey: naturaliste et anthropologue* (Paris, 1988)

74 J.-J. Virey, *De la puissance vitale, considérée dans ses fonctions physiologiques chez l'homme et tous les êtres organisés* (Paris, 1823), pp. xviii–xix.

75 J.-J. Virey, *Hygiène philosophique, ou de la santé dans le régime physique, moral et politique de la civilisation moderne* (2 vols, Paris, 1828), vol. 1, pp. xxi–xxii, 164. Virey used the expression 'macrobiology' in his *De la puissance vitale*, p. 425; this neologism was originally introduced by Christophe-Wilhelm Hufeland, *L'art de prolonger la vie humaine, ou la Macrobiotique* (1796), to denote the large-scale regimen to reform the health of populations.

76 Virey, *Hygiène philosophique*, vol. 1, pp. 174–75 (at p. 177 n. 1).

77 See especially J.-J.Virey, *De la femme, sous ses rapports physiologique, moral et littéraire*, 2d edn (Paris, 1825).

78 J.-J. Virey, *Des métamorphoses physiologiqes de l'homme dans l'éducation* (Paris, n.d. [1845]), p. 3.

For Virey, physical healing also meant political change. Even under the Restoration and July monarchies, Virey never abandoned his revolutionary roots, insisting that 'the republican economy, with its bodily activity, offers more assistance to health and happiness than the ostentation of all our forces with the idle dignities of monarchies, which weaken the organism with luxury and feebleness'. For him, republican values were in fact *bourgeois* values, implying that the post-revolutionary regime was clearly incapable of providing the kind of environment needed to maintain health, moral virtue and national grandeur. He explained, 'With the equilibrium established by [the middle classes], they preserve order and respect for law; they guarantee the stability of empires and resist anarchy and despotism'.[79] These values – like ascetic principles and civic virtue – toughened the nerves and fortified the male semen. Therefore, in bourgeois republics, citizens were filled with civic pride, their marriages were loving and fertile, and children were happy and healthy. People cultivated the arts, and these virtuous and talented men made better teachers and workers for the nation.[80]

Whereas Virey was steeped in the sentimental values of the previous century, other medical activists looked to new philosophic and political ideas brewing in Restoration society. In the early 1800s, new forms of cutting-edge social thought flowered in France and helped stimulate new forms of philosophic engagement and political activism. The best-known examples, of course, are Henri de Saint-Simon, Charles Fourier and Auguste Comte. Often, these socially engaged intellectuals combined medicine and political theory in their projects to overhaul society: from medical science, in particular, they borrowed key ideas about physical and moral relations and so-called 'positive' socio-scientific techniques such as observation and induction. They were particularly inspired by the nascent field of experimental physiology (associated with Xavier Bichat and François Magendie). For these social thinkers, a physiological analytic approach meant that the dispassionate observer 'decomposed' an object into its constituent parts to understand how the whole operated. By the 1820s, this socio-scientific approach had even acquired an aesthetic status with the publication of books such as J.-A. Brillat-Savarin's *Physiologie du goût* (1826) and Honoré de Balzac's *Physiologie du mariage* (1829).[81] Like a reverse feedback mechanism, physicians such as the popularizer Dr Morel de Rubempre then exploited this aesthetic meaning when composing popular medical books, like his manuals on procreation (*Les secrets de la génération* [1829]), politics (*La physiologie de la liberté* [1830]) and prostitution (*La pornologie* [1848]).

Perhaps the best-known important proponent of this applied physiological approach was the utopian socialist, Henri de Saint-Simon. Historians have long noted Saint-Simon's intellectual debt to medical practitioners such as Xavier Bichat and Félix Vicq d'Azyr, and his writings were steeped in the language and ideas of physiological science and natural history.[82] In his political theories, Saint-Simon

---

79 Virey, *Hygiène philosophique*, vol. 1, pp. 244, 268.

80 Ibid., vol. 2, pp. 22–24, 27–29.

81 Brillat-Savarin, *Physiologie du goût* (2 vols, Paris, 1826).

82 Frank Manuel, 'From Equality to Organicism', *Journal of the History of Ideas* 17 (1956): 54–69; Barbara Haines, 'The Inter-Relations between Social, Biological and Medical

imagined society in organic and symbiotic terms and thus rejected liberal and atomist ideas about conflict and competition as a driving force in human progress. Rather, he thought that greater social advancement was caused by cooperation and interdependence, and he hoped that scientific and technical expertise could better manage unnecessary conflict in a rapidly changing world. To achieve this technocratic utopia, Saint-Simon looked to biomedical science to explain human nature and provide solid insights about managing and improving society. He took the individual body as a social model, claiming that society was a 'macrobiological' projection of the single organism.[83] He wrote: 'The history of civilization is only the history of the life of the human species, that is, the physiology of its different ages, just as [the history] of its institutions are only the exposition of the health knowledge that it uses for the conservation and melioration of general health.'[84] Accordingly, Saint-Simon differentiated between instruction and education when discussing 'physical and moral amelioration': the former assured literacy and technical skills, but it was the latter that transformed mind and body. At this juncture, Saint-Simon insisted, doctors and physiologists could make *les hommes valides* (in contrast to revolutionary doctors such as L.-J.-M. Robert, who wanted to make *grands hommes* worthy of the Panthéon).[85]

In his political blueprint, Saint-Simon returned to physical and moral hygiene. Like Virey, Saint-Simon also sought a 'transcendent physiology' that would remake humankind, but he wanted to improve the 'lot of the human species' and make them happy in mind and body, looking to a future progress rather than an idyllic pastoral past.[86] According to him, biology shaped human nature in significant ways and helped mould social organization. He wrote, 'One of the important points of physiology … is to demonstrate that the intelligence of each animal is proportionate to its organization, [and that] the intellectual scale is the same as the organic scale'.[87] But unlike Bichat and Alibert, Saint-Simon never claimed that biology absolutely limited human aptitude – it might limit faculties, but it did not create them *a priori*

Thought, 1750–1850: Saint-Simon and Comte', *British Journal for the History of Science* 11 (1978): 19–35; and John V. Pickstone, 'Bureaucracy, Liberalism and the Body in Post-Revolutionary France: Bichat's Physiology and the Paris School of Medicine', *History of Science* 19 (1981): 115–42.

83 See the classic studies by Frank Manuel, *The New World of Henri Saint-Simon* (Cambridge, MA, 1956), and *The Prophets of Paris* (Cambridge, MA, 1962). See also Robert B. Carlisle, *The Proffered Crown: Saint-Simonianism and the Doctrine of Hope* (Baltimore, 1987), 9–23.

84 C.-H. de Saint-Simon, 'De la physiologie sociale', *Oeuvres*, ed. E. Dentu (6 vols, Geneva, 1977), vol. 5, pt 1, p. 178. Saint-Simon further argued that 'political economy, legislation, public morality, and everything which constitutes the administration of the general societal interests are only a collection of hygienic rules of which nature ought to vary according to the stage of civilization' (ibid., p. 178).

85 C.-H. de Saint-Simon, 'De l'organisation sociale: fragments d'un ouvrage inédit', *Oeuvres*, vol. 5, pt 1, pp. 113, 128, 147.

86 C.-H. de Saint-Simon, 'Mémoire sur la science de l'homme', *Oeuvres*, vol. 5, pt 2, pp. 41–43, 47, 190.

87 Ibid., pp. 49, 55–56.

– and they could always be improved by education and habit. Humans must learn and develop through learned 'conventional signs', beyond innate ideas or physical organization – as the renowned wild boy of Aveyron demonstrated. By understanding physical limits and opportunities, an enlightened elite could study human relations and help reorganize society along more natural and efficient means. Progress was possible.[88]

Inspired by Saint-Simon's message of social melioration, politically conscious doctors used his social-physiological insights in service of health reform. One of the most significant of these pupils was the physician and utopian socialist, Philippe Buchez. In his youth, Buchez joined the Carbonist movement and immersed himself in Restoration counterculture, and he drifted toward the Saint-Simonian circle. A dedicated metaphysician, Buchez broke with Prosper Enfantin and Eugène Rodrigues over Christian teachings; and after the 1830 Revolution, he joined working-class organizations and taught courses on hygiene at the Athénée des Ouvriers. In the 1848 Revolution, he was elected to the National Assembly and briefly served as president, where he showed political indecision and administrative inexperience.[89]

In 1825, Buchez first combined his faith in hygiene and social activism in his *Précis élémentaire d'hygiène*, a work he co-authored with Ulysse Trélat. In the early nineteenth century, health manuals were still an important medical genre, as evidenced by texts such as J.-M. Audin-Rouvière's *La médecine sans médecin*, which first appeared in 1823.[90] But unlike competing books on domestic hygiene for special-interest groups (such as beauty manuals written for people of fashion), Buchez and Trélat wanted to use biomedical science in a utopian project to transform society: they effectively appropriated the traditions of the health manual in order to advance a sociopolitical agenda. In this manner, they echoed Enlightenment and revolutionary doctors – ranging from Samuel Tissot to Robert and Millot – who wanted to use exploit their readers' interest in private health and hygiene, but they applied these projects to the social world of early industrial France.[91]

In this text, Buchez and Trélat divided medicine into three branches: hygiene, pathology and therapeutics. Whereas the latter two required specialized study and skills, hygiene had universal appeal because 'its principles are accessible by everyone, and its precepts are of simple observation'. In a further distinction from prevailing clinical or nosological approaches, hygiene also demanded a more total understanding of the human condition, one rooted in a broad physiological model of man and then combined with a deep sense of social commitment. According to them, the individual did not contain 'all conditions of existence within himself', so health regimen had to be 'founded upon an understanding [*connaissance*] of man and the

---

88 Ibid., pp. 113, 118–19, 126, 153.

89 On social-Christian medicine and the science of man, see Williams, *Physical and the Moral*, pp. 213–24.

90 J.-M. Audin-Rouvière, *La médecine sans médecin, ou moyens préservatifs et curatifs d'un grand nombre de maladies, par une méthode purgative, perfectionnée* (Paris, 1823).

91 M.-J. Lavolley, *Manuel d'hygiène, ou l'art de prolonger la vie et de conserver la santé* (Paris, n.d.); and E. Sarrau de Montmahoux, *Considérations médicales sur les moyens employés pour conserver la beauté* (Paris, 1815).

relations that exist between him and the exterior world'.[92] In Saint-Simonian fashion, the key was socal interdependence.[93]

In light of these observations, Buchez and Trélat proceeded in three directions. The first part briefly explained human nature, which they thought should inform all health knowledge. In the second part, Buchez and Trélat explored what factors caused disease and provided an overview of recent aetiological and physiological theories. In the final part, they explained how to avoid disease and maintain a productive life. In truth, this extended analysis basically reworked the many earlier health manuals based upon the 'six things non-natural' (a classic example is Achille Le Bègue de Presle's *Le conservateur de la santé*); however, they also incorporated new physiological insights borrowed from Pierre Cabanis and Xavier Bichat by emphasizing bioanthropological categories of age, life cycle, sexuality and innate or acquired circumstances.[94] After each category, Buchez and Trélat detailed how particular temperaments determined health regimen and urged public officials to take these measures to reform health conditions in French society. In this manner, Saint-Simonianism made them think about public health in radical new ways, forcing them to rework the Idéologue tradition of moral hygiene and apply these ideas in the early industrial context.

Buchez and Trélat also worried how immorality affected urban health and hygiene. Unlike anti-luxury pastoralists such as Tissot and Virey, they did not believe that civilization itself had made people weak in mind and body. Still, they thought that urban and industrial change had significantly transformed health and hygiene in urban areas, thereby increasing promiscuity and deviance amongst the labouring poor. For them, the greatest threats were libertinism and onanism – especially for teenage boys – and doctors and public officials needed to help eradicate these habits. Still, Buchez and Trélat believed that the poor could improve, by their own efforts and initiative, their moral and physical health. As they put it, 'The only means of making people moral is to make sure that they understand their durable interests, because morality does not want to say anything else. Therefore, we must enlighten [the labouring classes], or rather, allow them to enlighten themselves, instead of keeping them like children'.[95]

Throughout the 1810s and 1820s, reforming doctors tried to explain human nature in broad terms and thus plan social reform. Though influenced by Eclectic philosophy, doctors such as Virey and Buchez sought to change social morals and manners by changing mind–body relations. For Virey, moral hygiene could make people happier and more virtuous while rendering a conflict-ridden society more peaceful and harmonious. For Buchez and Trélat, hygiene could alleviate poverty and social injustice, thereby promoting greater social cohesion and interdependence between antagonistic social classes. In both cases, these ideas about social hygiene potentially threatened the more moderate and conservative members of the Parisian medical elite, who wanted to avoid political debate by focusing upon the pragmatic

---

92 Philippe Buchez and Ulysse Trélat, *Précis élémentaire d'hygiène* (Paris, 1825), p. i.
93 Ibid., p. ii.
94 Ibid., pp. 29–30.
95 Ibid., pp. 107, 219–20, n. 2.

aspects of social medicine, or whose philosophical commitment to radical materialism did not translate into a radical political agenda.

The 'new sanitarians' and early statistical inquiry in the 1820s

In the 1820s, Buchez and Trélat were not alone in their thinking about changing conditions in the factories and cities. At this time, a number of prominent physicians and fellow men of science also interested themselves in the health of the labouring and migrant populations of Paris and the northern industrializing sectors of France. These figures included Adolphe Quetelet, Louis-René Villermé, Alexandre Parent-Duchâtelet, Louis-François Benoiston de Châteauneuf, Edouard Mallet and Francis d'Ivernois.[96] In many ways, these health activists formed a coherent medical movement, something that William Coleman first labelled as the *parti d'hygiène* and what Ann La Berge has more recently called the 'community of hygienists'. For our purposes, I shall simply refer to them here as the 'new sanitarians'. These physicians radically reconceptualized sanitary approaches in two basic ways. First, they insisted that urbanization and industrialization had created new and unprecedented health problems, and studying these new problems required new tools and methods. To meet these challenges, these doctors applied full-scale statistical and socio-scientific methods for the first time in medical research. In so doing, they moved public hygiene from older medical police models associated with Mahon and Fodéré and formalized what medical historians now call the social theory of disease causation. Second, these sanitarians approached sexuality and fertility in markedly new ways. Previously, doctors had feared depopulation. But by the early 1800s, however, this fear had begun to disappear. For these new sanitarians, the new pestilence was in fact overpopulation.[97]

These health activists announced their methodological approach in their journal, *Annales d'hygiène publique et de médecine légale* (1829), in which they drew upon a burgeoning interest in probability calculations and applied these insights to health conditions.[98] Though this approach was novel in some senses, it should be noted that these hygienists had substantial pedigree. Since the mid-1700s, public officials and intellectuals had been using socio-statistical methods in demographic

---

96 See Erwin H. Ackerknecht, 'Hygiene in France, 1815–1848', *Bulletin of the History of Medicine* 22 (1948): 117–53. For more recent treatments, see Coleman, *Death is a Social Disease*, pp. 3–33, 205–38; and La Berge, *Mission and Method*. The classic overview of this period remains Louis Chevalier's controversial *Classes laborieuses et classes dangereuses à Paris pendant la première moitié du XIXe siècle* (1958; Paris, 1984).

97 See *Annales d'hygiène publique et de médecine légale* 1 (1829): 'Prospectus' (pp. v–viii) and 'Introduction' (pp. ix–xxxix); and L.-R. Villermé, 'Sur l'hygiène morale, considérée particulièrement dans le royaume des Pays-Bas', ibid., 4, pt 1 (1830): 25–47.

98 See Edmonde Vedrenne-Villeneuve, 'L'inégalité sociale devant la mort dans la première moitié du XIXe siècle', *Population* 16 (1961): 665–99; Bernard Lécuyer, 'Démographie, statistique et hygiène publique sous la monarchie censitaire', *Annales de démographie historique* (1977): 215–45; and Terence D. Murphy, 'Medical Knowledge and Statistical Methods in Early Nineteenth-Century France', *Medical History* 25 (1981): 301–19.

and fiscal inquiries, and mathematicians such as Pierre Simon de Laplace and A. N. de Condorcet had first introduced probability models in the emerging human sciences.[99] In the eighteenth century, this socio-statistical approach was often inspired by demographic anxieties: the royal government wanted to know precise demographic patterns and it demanded that formal institutional bodies such as the Académie des Sciences research these problems. Consequently, intellectuals such as Laplace, Condorcet and A.-L. de Lavoisier submitted a detailed probability calculus that correlated demography, wealth, geography and human resources.[100]

Despite powerful fears about depopulation and decline, many Western states – including France – did not start keeping vital records until the mid-1830s. In France, initial steps to address this lacuna were taken during the French Revolution and Napoleonic era. At this point, public officials promoted demographic research by creating the Bureau de Cadastre in 1794 and the Bureau de Statistique in 1800 (the latter of which conducted the first census of France in 1801). Because a national statistics bureau seemingly smacked of Jacobin centralization, the Restoration government avoided demographic inquiries and did not regularly conduct censuses until Adolphe Tiers created a national statistical bureau under the July monarchy in 1833.[101] Despite this reactionary hostility, vital records were kept by Paris authorities (supported by mathematicians at the École Polytechnique), and in 1821–23, the Seine prefecture compiled and published its annual *Recherches statistiques sur la ville de Paris et le département de la Seine*. By the early 1820s, these statistical and demographic studies inspired new models of health inquiry and provided sanitarians with raw data upon which to base their studies.[102]

Despite these new mathematical influences, the new sanitarians still borrowed from the older traditions of philosophic medicine associated with the Montpellier vitalists and the Idéologues. In many ways, these hygienists used the older analytic categories found in the science of man, and focused upon age, sexuality, class, race and habitat as crucial elements of human health and morality.[103] However, the

---

99 Theodore M. Porter, *The Rise of Statistical Thinking, 1820–1900* (Princeton, 1988); and Ian Hacking, *The Taming of Chance* (Cambridge and New York, 1990).

100 See Pierre Simon Laplace, 'Mémoire sur les probabilités', *Oeuvres complètes*, ed. Académie des Sciences (14 vols, Paris, 1878–1912), vol. 9, pp. 383–485; and A.-L. de Lavoisier, 'Résultats extraits d'un ouvrage intitulé "De la richesse territoriale du royaume de France"', in *Oeuvres*, ed. Eduard Grimaux (6 vols, Paris, 1864–93), vol. 6, p. 405, cited in Charles C. Gillispie, *Science and Polity in France at the End of the Old Regime* (Princeton, 1980), pp. 45–50.

101 The first director of the bureau was statistician Alexandre Moreau de Jonnès, who was abhorred in medical circles for his staunch contagionist policies. For his fundamental study, see Alexandre Moreau de Jonnès, *Eléments de statistique*, 2d edn (Paris, 1856).

102 See Coleman, *Death*, pp. 124–48; and La Berge, *Mission and Method*, pp. 49–81.

103 Indeed, this categorical logic can be found, for example, in the spatial organization of prisons and hospitals, which divided their respective populations according to sex, age, class, disease and offense. For example, the first two articles of the first volume of the *Annales d'hygiène publique et de médecine légale* provided a statistical accounting of prison and hospital conditions; see L.-R. Villermé, 'Mémoire sur la mortalité dans les prisons', *Annales d'hygiène publique et de médecine légale* 1, pt 1 (1829): 1–100; and Esquirol, 'Rapport

new sanitarians moved beyond these more holistic approaches by studying these anthropological categories in empirical and statistical terms. The best example appears in the Belgian statistician Adolphe Quetelet's important book, *De l'homme* (1835), which tried to quantify the different dimensions of human nature. By using rigorous statistical methods, Quetelet insisted, social thinkers could identify 'normal' or average types and therefore identify and cure pathological anomalies.[104] This pioneering study was roundly praised by the new sanitarians, who wanted to apply Quetelet's insights and methods into health inquiry, and who ultimately counted him as one of their members.

In these works, the new sanitarians wanted to make hygiene into a true social science and emphasized that hygienists should adopt the same observational and empirical rigor found in clinical research.[105] If clinicians should study disease in the hospital, they said, hygienists needed to study social diseases in their natural habitat – the urban and industrial setting. Consequently, the new sanitarians turned their focus upon the marginal and destitute elements of French society. Hygienists such as Benoiston de Châteauneuf, Parent-Duchâtelet and Villermé recorded the dark underside of early industrial France and focused upon topics such as housing conditions, prisons, prostitution, illegitimacy, alcoholism and poverty.[106]

To put their health inquiries into a broader theoretical context, the new sanitarians often looked to the science of political economy, which used models of money, goods and exchange to understand the gamut of human experience.[107] By the early 1800s, liberal political theory had come to rather bleak conclusions about economic exchange and human progress, earning it the moniker of the 'dismal science'. Influenced by Thomas Malthus, liberals such as J.-B. Say, Charles Ganilh, Michel Chevalier, Charles Dunoyer and Jospher Garnier now saw population growth – what eighteenth-century economists had seen as an ideal – as a danger to society.[108]

---

statistique sur la maison royale de Charenton, pendant les années 1826, 1827 et 1828', ibid., 1, pt 1 (1829): 101–51. On this phenomenon, see the classic analysis in Michel Foucault, *Discipline and Punish: The Birth of the Prison*, trans. Alan Sheridan (New York, 1977).

104 Adolphe Quetelet, *A Treatise on Man and the Development of his Faculties* (1842; New York, 1968), pp. v–vi, 5, 7.

105 La Berge, *Mission and Method*, p. 51.

106 Alexandre Parent-Duchâtelet, *De la prostitution dans la ville de Paris* (2 vols, Paris, 1836); and L.-R. Villermé, *Des prisons telles qu'elles sont et telles qu'elles devraient être* (Paris, 1820). See also d'Arcet et al., 'Rapport sur le curage des égouts Amelot, de la Roquette, Saint-Martin et autres, ou exposé des moyens qui ont été mis en usage pour exécuter cette grande opération, sans compromettre la salubrité publique et la santé des ouvriers qui y ont été employés', *Annales d'hygiène publique et de médecine légale*, 2, pt 1 (1829): 5–159; and 'Plan de la prison-modèle que l'on élève à Paris sur le terrain dit La Roquette, et observations sur ce plan [par le Comité de la société de Londres pour l'amélioration des prisons]', ibid., 2, pt 2 (1829): 347–52 (including plates).

107 See Katherine A. Lynch, *Family, Class, and Ideology in Early Industrial France: Social Policy and the Working-Class Family, 1825–1848* (Madison, 1988), Ch. 2.

108 Angus McLaren, *Sexuality and the Social Order: The Debate over the Fertility of Women and Workers in France, 1770–1920* (New York, 1983), pp. 73–74, 80–81.

Within hygienist circles, two distinct groups emerged: the 'social economists' and 'moral economists'. Inspired by liberal political economy, these economic theorists thought that the best public policy was to have no public policy, though each 'school' saw population growth and social improvement in different ways.[109] For their part, social economists believed that immorality caused poverty, in that personal laziness and vice dragged labouring people into poverty and misery, and they concluded that public officials could not improve society simply because there were too many people and too few resources. Therefore, society couldn't avoid human disaster and tragedies. At best, social reformers could reduce poverty by teaching the poor the values of hard work, sobriety and cleanliness.[110]

By contrast, the 'moral economists' such as Joseph-Marie Degérando saw class and personal morality in less stark terms.[111] Whereas the social economists believed the immorality caused poverty, the moral economists thought that poverty itself had dragged working-class people into the cesspool of vice and iniquity, making it impossible for them to pull themselves out of the cycle of misery. For these reasons, society could improve personal morality by meliorating poverty, and they urged philanthropic societies and religious charities to help needy families. At the same time, the moral economists doubted that public welfare provided a lasting solution because outdoor relief undermined the moral foundations of self-discipline and personal reliance.[112]

Despite these formal differences, both the social economists and the moral economists projected a powerful image of urban malaise and suggested that poverty and immorality were contagious, jumping back and forth from the shopfloor to the hearth. Usually rejecting statist initiatives – an important exception was Parent-Duchâtelet – both groups urged manufacturers to implement paternalistic programmes in order to manage the health of the labouring poor. For them, this kind of 'physical and moral hygiene' could maintain morality and the social order in urban and other industrial areas without incurring public expense.

In this debate, social economists and moral economists forced doctors to ask pressing questions about the relationship between sickness and poverty, and telescoped unprecedented public attention upon urban conditions. In this analysis, the social economists turned to statistical data – provided by the department of the Seine, parishes, genealogies, census inquiries and conscription records – and they directly observed worker households and shop floors.[113] Their socio-statistical

---

109 See Coleman, *Death*, pp. 59–92; and Rachel G. Fuchs, *Poor and Pregnant in Paris: Strategies for Survival in the Nineteenth Century* (New Brunswick, 1992), pp. 39–51.

110 See Thomas J. Duesterberg, 'Criminology and the Social Order in Nineteenth-Century France' (PhD thesis, Indiana University, 1979), ch. 2. The term *les classes dangeureuses* comes from Honoré Frégier's prize-winning work, *Des classes dangereuses de la population dans les grandes villes et les moyens de les rendre meilleures* (2 vols, Paris, 1840). See Chapter 6 below.

111 Joan W. Scott, *Gender and the Politics of History* (New York, 1988), p. 147.

112 Rachel G. Fuchs, *Abandoned Children: Foundlings and Child Welfare in Nineteenth-Century France* (Albany, 1984), pp. 34–40.

113 For a good example, see L.-R. Villermé, 'Mémoire sur la taille de l'homme en France', *Annales d'hygiène publique et de médecine légale*, 1, pt 2 (1829): 351–99.

methods demonstrated, in graphic detail, health inequalities in French society. The initial results galvanized the medical establishment and forced doctors to ask new questions about sanitary reform and public welfare. Two examples of this approach appear in the early writings of L.-R. Villermé and L.-F. Benoiston de Châteauneuf.

According to Villermé, there was a powerful correlation between health and socioeconomic status. Previously, medical crusaders had debated whether indigence or luxury made people sick, but Villermé flatly rejected the anti-luxury pastoralism of earlier hygienists such as Samuel Tissot and J.-J. Virey.[114] By using socio-statistical methods, he proved the hypothesis that affluent people enjoyed a long life and good health, whereas the poor became sick more often and died in greater numbers. Drawing upon Parisian vital records, Villermé demonstrated that class and wealth influenced rates of sickness and mortality.[115] For example, the average mortality among the Parisian middle classes remained 1/50 per year. By contrast, people who lived in the poor and densely populated and impoverished twelfth arrondissement died at a rate of 1/14 per year. In his population sample, Villermé found that the death rate was highest amongst the aged and extreme poor, and abandoned children suffered most of all. As a prominent social economist, Villermé kept a liberal faith in industrial progress and industrial paternalism. Self-help and private initiative, he believed, could eradicate poverty and sickness. These reforms could come either from manufacturing elites or self-help techniques.[116]

Benoiston de Châteauneuf explored class and disease in similar fashion. As he saw it: 'At every cycle of life, but above all during infancy and old age, the rich do not die as much the poor.'[117] For him, the poor presented a statistical conundrum: they were born, lived and died, and were ignored or forgotten by all – unless, of course, the government kept vital records. For socio-statistical inquiry, however, the rich provided the most useful data, thanks to abundant genealogical records. When he juxtaposed average life expectancy in this population with mortality rates in the twelfth arrondissement of Paris, Benoiston de Châteauneuf discovered: 'While death is scarcely known amongst the rich, the poor already see it decimate and carry off more than double of those that it spares during the same age in the opulent classes.'[118] Nevertheless, Benoiston de Châteauneuf did not advocate policy reforms. Rather, he hoped that educational projects could inculcate 'instruction, work and liberty'. These

---

114 L.-R. Villermé, 'Mémoire sur la mortalité en France dans la classe aisée et dans la classe indigente', *Mémoires de l'Académie royale de médecine* 1 (1828): 51–98 (at p. 51).

115 See also L.-R. Villermé, 'De la mortalité dans les divers quartiers de la ville de Paris, et des causes qui la rendent très différente dans plusieurs d'entre eux, ainsi que dans les divers quartiers de beaucoup de grandes villes', *Annales d'hygiène publique et de médecine légale*, 3, pt 2 (1830): 294–341.

116 Villermé, 'La mortalité en France', pp. 80–81.

117 L.-F. Benoiston de Châteauneuf, 'De la durée de la vie chez le riche et chez le pauvre', *Annales d'hygiène publique et médecine légale*, 3, pt 1 (1830): 5–15. Benoiston de Châteauneuf's first study involved differential mortality among men and women; see his *Mémoire sur la mortalité des femmes de l'âge de quarante à cinquante ans* (Paris, 1822), pp. 4–5.

118 Benoiston de Châteauneuf, 'De la durée', p. 11.

reforms could produce 'industry', 'affluence', 'morals', 'virtue' and 'happiness' amongst the labouring poor.[119]

Not all doctors supported these socio-scientific methods and political beliefs. The greatest sceptics were those physicians who had long worked within the physiological tradition of the science of man, and who thought that hygienists could not reduce complex phenomena such as individual sickness and health to mathematical abstractions. The fiercest critics were Montpellier Eclectic vitalists such as Frédéric Bérard, François Ribes and Fulcrand-César Caizergues.[120] But these doctors didn't totally reject quantitative methods, and they pointed to the long tradition of using statistical research in physiological and anthropological studies. For example, G.-L. Leclerc de Buffon used Parisian demographic figures in his classic *De l'homme* (1749); P.-J. Barthez and Xavier Bichat made use of Peter Camper's facial angle; and Philippe Pinel measured cranial structure to discuss mental disease. Moreover, the Académie Royale de Médecine had started compiling demographic data in the 1820s and published detailed reports in 1826.[121]

In this manner, as Elizabeth A. Williams points out, physicians were not simply resisting new and unfamiliar quantitative methods. On the contrary, for these doctors, socio-statistical research undermined deeply held beliefs about free will and individual autonomy (issues that had motivated Eclectics such as Maine de Biran in the early 1800s). Originally, physiologists claimed to study organismal diversity and specificity, and they emphasized that scientists could not reduce living phenomena to physical, chemical and mathematic laws. What mattered was individuality and difference.[122] However, these beliefs were challenged by statistical research, in which the biological individual seemed to disappear into a new and abstract idea of the normative type. Ironically, these new statistical 'types' created by Quetelet and his followers were directly taken from these earlier physiological categories: age, sex, temperament, occupation, race, and so on. Though these medical concepts persisted, the new sanitarians expressed them in quantitative, not qualitative, terms. Holistic physiology gave way to figures and computations.

Conclusion

Between 1804 and 1830, doctors charted their ideas about 'physical and moral hygiene' through an uncertain and fragmented intellectual landscape. As we have seen, doctors were divided by a plurality of political, religious and social interests, as the new political ideologies created by the French Revolution – ranging from conservatism to liberalism and socialism – entered medical thought and practice in new and striking ways. These differences appear in Mahon and Fodéré's medico-legal practice, Alibert's Eclectic sympathies, Virey's moral hygiene, Buchez's Christian

---

119 Ibid., p. 15.

120 Williams, *Physical and the Moral*, p. 157.

121 'Discussion sur la statistique médicale', *Bulletin de l'Académie royale de médecine*, no. 13 (April 15, 1837): 684–714; and 'Avant-propos', *Mémoires de la Société médicale d'observation* 2 (1844): xv–xxxv.

122 Williams, *Physical and the Moral*, pp. 155–56.

socialism and Villermé's liberalism. But the various social medical agendas often shared a common rhetorical thread. The partisan attachments aside, medical activists generally tried to justify their agendas by claiming they served public interests and law-and-order programmes, and they carefully crafted their works to meet specific constituencies in the highly charged political context of Restoration society.

In this regard, doctors were not alone. In the post-revolutionary period, political uncertainties and antagonisms weighed heavily upon general scientific discourse. This was because scientific thinkers often lacked a firm professional or institutional footing and this raw uncertainty deeply influenced their public and private experiences and self-perceptions. Consequently, they controlled their public personas as best as possible in order to advance their careers and research agendas; and this was doubly true when their ideas ran against the conventional opinion of the ruling elites. The best example is the naturalist Georges Cuvier, who found himself overseeing a complex network of familial and naturalist personalities and investing inordinate amounts of personal energy to control this patronage system.[123]

In contrast to other scientific practitioners, however, physicians were less sensitive about their public personas and reputation outside the medical marketplace, and this attitude gave them more confidence and latitude to discuss potentially contentious political and social issues. There were a number of reasons for medical confidence: doctors enjoyed a private source of income; they had a more secure professional status thanks to government licensing; medical institutions had become the envy of Europe and the Americas; and diverse and far-flung medical networks and associations allowed them to express opinions and agendas in a variety of fora. It is important to emphasize, however, that this medical status and security sometimes proved a double-edged sword. Like other scientific practitioners, the politics associated with privilege and prestige could potentially comprise medical independence: these entanglements either led doctors to support the government regime and its policies as a matter of personal interest, or inhibited them from expressing their true political beliefs and values because they knew they in some senses represented the prevailing political order and some form of professional shunning could follow. Despite these conflicting loyalties, however, an overall sense of professional stability allowed various medical activists to bring political and social agendas to the table – some of them, such as Virey and Buchez, still radical in scope – and to push these ideas in the public sphere.

In many ways, the dynamics of post-1800 health activism reflected the changing status of doctors themselves. During the French Revolution, medical reforms had given doctors unprecedented cultural authority, though the sources of this authority weren't entirely derived from professional power or economic status in terms of wealth. For example, the medical profession neither grew in overall numbers nor did it manage to penetrate the countryside to a greater degree.[124] Nevertheless, something quite profound was changing about the doctor's persona, giving him a new and

123 Dorinda Outram, *Georges Cuvier: Vocation, Science, and Authority in Post-Revolutionary France* (Manchester, 1984), especially pp. 189–202.

124 Ramsey, *Professional and Popular Medicine*, pp. 71–125; and Jean-Pierre Goubert and Bernard Lepetit, 'Les niveaux de médicalisation des villes françaises à la fin de l'Ancien

powerful mystique: medical knowledge could be consulted and used by a variety of historical agents, and it was not something just commanded by doctors alone. Consequently, the physician appeared as an important social and moral influence, and this authority persuaded contemporaries that medical knowledge spoke to a wide range of human experience.[125]

At the same time, medical practitioners saw their profession as contributing to public life by promoting both high-level scientific discourse and meaningful social change, and characterized themselves as proud but well-meaning members of the social elite. Medical science, they told sympathetic audiences, could contribute to the public and private well-being, and could improve French society, within certain limits, for the better. This does not suggest that the medical profession had any definite sense of ideological coherence, or that practitioners followed a set social agenda. Despite a shared Enlightenment and revolutionary background, it must be emphasized that these doctors were deeply divided in their political beliefs and they were carefully attuned to the political and socioeconomic realities of the period. Consequently, post-revolutionary hygienists often espoused a pragmatic if not hard-nosed realism, and they positioned themselves as defenders of a moderate status quo rather than instruments of radical change. These views, as we shall see, hardened after the terrible cholera epidemic of 1832, an event that gave new socio-statistical approaches an unprecedented voice in health activism.

Régime', in *La médicalisation de la société française, 1770–1830* (Waterloo, 1982), pp. 45–67.

125 My comments on medical authority draw upon Paul Starr, *The Social Transformation of American Medicine: The Rise of Sovereign Profession and the Making of a Vast Industry* (New York, 1984).

CHAPTER SIX

From Cholera to Degeneration, *c.* 1832–1852

Between the Napoleonic Empire and the Revolution of 1830, medical crusaders responded to new social, institutional and political transformations, and created new and diverse socio-medical ideologies that included pragmatic scientism, conservative Eclectic philosophy, Christian socialism and Malthusian demography. In the post-revolutionary years, these new socio-medical views undermined a previous medical faith in an integrated, *regenerated* national identity, whose universalism had transcended social distinctions, and instead steered social medicine into an apolitical realm to service the ever-changing status quo. But radical dreams of physical and moral hygiene truly collapsed after the disastrous cholera epidemic of 1832. In the contradictions of the so-called *juste milieu*, that moderate, middle-of-the-road political realm of the July monarchy, health activists turned against the urban labouring classes and revealed an ocean of seething class hatreds. According to Catherine J. Kudlick, members of the bourgeoisie saw cholera 'not just as an inexplicable natural disaster but also a crisis inherently bound up with the general malaise that many felt toward the Paris environment and its growing legions of poor'.[1] As this chapter demonstrates, health activists explained this cultural malaise and emerging social antagonisms by evoking a new and powerful force of hereditary degeneration.

'La mort de chien'; or, death comes in black and blue

The final part of this story begins with an intercontinental disease exchange between Europe and Asia. Cholera is caused by the bacterium *Vibrio cholerae*, a water-born microbe that invades the body by ingesting cholera-infected faecal matter. In cases of infection, the disease selects a disproportionate number of young and middle-aged adult men and women, depending upon current (and chronic) well-being. Healthy, active and well-fed individuals can produce alkali and acids that may offset the vibrio and prevent the person from getting sick; however, people who suffer from malnutrition, intestinal worms, chronic illness, long-term deprivation or severe mental depression often lack these counteractive secretions. Put in blunt terms, cholera has traditionally killed the poorest people across the globe – an observation demonstrated by the fact that in Britain during the nineteenth century some 130,000

---

1   Catherine J. Kudlick, *Cholera in Post-Revolutionary France: A Cultural History* (Berkeley, 1996), p. 213.

native residents died of cholera (chiefly amongst the poor), whilst in India the disease has killed over 25 million people in roughly the same century and a half.[2]

Cholera had a long history before reaching France in 1832. Endemic to India's Gangi river valley, cholera left its muggy banks in 1817 and spread all across the globe, crawling along trade routes and colonial outposts throughout the Russian hinterlands and Near East.[3] In 1817, the French archives first mention the disease when it appeared on the Île de Bourbon and the Île de France, and observers initially blamed the disease upon black slaves.[4] The first pandemic reached China, Japan, South-East Asia, Madagascar and the East African coasts before sputtering out on the doorstep of the Caucuses and Anatolia in 1823. But this was only a respite. In 1826, cholera again went on the offensive. It first infected the Caspian and Siberian regions and struck St Petersburg in 1830; immediately afterwards, it infiltrated most of eastern Europe, devastating Prussia, Hungary, Austria and Bohemia.

For obvious reasons, cholera was anxiously observed by French sanitary officials.[5] In 1830–31, the government sent Parisian doctors to observe the outbreaks in Russia and Poland and doctors debated disease aetiology in the Académie Royale de Médecine. At this juncture, physicians such as F.-J. Doublet and D.-J. Larrey promised public authorities that this colonial disease couldn't permeate France's *juste milieu*.[6] According to Dr Sarazin, cholera was 'an exotic production; its yeast was born or developed in the uncultivated, arid plains of Asia and in the rotting algae deposited by the flooding Nile; it ferments and warms itself amidst the residue of poisonous plants burned by the sun'.[7] The *haute culture* of France would resist a disease bred in Oriental despotism, misery and superstition.

---

2   See Sheldon Watts, *Epidemics and History: Disease, Power and Imperialism* (New Haven, 1997), p. 167; for a thorough account, see the standard treatment in R. Pollitzer, *Cholera* (Geneva, 1959).

3   On cholera in France, see especially George D. Sussman, 'From Yellow Fever to Cholera: A Study of French Government Policy, Medical Professionalism, and Popular Movements in the Epidemic Crises of the Restoration and the July Monarchy' (PhD thesis, Yale University, 1971); Patrice Bourdelais and Jean-Yves Raulot, *Une peur bleue: histoire du choléra en France, 1832–1854* (Paris, 1987); and Kudlick, *Cholera*. The most controversial study remains François Delaporte, *Disease and Civilization: The Cholera in Paris, 1832*, trans. Arthur Goldhammer (Cambridge, MA, 1986).

4   AN F⁸11, fol. II, Copie d'une lettre écrite de St Denis (Île de Bourbon), le 4 décembre 1819 ... par M. le Baron Milius (n.d.); Rapport présenté à Son Excellence le Ministre Secrétaire d'État au Département de l'Intérieur, Paris, 12 May 1820; and Ministre de la Marine et des Colonies, à Son Excellence le Ministre Secrétaire de l'Intérieur, Paris, 17 May 1820.

5   On comparative responses to cholera in nineteeth-century Europe, see Richard J. Evans, 'Epidemics and Revolutions: Cholera in Nineteenth-Century Europe', in Terence Ranger and Paul Slack (eds), *Epidemics and Ideas: Essays on the Historical Perception of Pestilence* (Cambridge and New York, 1992), pp. 149–73; the classic account remains Asa Briggs, 'Cholera and Society in the Nineteenth-Century', *Past and Present*, no. 19 (1961): 76–96. See also Charles E. Rosenberg, *The Cholera Years: The United States in 1832, 1849, and 1866* (Chicago, 1962).

6   Delaporte, *Disease*, pp. 15–22.

7   J. Sarazin, *Le choléra pestilentiel* (Paris, 1831), 19–20, quoted in Delaporte, *Disease*, p. 17.

Of course, some doctors objected. Playing upon Orientalist phobias, statistician Alexandre Moreau de Jonnès characterized cholera as the new 'yellow horde'. As he saw it, 'one can scarcely believe that the rest of Europe shall escape [cholera's] ravages … . [O]ne cannot doubt that this flu, similar to the barbaric invasions of the Middle Ages, shall not decimate peoples, disorganize society, crush commerce and degrade civilization'.[8] Similarly, F.-E. Fodéré denounced the medical establishment for keeping silent about cholera. Like Moreau de Jonnès, he called the disease 'an enemy who knows neither cannons, nor ruse, nor intrigue; who is stopped by neither cold nor heat; and who advances hardily to the centre of Europe'. Judging from recent medical journals, Fodéré said, medical elites preferred to discuss less important issues regarding adolescent behaviour and gelatine supplements for the poor. Cholera received short shrift. Doctors, he said, should stop debating whether the disease was contagious or not, and push public authorities to establish quarantines and clean the cities.[9]

At first, Moreau de Jonnès and Fodéré seemed like Casandraesque soothsayers. But all that changed when cholera hit England in October 1831. Even liberalism, it seemed, couldn't stop this disease. Immediately, French doctors fell into frenzied action. Royal ordinances established sanitary cordons, reinforced quarantine regulations and allocated emergency funds from the Chamber of Deputies. Meanwhile, Paris braced itself for the epidemic. The government created health commissions in each quarter in Paris. Physicians and volunteers inspected insalubrious habitations. Charities collected donations. Authorities expanded hospital services.[10] Much to their surprise, doctors now discovered that the *juste milieu* was an infected cesspool, and that much work had to be done. But they accomplished little. Well-meaning physicians and officials bemoaned neglected health measures. Liberal politicians did not want to spend public funds. Working people didn't trust new government regulations.[11] No matter, perhaps. In March 1832, 'king cholera' crossed the English Channel at Calais. On March 26, it entered Paris and killed four victims by nightfall.[12]

After having ravaged most of the globe, cholera seemed to have saved its final wrath for the French capital. Within seven days of its initial appearance, the Paris death rate jumped from four to 100 per day. On April 9, some 1,200 inhabitants fell ill and 814 died by nightfall. Eighteen days after the epidemic had hit Paris, between

---

8   Alexandre Moreau de Jonnès, *Rapport au Conseil supérieur de santé sur le choléra-morbus pestilentiel* (Paris, 1831), pp. 340–41.

9   F.-E. Fodéré, *Recherches historiques sur la nature, les causes et le traitement du choléra-morbus* (Paris, 1831), pp. 2, 17–19, 333–77. Urban hygiene did not impress all observers; see BN 4° Z. Le Senne. 2273 (9): 'Projet sur le nétoiement de la ville de Paris, adressé à Mr. le Préfet de police le 12 mars 1828' (ms.).

10   AP 20 Foss, 'Tableau du mouvement des hospices et hospices civils de la ville de Paris, de 1805 à 1832', n.d.; and AP 708 Foss 18, Hôpital St.-Louis, Administration générale des hôpitaux, hospices et secours à domicile à Paris, letter of May 3, 1832. See also 'Mesures hygiéniques', *Gazette médicale de Paris* 3, no. 13 (31 Mar. 1832), p. 139.

11   Delaporte, *Disease*, pp. 22–33; and Kudlick, *Cholera*, pp. 65–103.

12   The expression is from Norman Longmate, *King Cholera: The Biography of a Disease* (London, 1966).

12,000 and 14,000 people lay sick and at least 7,000 were dead. The Paris prefecture closed all cesspools and ponds, barricaded infected streets and submerged waste depositories. There wasn't enough room in the hospitals, so the government created ambulant stations to transport the sick and dead. Philanthropic citizens offered their homes as temporary hospices; others served as volunteer nurses. The administration finally gave up on printing daily mortality lists and thus increased public paranoia. To add to this disaster, typhus now swept the hospitals. The results were horrific. The bureau of vital statistics was so swamped it couldn't process death certificates. There weren't enough graves in the cemeteries. Decaying corpses were piled up to be scavenged by dogs – hence, that grim euphemism for death from cholera: 'la mort de chien' (a dog's death). In late spring, the disease lulled, but this respite proved illusory, and it returned throughout the summer and early autumn. On 25 September, the administration officially declared that the epidemic was over, although people continued to die from cholera until early October. All in all, the cholera epidemic lasted about seven months and it doubled the average annual mortality in Paris – that is, if one accepted the official government statistics, which many contemporary observers doubted anyway (some sources claimed over 40,000 deaths).[13]

During the epidemic, pandemonium reigned. There were widespread rumours that either reactionary aristocrats or the bourgeoisie had invented the disease as a form of class-based biological warfare. The people blamed either the liberal economists (who wanted to poison the poor to prevent famine) or the vengeful Carlists (who wanted to bring the Bourbons back to the throne). People panicked following stories that cholera victims were being buried alive; popular riots broke out at the Île de la Cité and the Place de Grève and authorities used force to put them down.[14] Indeed, the upper classes abandoned all the carnivalesque stories traditionally told about epidemics and they became hysterical about the labouring classes, the group that seemed to suffer most from the disease. In the contemporary mind, cholera presaged social revolution.[15]

Cholera had a terrifying effect. Fifty percent of those afflicted die, often within the course of a day.[16] Ordinary people might be going about their daily affairs when suddenly stricken with gross disorientation. They then suffered uncontrollable diarrhoea and vomiting and voided faecal matter that looked like soapy water or

---

13   E. Hellis, *Souvenirs du choléra en 1832* (Paris and Rouen, 1833), pp. 80–85.

14   'Que croira que Paris, la première ville du monde civilisé, Paris, le foyer des lumières, sur lequel l'Europe entière a les yeux fixés, renfermait encore dans son sein des hommes assez barbares pour massacrer leurs concitoyens sur les soupçons aussi absurdes, oubliant qu'il est des lois pour punir les coupables, et qu'à la justice seule appartient le droit de les juger'; H. Paillard, *Histoire statistique du choléra morbus qui a régné en France en 1832* (Paris, 1832), pp. 30–31.

15   On the connection between cholera and revolution, see Kudlick, *Cholera*, pp. 31–64; and Delaporte, *Disease*, pp. 47–72. On carnivalesque subversion in plague accounts, see Colin Jones, 'Plague and Its Metaphors in Early Modern France', *Representations*, no. 53 (1996): 97–127.

16   AP 712 Foss 1, 'Relevé numérique et par jour des personnes atteintes du choléra-morbus, qui ont été admises dans les hôpitaux et hospices civiles de Paris depuis l'invasion de la maladie' (n.d).

boiled rice.[17] Quickly dehydrating, the victim experienced unbearable cramps and convulsive pain. Within twelve hours, the person fell into a near-comatose, apathetic state – a condition that doctors such as the famed physiologist François Magendie described as 'cadaveresque'. The eyes shrunk, the teeth protruded and the skin faded to a blue-grey hue. Even after the victim had apparently died, the body could still become convulsed. These events horrified loved ones holding vigil over the body, whilst doctors and coroners complained they sometimes could not distinguish between the living and the dead.[18]

Cholera shocked the upper classes, and it became, as Giacomo Leopardi aptly points out, a devastating 'symbol of modernity'.[19] In her cultural study of the epidemic, Catherine J. Kudlick has demonstrated that this discourse contained powerful concerns over bourgeois identity itself, an identity that seemed so tenuous and fragile after the French Revolution.[20] In powerful ways, cholera overturned cherished bourgeois ideals about the beautiful and disciplined body, that self-contained vision of *homo clausus* described in Norbert Elias's sociological study.[21] According to Richard Evans, the choleric patient's pain, loss of control and convulsions violated the bourgeoisie's most valued ideas about poise, polish and self-control, opening up these markers of class to substantial public scrutiny.[22] It even overturned the prevailing aesthetics of death. Before the cholera, the genteel classes celebrated the individual's 'beautiful death'. In fashionable Romantic circles, painters and poets were fascinated by diseases such as typhus and tuberculosis, because they seemed to substantiate their fantasies about a sublime and convulsive beauty. For these thinkers, these sicknesses enhanced sensuality and sexuality, particularly at the moment of death.[23] Cholera's faecal wash, distortions and discoloration violated all these upper-class aesthetics of an idyllic, erotic death – and possibly forced social elites to consider, in sustained ways, the real world of death amongst the poor and labouring classes.

Cholera also shattered faith in European superiority. Elites could scarcely believe that an 'Oriental' disease, a pathological by-product of colonial commerce, had decimated the civilized and liberal West. Cholera had gone from the banks of the Gangi to the quays of the Seine, advancing upon Europe like a colonial 'return of the repressed'. Even yellow fever could not compare. And in the wake of the disease, the public wanted answers. But the government wanted to avoid the minefield of public scrutiny; nor did they want to provoke a medical debate and further undermine confidence. For this reason, authorities asked the new sanitarians – such as Louis-François Benoiston de Châteauneuf, Alexandre-Jean-Baptiste Parent-Duchatelet

---

17   J. Le Couer, *Précis sommaire sur le choléra-morbus épidémique, ses premiers symptoms, et les moyens les plus propres à les combattre* (Caen and Paris, 1832), p. 11.

18   See Watts, *Epidemics*, p. 173; and Evans, 'Cholera', pp. 153–54.

19   Giacomo Leopardi, *Pensieri* (Milan, 1987), p. 27, qtd. in Eugenia Tognotti, *Il mostro asiatico: storia del colera in Italia* (Rome, 2000), p. 342.

20   Kudlick, *Cholera*.

21   Norbert Elias, *The Civilizing Process: The History of Manners and State Formation and Civilization*, trans. Edmund Jephcott (Oxford, 1994).

22   Evans, 'Cholera', p. 154.

23   Philippe Ariès, *The Hour of Our Death*, trans. Helen Weaver (New York, 1981), pp. 409–72; and Susan Sontag, *Illness as a Metaphor* (Harmondsworth, 1983), p. 41.

and Louis-René Villermé – to investigate the epidemic. These sanitarians had earned a reputation for dispassionate observation and they avoided careless aetiological speculation. In empirical terms, the sanitarians could also draw upon an enormous body of data collected by the special health commissions established in 1831, data that showed infection levels, housing conditions and clinical experiences. According to Ann F. La Berge, these health commissioners had approached the epidemic as though Paris was a living 'laboratory' and they used these data to test the socio-statistical methods of the *Annales d'hygiène publique et de médecine légale*.[24] Over the next year, the cholera inquest made substantial use of these social observations and statistics.

The results were impressive. In 1834, Benoiston de Châteauneuf published the final report, called *Rapport sur la marche et les effets du choléra-morbus dans Paris et les communes rurales du département de la Seine*. This extensive epidemiological study was a landmark in socio-medical activism, ranking alongside Edwin Chadwick's renowned *Report on the Sanitary Condition of the Labouring Population of Great Britain* (1842). The doctors wanted to pioneer a new way to study epidemics and thus solidify public support for the socio-scientific approach associated with the *parti d'hygiène*.

In systematic fashion, the commission entertained traditional disease hypotheses and then discounted each. The book first provided a thorough medical topography of Paris on the eve of the cholera outbreak (whose details, the authors claimed, provided little insight into the epidemic) and then examined disease incidence according to sex and age, finding nothing more than inconclusive mortality rates. The commission then looked at environmental factors. Here again, the statistical evidence failed to show convincing analogies, because the weather didn't really influence disease incidence and mortality. Mortality was highest within filthy and poorly aired quarters; but it also varied in astonishing ways according to what apartment level people lived in. The doctors then examined mortality in rural regions, prisons and military barracks.[25]

In the end, the commission offered few conclusions. As they noted, cholera had simultaneously invaded urban and rural localities in the department of the Seine. In the city and in the countryside, its development, path, ferocity and tapering appeared identical. In general, the very young, middle aged and the elderly were particularly affected, though the young survived because of their 'force of age'.[26] In Paris, Sunday debauchery amongst the working population caused higher mortality on Mondays. As for isolated communities, prison deaths were lower than in the 'domiciled' population; hospital mortality was roughly even with that of the sixty-

---

24   The expression is from Ann La Berge, *Mission and Method: The Early Nineteenth-Century French Public Health Movement* (New York, 1992), p. 185. Note also that contemporary doctors viewed the epidemic as a testing ground for young medical personnel; see AN AJ[16]929 ('correspondance relative au choléra').

25   L.-F. Benoiston de Châteauneuf et al., *Rapport sur la marche et les effets du choléra-morbus dans Paris et les communes rurales du département de la Seine* (Paris, 1834), pp. 65, 75–76, 90, 99, 105.

26   Ibid., p. 188.

plus Paris age group. Soldiers suffered the highest comparative mortality (15.66/1000 in contrast to the 21.83/1000 rate for the civilian population). Although the report doubted environmental causes, it noted cholera was most vicious where people were exposed to winds. Most revealingly, the commissioners claimed, 'Finally, in several places infected by putrid emanations, cholera demonstrated itself to be neither more formidable nor mortal than in other localities.'[27] As the *Rapport* suggested, traditional epidemic inquiry – the older topographic or constitutional medicine used for diagnosing yellow fever – could not explain cholera.

As a result of this maddening aetiology, cholera forced doctors to consider epidemic determinants in novel ways. In 1831, Fodéré first called cholera a gross nervous disorder,[28] but by 1832, physicians flatly conceded they didn't know what caused it.[29] However, they were relatively sure that cholera wasn't contagious.[30] For this reason, many historians believe that the European cholera outbreak of 1831–32 and its successor pandemic of 1848–49 (which was more lethal) changed aetiological theory, which had alternated between models of contagion and infection. As Erwin H. Ackerknecht argued, the failure of sanitary cordons and quarantine policies during the 1831–32 pandemic confirmed the anticontagionist outlook of liberal doctors and officials, which had been steadily growing since he 1820s. These men believed that the environment or miasma made people sick (that is, disease did not spread from person to person) and thus rejected quarantines. Instead, these doctors and policy-makers, such as the British Erwin Chadwick, wanted to remove the urban filth that made disease-provoking miasma or other exciting causes.[31] Medical historians have claimed that anticontagionists promoted optimistic activism over stodgy conservatism. Although anticontagionism was an incorrect aetiological explanation, it nevertheless motivated authorities to help meliorate desperate social conditions.

However, cholera does not fit neatly into the classic contagionist–anticontagionist polarity. In her brilliant work on English cholera, Margaret Pelling showed that the epidemic was less important for doctors than chronic health problems such as fevers and tuberculosis. In her view, the aetiological debates over infectious diseases (such as yellow fever and cholera) simply did not influence general practitioners.[32] More recently, Christopher Hamlin and John V. Pickstone have built upon Pelling's insights, revealing that British physicians worked within a confused and conflicted aetiological scene: for example, prominent contagionists advocated

27 Ibid., p. 189.

28 Fodéré, *Recherches*, p. 391; and Le Couer, *Précis*, p. 13.

29 Benoiston de Châteauneuf, *Rapport*, p. 12. See also Hellis, *Souvenirs*, pp. 25, 26–27, 28, 30–31; and Dr Lejumeau de Kergaradec, *Quelques mots sur le choléra-morbus épidémique et sur les moyens de s'en préserver* (Paris, 1832).

30 AP B-4822², *Observations sur le choléra-morbus, recueillies et publiées par l'ambassade de France en Russie* (Paris, 1831), pp. 22–23, 28–31.

31 Erwin H. Ackerknecht, 'Anticontagionism between 1821 and 1867', *Bulletin of the History of Medicine* 22 (1948): 562–93. For a recent historiographical review, see William Coleman, *Yellow Fever of the North: The Methods of Early Epidemiology* (Madison, 1987), pp. 173–94.

32 Margaret Pelling, *Cholera, Fever and English Medicine, 1825–1865* (Oxford and New York, 1978).

Edwin Chadwick's sanitary plans or acknowledged environmental factors in disease causation. Overall, however, the vast majority of medical practitioners generally saw contagionist and anticontagionist principles more or less compatible, as some diseases manifested qualities of both; and conversely, as James C. Riley points out, anticontagionists sometimes pessimistically concluded that health reforms were worthless in an inescapable pathological environment.[33] Finally, as Roger Cooter has inveighed, anticontagionism showed signs of being an elite social movement, one that wanted to deprive the lower classes of control over their own health and implement reforms that did not challenge prevailing power structures.[34] As historians now think, the Chadwickian movement largely trampled over established notions of disease predisposition, dearth and fever sickness and caused physicians to stop seeing poverty as a cause of disease.

Despite these important insights, historians such as Pelling and Richard Evans have gone further and claimed that cholera didn't substantially influence European health policy before John Snow's and Robert Koch's discoveries, better state services and 'higher standards of personal hygiene'.[35] This may be true in terms of state actions, but this analysis ignores how cholera transformed broader cultural mentalities – something as tangible as social policy itself. This was particularly true in France. The cholera outbreak challenged medical practitioners, intellectuals and public authorities on three fronts: first, they expressed a more pointed scepticism about the general optimism and faith in progress found in advanced social thought (though they did not entirely relinquish these beliefs); second, they questioned both traditional and more liberal 'do nothing' attitudes towards charity and public assistance; and, finally, they moved beyond the anti-contagionist/contagionists debates that rocked the Royal Academy of Medicine in 1827 and 1828. As a consequence of these new attitudes, physicians asked whether poverty caused epidemic disease and whether social reform could reduce disease. Ackerchknecht has called this insight the 'social theory of disease'.[36] These ideas were not entirely new: in the 1770s and 1790s, as we have seen, the Royal Society of Medicine had first discussed the relation between poverty and disease in its health police projects; and in the 1790s, revolutionary legislators in the health and poverty committees had passionately debated the poor's 'right to health' and the need for subsistence. Despite these important antecedents, as François Delaporte has argued, cholera was still the predominant factor that caused the social theory of disease to sink into the medical mind.[37] But these insights raised

---

33   See Christopher Hamlin, 'Predisposing Causes and Public Health in Early Nineteenth-Century Medical Thought', *Social History of Medicine* 5 (1992): 43–70, especially pp. 45–50; and John V. Pickstone, 'Dearth, Dirt, and Fever Epidemics: Rewriting the History of British "Public Health", 1780–1850,' in Terence Ranger and Paul Slack (eds), *Epidemics and Ideas: Essays on the Historical Perception of Pestilence* (New York, 1992), pp. 125–48. On medical resignation in the face of hostile environments, see James C. Riley, *The Eighteenth-Century Campaign to Avoid Disease* (London, 1987), pp. x, 36.

34   Roger Cooter, 'Anticontagionism and History's Medical Record', in P. Wright and A. Treacher (eds), *The Problem of Medicial Knowledge* (Edinburgh, 1983), pp. 87–108.

35   Pelling, *Cholera*, pp. 3–6; Evans, 'Cholera', pp. 153, 172.

36   Ackerknecht, 'Anticontagionism', pp. 592–93.

37   Delaporte, *Disease*.

further questions for doctors. If poverty caused disease, then what caused poverty? Like some sicknesses, did 'lifestyle' cause poverty? And, if people could cure poverty through self-control, was the same true for disease? Doctors wondered what natural laws caused social inequalities and, by extension, disease itself.

In the cholera report, the commission zeroed in on what they called the 'conditions of existence', 'modes of existence' or the 'genre of life' in the urban environment.[38] These terms were carefully borrowed from comparative anatomy. Medical observers had noticed that the affluent largely escaped the cholera, even when they had been in close proximity to the sick.[39] To explain this phenomenon, the commission turned to naturalist studies about how organisms lived under specific habitat conditions. In different ways, the most important insights came from biologists such as Georges Cuvier and Jean-Baptiste Lamarck, who, despite their differing views on species change, shared similar beliefs about the power of habitat.

According to Cuvier, all living beings had a specific ecological niche. In his view, the organism's form and function reflected predetermined ends (his ideas of species remained essentialist or neo-Platonic) and these ends put heavy limitations or 'conditions' upon the organism. As a consequence, the living being must always harmonize with its pre-established environment. In biological terms, Cuvier's 'correspondence of parts' made it impossible for organisms to progressively adapt to their environment, since radical habitat changes caused an internal structural catastrophe, a biological event he called a 'revolution'.[40] The result was death or extinction.

By contrast, Lamarck saw the relationship between organism and environment in more dynamic terms. When discussing organic adaptation, Lamarck rejected easy ideas about ecological symbiosis or environmental determinism. Under his gaze, the organism enjoyed no pre-established symbiosis with its habitat; rather, the living being must always readjust its internal equilibrium to accommodate powerful exogenous conditions, conditions which he called *circonstances influentes* or 'milieux' (he introduced the plural form of this noun). Change, in this way, was a central part of organic life.[41] According to Paul Rabinow, 'Climate and place were thus dethroned as major categories (at least in their classical senses) during the nineteenth century, whilst milieu progressively gained importance (both as a concept and as a metaphor), and it spread across a large and disparate group of disciplines, from biology to sociology.'[42] Though Cuvier and Lamarck had markedly different ideas about species evolution and extinction, they both emphasized the overwhelming power of habitat over living beings – and sanitarians eagerly applied these insights to their social analysis.

---

38 Benoiston de Châteauneuf, *Rapport*, pp. 121, 123, 137.

39 'Hôpital de Val-de-Grace', *Gazette Médicale de Paris* 3, no. 17 (10 Apr. 1832), p. 163.

40 On Cuvier, see William Coleman, *Georges Cuvier, Zoologist: A Study in the History of Evolution Theory* (Cambridge, MA, 1964), Ch. 2; and Dorinda Outram, *Georges Cuvier: Vocation, Science and Authority in Post-Revolutionary France* (Manchester, 1984).

41 Georges Canguilhem, 'Le vivant et son milieu', in *La connaissance de la vie*, 2d edn (Paris, 1969).

42 Paul Rabinow, *French Modern: Norms and Forms of the Social Environment* (Cambridge, MA, 1989), 133–37, quote at 134.

For doctors, the cholera outbreak showed that people became sick because of underlying biological 'conditions of existence' associated with urbanization and industrialization. In order to understand these new economic conditions, physicians invoked theories of social economy (as seen in Chapter 5 below), which generally attributed poverty to lower-class immorality and laziness (indeed, the cholera inquest boasted prominent social economists such as L.-R. Villermé). These physicians and administrators shifted the social theory of disease, and turned epidemic disease – rather than poverty itself – into a symptom of physical and moral degeneracy. The Royal Academy of Medicine concluded, 'The disease first took those classes which are poorly housed, poorly clothed, poorly fed and, moreover, exhausted by all kinds of excess' – and sanitarians now set out to better understand these social pathologies.[43]

These beliefs appear in a number of writings on cholera. Contrasting working-class debauchery to bourgeois prudence, J.-P.-F. Marie de Valognes explained, 'That is why the *juste milieu* is healthy: one must always ... [consider] the season, age, constitution, genre of work and the regimen of the subject.'[44] For his part, Dr Tacheron argued that sickness varied according to class and milieu. In his examination of cholera in the eleventh arrondissement of Paris, he found that disease struck five levels of people: the very poor and destitute (171 deaths); those who indulged in an 'excessive' and drunken lifestyle (55 dead); patients who suffered from flu symptoms before the arrival of cholera (50 dead); enteritis victims (25 dead); and the physically and morally healthy (only 18 dead). This cursory tabulation, in his eyes, linked cholera with class status. He wrote, 'An incontestable fact is that intemperance and irregularities of every genre in regimen, in the working classes just as in the affluent classes, were the two principle causes in the development of mortality'.[45]

As Tacheron's comments make clear, many observers believed that cholera was caused by immorality, and they were willing to lay the blame squarely in the lap of the labouring classes. Dr Marie de Valognes and Dr Paillard identified the worst culprits: 'venereal pleasures', 'prolonged voluptuous contacts', 'debauchery', 'misery', 'excesses of every species' and 'slovenliness'.[46] As in cases of chronic gastrointestinal maladies, G.-A.-L. Buard d'Agen said, immorality shaped the individual's physical and moral constitution, causing perturbations in the 'intestinal tube' and choleric symptoms.[47] For Dr Fougnot de Clisson, urban degeneracy caused choleric susceptibility; he identified 'insalubrious habitations', poorly ventilated streets, drunkenness and rambunctious behaviour amongst labourers on Sundays as potential causes.[48] As A.-N. Gendrin explained, the working-class home bred disease

---

43 AP B-4822³, *Rapport et instruction pratique sur le choléra-morbus, rédigés et publiés d'après la demande du gouvernement* (Paris, 1832), p. 2.

44 J.-P.-F. Marie de Valognes, *Quelques propositions de médecine, et en particulier sur l'hygiène prophylactique du choléra épidémique* (Paris, 1832), pp. 10–11.

45 Dr Tacheron, *Statistique médicale de la mortalité du choléra-morbus dans le XIe arrondissement de Paris* (Paris, 1832), pp. 1–2, 46–47, 56, 58–59.

46 Marie de Valognes, *Quelques propositions*, p. 9; and Paillard, *Histoire statistique*, p. 78.

47 G.-A.-L. Buard d'Agen, *Du choléra-morbus épidémique* (Paris, 1832), p. 11.

48 F. Fougnot de Clisson, *Dissertation sur le choléra-morbus épidémique* (Paris, 1832), p. 9.

because of endemic debaucheries and unsanitary conditions.[49] However, not all physicians dismissed working-class lifestyle. As Dr Hellis argued, doctors criticized working people because of their own class prejudices and couldn't empathize with them.[50]

Hellis was exceptional. Prominent hygienists often suggested that the poor somehow deserved to get cholera. Benoiston de Châteauneuf's *Rapport* underscored this belief. 'In light of these facts and many others … it was impossible for the commission not to believe that there exists a certain species of population, just like a certain nature of places, that favours the development of cholera, and renders it more intense and murderous.'[51] As F.-J.-V. Broussais explained, cholera's bizarre epidemiological pattern had forced clinical practitioners to reconsider some of their fundamental aetiological presuppositions. For example, the interior of an isolated building might demonstrate an odd morbid quilting; even should the doctor consider the house as a prescribed 'milieu', cholera was still manifest 'in different families of which the genre of life was not the same'. Crucially, these data suggested that '*something* particular existed in affected houses that was predisposed to cholera'. Indeed, this unknown *something* became a leitmotif for concerned doctors. They searched for predisposing causes beyond sociological or environmental determinants, because moral, climatic, miasmic and zymotic determinants seemed inconclusive. As Broussais stated, 'What is positive, is that a *predisposition* to cholera exists; it is here that we must focus our research'; and he reiterated that the disease constituted a 'species of infection' that 'acted only upon predisposed persons' with an 'extraordinary irritability or a morbid irritation of the digestive canal'.[52]

In this discourse about cholera and predisposition, clinicians and sanitarians were groping towards a new way of understanding disease susceptibility. Predisposition, here, was acquiring a different signification. Not only had it been the centrepiece of the so-called 'bedside' medicine associated with humoral balance and temperament, but it was also the key to projects of physical and moral hygiene: from the 1750s onwards, physicians had believed that they could use knowledge of patient predisposition – that is, the unique health profile and disease susceptibility shaped by the seasons, geography, occupation, health, sex, age, and so on – to reform the internal and external factors that determined human nature itself and remake society for the better.

Cholera, however, helped reinforce another idea that was taking shape in the medical mind: namely, that predisposition might involve either some kind of *internal* predetermining force, or even some inescapable environmental influence that ultimately overturned all other aetiological considerations. Predisposition, in this sense, was becoming an insurmountable factor in terms of disease prevention

---

49 A.-N. Gendrin, *Monographie du choléra-morbus épidémique* (Paris, 1832), pp. 283–84, 287.

50 Hellis, *Souvenirs*, p. 65.

51 Benoiston de Châteauneuf, *Rapport*, pp. 124–25.

52 F.-J.-V. Broussais, *Le choléra-morbus épidémique, observé et traité selon la méthode physiologique* (Paris, 1832), pp. 9–10, 14–15, 42–43 (my emphasis); also Paillard, *Histoire statistique*, pp. 73–74, 74 n. 1.

and avoidance, one that offered health activists more of a stumbling block than opportunity. This stumbling block challenged, on the one hand, long-standing hopes about physical and moral hygiene, and the rhetoric about pro-natalist policies, on the other, because it suggested that medical practitioners could not surmount innate predisposing conditions. Biology, in other words, was destiny.

To sum up, then, the 1832 cholera epidemic shifted medical views about organism and habitat. For doctors, cholera undermined the older environmental medicine and its attendant medical police responses; neither anticontagionist nor contagionist insights could explain this horrible epidemic. Beneath these socio-scientific debates was an anxious image of the urban underclass, which seemed to be a source of disease and disorder. Levels of cholera incidence within this group suggested a biological susceptibility, as though something alien and preordained contaminated their bodies and habitat.

Following this belief, hygienists moved in two closely interrelated directions. First, doctors examined sociological factors that caused the physical and moral degradation of the labouring classes. Second, they turned to the question of disease predisposition – in other words, why the working population seemed to succumb to diseases like cholera. Both social conditions and predisposition suggested that some underlying degenerative 'force' might make labouring people sick and immoral. Doctors looked closely at two things: habitat and heredity.

Cruel discoveries

'Cholera', wrote Dr Émile Littré, 'by the visitations it caused, has made cruel discoveries'.[53] By 'cruel discoveries', Littré meant something specific: France had serious social problems. Thanks to these discoveries, physicians now openly recognized the labouring classes' infectious and degraded 'conditions of existence' and suggested that something ought to be done about them.[54] But when doctors acknowledged these problems, they raised broader questions about politics and society. By comparing rich and poor, doctors entertained broad existential questions about shared bodily experience, suggesting that the lower classes were totally different from the upper-class world. Several doctors said that this alien working-class element might constitute, under some circumstances, an expendable vital mass, one obviously needed for the production process but potentially dangerous in large numbers or in high density. The cholera report identified this parasitic population:

> Placed at the lowest level of the social scale, this class is incessantly created in our populated and manufacturing towns by industrial reversals, miscalculation, disorders of misconduct, [and] is nowhere more numerous than in Paris, where it grows incessantly from the crowd of vagabonds that are attracted to the city by the lures of its bait. Without fixed domicile [*sans domicile fixe*], without assured work, this class, which possesses

---

53 Émile Littré, *Médecine et médecins*, 3d edn (Paris, 1875), p. 194.

54 AP 712 Foss 1, 'Choléra-morbus: résumé basé sur 150 observations suivies depuis le début ou depuis le moment où les secours de l'art ont été réclamés jusqu'à la terminaison, tant en ville qu'à l'hospice temporaire de la rue de Clichy', 12 May 1832.

nothing in its own right but its poverty and vices, having wandered all day through public places, returns during the night to *maisons garnies* [provisional working-class accommodation] in the different quarters of the capital, which seem to be forever destined to receive these types.[55]

Elites had a name for 'this class' of people: the dangerous classes. Since the Restoration, authorities had been nervously tracking the indigent population of Paris and they worried about the problems they might pose to public health and order.[56] But the cholera epidemic changed everything and gave public officials and medical authorities new urgency in studying lower-class conditions.[57] As a consequence, in 1832, the July monarchy encouraged the new Académie des Sciences Morales et Politiques at the Institute of France to study public health and morality from the perspective of political economy.[58] As the Academy's members saw it, scientific elites must study the Parisian 'dangerous classes', so the 'administration, rich or affluent men, intelligent and industrious workers' could better meliorate this 'depraved class'. Previously, public officials and philanthropists had merely tried to tabulate the numbers of indigent and the costs of charity and welfare services. Now, a more holistic approach was needed.[59]

In response, the police prefect and social economist H.-A. Frégier published an enormous socio-statistical study of Paris crime, employing the new sanitarians' observational and empirical techniques. Although he praised the moral rectitude of some segments of the labouring classes, Frégier often saw all working people as part of the so-called 'mobile and mysterious class' – those types he labelled 'gamblers', 'speculators', 'vagabonds', 'prostitutes', 'frauds', 'swindlers', 'robbers', 'pickpockets' and 'dealers in stolen merchandise'.[60] For him, 'corruption propagates itself most easily' amongst urban labourers; and fallen women figured heavily in their midst.[61] Their moral degradation was a biological phenomenon: the urban labouring classes had a 'distinct physiognomy' and their 'physical constitution' caused immorality and disorder. Moreover, their 'bad habits' and moral 'vice' were 'contagious' and were transmitted to children like any other hereditary disease.[62]

---

55   Benoiston de Châteauneuf, *Rapport*, pp. 191–92.

56   AP F11 Foss 2, Extrait du Moniteur, 27 Nov. 1828.

57   AP 127 Foss, Administration générale des hospices, hospices civils et secours à domicile de la ville de Paris, 'État numérique de la population indigente de Paris, et renseignements statistiques sur cette population' (1841).

58   See 'Histoire de l'Académie', *Mémoires de l'Académie des Sciences Morales et Politiques*, nouvelle série (Paris, 1837), vol. 1, pp. i–xxv. The original 'second class' of Moral and Political Sciences of the Institute of France was dissolved in 1803 by Napoleon Bonaparte on account of its Idéologue sympathies. See Martin S. Staum, *Minerva's Message: Stabilizing the French Revolution* (Montreal, 1996).

59   AP 170 Foss 1, Neizey, 'Recherches sur moyens d'améliorer le sort des indigents de la ville de Paris, suivies de tableaux de population' (1819).

60   H.-A. Frégier, *Des classes dangereuses de la population dans les grandes villes, et des moyens de les rendre meilleures* (2 vols, Paris, 1840), vol. 1, pp. 9, 44.

61   Ibid., vol. 1, pp. 9–10, 14.

62   Ibid., vol. 1, pp. 11, 40, 79, 82, vol. 2, p. 222.

Though he saw social problems in medical terms, Frégier provided few concrete policy solutions. Following the Academy's liberal sensibilities, he rejected government intervention into private industry; rather, he encouraged manufacturers to implement moral programmes that would prevent the 'true' labouring populations from being infected. But workers must also use individual initiative to help transform their lives. 'The amelioration of the worker's lot depends primarily upon his own will power', he said. 'Before demanding the regeneration of the rich, might he begin by regenerating himself. In showing himself prudent, sober and temperate, he will have made half the journey himself.'[63]

As these social critics claimed, urban sickness and death showed that the lower classes had overrun the natural 'conditions of existence'.[64] Cholera, for example, simply purged a parasitic group that had lived beyond its socioeconomic means. These problems, explained Louis-René Villermé, could not be solved by modern civilization. Progress meliorated some diseases but left behind the 'miserable and indigent'. This was the natural order. Citing Thomas Malthus, Villermé wrote that 'everywhere they frequently recur, epidemics indicate the poverty [*misère*] of people, or, what is the same thing, an excess of population relative to the means of existence that it enjoys'. Nature thus marked poor workers for extinction.[65] After 1832, doctors suggested that cholera merely demonstrated Malthus's grim laws at work, something already suggested by J.-J. Virey in 1828.[66]

By the mid-1830s, Malthusian attitudes convinced the noted physiologist, Dr Balthasar-Anthelme Richerand, that the government needed a new population policy. For him, demographic growth and dwindling resources were causing Europe's chronic sociopolitical crises. To restore civil harmony, he argued, the government needed to enforce paternal authority and sexual restraint in working families (he also entertained programmes for marriage limitation, colonization, infanticide and so on).[67] Throughout, Richerand moved from the 'physiological order' to the 'political order', showing that Malthus's demographic laws remained a 'physical, material, incontestable fact' that undermined utopian beliefs in human progress and perfection.[68] Modern life, he felt, was a double-edged sword. The population grew

---

63   Ibid., vol. 1, p. 358.

64   Cf. Claude Lachaise, 'De l'influence de l'entassement de la population sur la mortalité des grandes villes; prouvée par les registres mortuaires de Paris de 1820 à 1840', *Bulletin de l'Académie royale de médecine* 5 (1840): 570–80, who primarily considered overpopulation within urban spaces.

65   L.-R. Villermé, 'Des épidémies sous les rapports de l'hygiène publique, de la statistique médicale et de l'économie politique', *Annales d'hygiène publique et médecine légale* 9 (1833): 5–58, especially pp. 14, 38–39, 41.

66   J.-J. Virey, *Hygiène philosophique, ou de la santé dans le régime physique, moral et politique de la civilisation moderne* (2 vols, Paris, 1828), vol. 1, pp. 370–71. See especially J.-R. Kerckhove, *Considérations sur la nature et le traitement du choléra-morbus* (Anvers, 1833), pp. vi–vii; and H. Boulay de la Meurthe, *Histoire du choléra-morbus dans le quartier du Luxembourg* (Paris, 1832), p. 116, as cited in Delaporte, *Disease*, pp. 52–54.

67   B.-A. Richerand, *De la population dans ses rapports avec la nature des gouvernements* (Paris, 1837), pp. 215–16, 297–98, 303–04.

68   Ibid., pp. 3–4.

because of temperate climate, the fertility of soil, religious toleration and enlightened policies; however, progress had outstripped subsistence, causing the population to become sick and degenerate. By the 1830s, social conditions were so dismal that even recent upheavals – notably political revolution, cholera and yellow fever – could no longer purge society of this surplus demographic mass.[69] To add to these problems, charity and public assistance encouraged the population to grow and thus increased degeneracy. Richerand could not imagine how elites could maintain respect for throne, altar and property in a society otherwise bursting at its vital seams.[70]

Not all physicians espoused such heavy-handed ideas. Reformist doctors, such as the hygienist and occupational specialist, Dr François Mélier, battled against Malthusian policies, and championed the health-care reforms for the labouring classes and urban poor.[71] The lesson these practitioners drew from cholera was that the government must expand public welfare and institutions such as the urban health councils, which had helped to prepare for the choleric deluge. As they saw it, authorities must learn to manage the nation's health in light of urban industrialization and new epidemic threats. In 1837, the Royal Academy of Medicine also emphasized that the state needed to take greater initiative in sanitary reform and 'moralizing' the lower classes:

> Unfortunately, government vigilance can only exercise its force over individual will in a restrained number of cases, and [individual] anomalies and whims are rarely within the competence of positive laws. Therefore, in order to combat prejudices, errors, and negligence, public hygiene must diffuse, within the diverse classes of society, hygienic ideas and suitable health instruction; it must, in a word, persuade where it is impossible to constrain.[72]

In this discussion, doctors said that their colleagues must start with the greatest public health problem: worker sickness. This important topic, which had been raised by Antoine Fourcroy in the 1770s for the Royal Society of Medicine, had largely been derailed in academic medical circles in the political chaos of the French Revolution. Nevertheless, medical interest in occupational disease had been increasing since the Napoleonic period, and new concerns about urban health and hygiene, as we have seen in Chapter 5 above, were being voiced with greater regularity in more traditional topographic inquiries. In 1807, for example, Dr Pierre Nysten petitioned the internal ministry to fund a four-year inquest into labouring conditions, and tried to justify this inquest by claiming that epidemic disease often affected specific social classes. The standard reference remained the Marseilles plague of 1720, in which entire occupations had been wiped out by the pestilence. By studying occupational

---

69   Ibid., pp. 70–71, 73, 82–83.

70   Ibid., pp. 102, 104, 148.

71   Coleman, *Death is a Social Disease: Public Health and Political Economy in Early Industrial France* (Madison 1982), pp. 301–02.

72   AN F^{8}174, dos. 2 (ii), [Dupay, Pariset, Villeneuve, Chevalier, Adelon, and Marc], 'Projet d'organisation des conseils de salubrité départementaux', 1 Apr. 1837.

disease, Nysten urged, medical practitioners could potentially explain both disease aetiology and lay the groundwork for new public health policies.[73]

Though Nysten's proposal was not accepted by the government, other physicians picked up the study of occupational disease and hazards.[74] In 1822, Philibert Patissier published a new book on artisan disease, a work that owed much to Bernardino Ramazzini's pioneering text from the previous century. Although Patissier generally attributed worker disease to personal immorality, he believed that reformers could meliorate factory and living conditions. Foremost, the government should prohibit dangerous professions, employing in their stead condemned criminals. Municipal authorities should create public baths to promote working-class cleanliness; and mutual-aid societies could help manage periods of morbidity and dearth.[75] In these analyses, however, Patissier used older nosological approaches and treated occupational diseases as 'genera' or 'classes' as though they were independent botanical entities.[76] A similar trend emerges, for example, in Parent-Duchâtelet's projected study of occupational disease, which he began in earnest with Alphonse Chevallier and Jean-Pierre d'Arcet in 1829 but was unfortunately interrupted by his death in 1836. Though Parent-Duchâtelet criticized traditional studies for lacking observational and statistical rigor, his focus still remained on more traditional forms of artisan production: butchers, dock workers, sewer cleaners, tobacco workers, and so on.[77] At this point, many doctors did not raise issues about exchange, circulation and management in treatises on occupational health, and some critics pointed that public funds would be better served by improving health care and sanitation in the rural environment.[78]

Cholera encouraged medical practitioners to reinterpret older approaches to 'the diseases of artisans' and think about occupational disease in light of urbanization and industrialization. After the public disturbances during the cholera epidemic, political

---

73   AN F^{17}2107, dos. 6, [Pierre] Nysten, 'Projet de recherches sur les maladies qui attaquent les ouvriers dans les manufactures, les ateliers et les travaux d'exploitation, et sur les moyens de prévenir ces maladies', 9 Dec. 1807. Nysten's petition was supported by Jean-Noël Hallé. See also the comments in SEM, carton T (dos. Topographie), Roger, 'Topographie de Thionville et des environs', 28 Brumaire, Year V.

74   *Encyclopédie méthodique ou par ordre des matières: médecine*, ed. Félix Vicq d'Azyr (13 vols, Paris, 1782–1832), s.v. 'Métier'; and *Dictionnaire des sciences médicales*, ed. Adelon et al. (60 vols, Paris, 1812–22), s.v. 'Professions'.

75   Philibert Patissier, *Traité des maladies des artisans et de celles qui résultent de diverses professions d'après Ramazzini* (Paris, 1822), pp. xlvi–liv.

76   See F.-J.-V. Broussais, *A Treatise on Physiology Applied to Pathology*, 3d American edn, trans. John Bell and R. La Roche (Philadelphia, 1832), pp. 579–80.

77   La Berge, *Mission and Method*, 155–59.

78   AM 242, M.-L. Moreau de Blaye, 'Aperçu moral et hygiénique sur les populations des compagnes; suivi de quelques recherches statistiques sur leurs constitutions, leurs tempéraments, leurs maladies et les traitements qui leur conviennent, avec quelques considérations sur le personnel du médecins de campagne', 19 Sept. 1835; AM 241, M.-L. Moreau [de Blaye], 'Considérations sur la nécessité de dresser la topographie médicale de tous les cantons, de tracer les préceptes hygiéniques qui leur sont applicables, en particulier sur le topographie médicale', 21 Oct. 1836.

authorities connected disease and radicalism, and they now began to track sickness from the workplace back into the home itself.[79] Alarmed by working-class sedition, in 1835, the Academy of Moral and Political Sciences asked Dr L.-R. Villermé to study health and working-class conditions. In response, Villermé conducted a detailed ethnographic and socio-statistical study of industrial health in the areas of the Haut-Rhin, Seine-Inférieure, Aisne, Nord, Rhône and Zurich. The result was his massive *Tableau de l'état physique et moral des ouvriers*, first published in 1840 to critical acclaim. This critical text decisively moved the focus of occupational disease from traditional manufacturing to the new production techniques found in factories and cities.

In many ways, Villermé's shocking exposé was the culmination of his long career in public health research for the *Annales d'hygiène publique*. Villermé's work was unlike previous medical topographies or occupational inquests. Rather, like a field biologist, he claimed to have directly observed workers in their natural habitat, and he tabulated carefully what he considered to be their true conditions of existence. In this endeavour, Villermé tried, as best he could, to seem like workers, to talk and to dress like them. He moved through slum streets and alleys, peered through windows, and listened to daily banter, all along jotting down his responses. In the opening of his work, he forcefully declared:

> I followed [the worker] from his workshop to his home; I entered [these places] with him; I studied him interacting with his family; I watched him at his meals. I did more: I had watched him in his labours and in his domestic arrangements, I wanted to see him in his pleasures, in the places of festivity. There, listening to his conversations, I often participated and mingled, I was … the confidant in his joys and complaints, his regrets and hopes, [and] the witness to his vices and his virtues.[80]

For good reason, Villermé's work has attracted much recent critical attention from cultural and social historians. In their studies of work and representations in nineteenth-century France, William Reddy and William Sewell, Jr have analyzed the images and narrative techniques that Villermé used to discuss the poor and mendicant classes. As they have shown, Villermé's images pervaded elite public discourse on social reform, and even appeared in writings that ostensibly championed the plight of the poor (such as Eugène Sue's and Victor Hugo's descriptions of outcast Paris). In their analyses, both Reddy and Sewell have reiterated that Villermé's work shows less the 'real conditions' of labour than how worker stereotypes – whether disparaging or romanticized – permeated all levels of intellectual discourse and potentially undercut real efforts at social change.[81]

---

79 AP 712 Foss 2, 'Observations sur l'insalubrité de la plupart des logements des ouvriers' (n.d.).

80 L.-R. Villermé, *Tableau de l'état physique et moral des ouvriers employés dans les manufactures de coton, de lane et de soie* (2 vols, Paris, 1840), vol. 1, p. vi.

81 William M. Reddy, *The Rise of Market Culture: The Textile trade and French Society, 1750–1900* (Cambridge, 1984), Ch. 6; William H. Sewell, Jr., *Work and Revolution in France: The Language of Labor from the Old Regime to 1848* (Cambridge and New York, 1980), pp. 223–32.

The point here is not to ascertain Villermé's true philanthropic motives or to uncover the 'real' ideological issues lurking behind his text. Rather, the analysis shows how Villermé explored ideas of physical degeneracy after the cholera outbreak and how he put these ideas into the established framework of 'physical and moral hygiene'. Worker health and hygiene were reprehensible, Villermé insisted, looking at their conditions of existence; yet his text also intimated that some deeper pathological cause was at work. Villermé linked three issues: poverty, disease and immorality. In Alsace, he wrote, 'Many [workers] completely neglect propriety. But the poorest have neither the taste, the time, nor the means of doing otherwise.'[82] In Lille, he described 'the excessive misery, uncleanness, vices and disgusting promiscuity in which so many workers of this city live',[83] and their children evidenced a scrofulous demeanour, appearing 'discolored' and 'thin'.[84] In Rouen, the weavers had a 'pale' and 'indolent' constitution, appearing 'stunted' and 'scrofulous'; and in this area he found many goitres and cretins.[85] Even those working communities whose health rectitude and self-respect earned his praise only later served as fodder to drive home the point of worker alterity. He wrote: '[T]he defects of order, lack of foresight and drunkenness often aggravates, by the increase of privations that they impose, the sad lot of the workers.'[86]

Degeneracy infected both shop floor and household. The proximity of men and women on the shop floor caused 'the greatest excesses' (as evidenced by degraded conditions in Lille), and 'illicit' and 'premature' sexual relations. Worker sex 'exhaust[ed]' the young people in the factories (rather than the work itself).[87] Among female labourers in Saint-Quentin, the 'love of luxury', 'common chambers' and the 'mixing of sexes' had 'relaxed' and 'depraved' their morals. In Villermé's estimation, the high levels of worker illegitimacy measured this perceived 'moral slackening'.[88] As a consequence, he praised Alsatian manufacturers who had instituted a sexual division of labour and policed worker sexuality outside the shop floor.[89] With abject fascination, Villermé described the bedding upon which working families writhed in filth and misery, imagining their carnal familiarity. His details on the lack of individualized family rooms, separate beds, toiletries and personal space speak volumes as to how Villermé viewed the labouring populations as quintessentially dehumanized and alien. In a notorious passage, Villermé even claimed that workers violated that primal taboo: incest. In his words:

> I would like to add nothing to this detailing of hideous things that set off, at first glance, the profound misery of the unhappy habitants; but I must say that, in many of the beds of which I have just spoken, I saw individuals of both sexes and of different ages laying together, the majority without clothing and in a repulsive dirtiness. Father, mother, the

82   Villermé, *Tableau*, vol. 1, pp. 30–31.
83   Ibid., vol. 1, p. 110.
84   Ibid., vol. 1, p. 103.
85   Ibid., vol. 1, pp. 70–71.
86   Ibid., vol. 1, pp. 128.
87   Ibid., vol. 1, pp. 161.
88   Ibid., vol. 1, pp. 54.
89   Ibid., vol. 1, pp. 58, 60–61.

aged, children, adults, they all squeeze against each other, and are piled upon one another. But I stop myself … [sic] the reader will finish this picture, but I warn him that if he is anxious to be faithful, his imagination mustn't recoil in front of the disgusting mysteries that are carried out on these impure beds, in the midst of darkness and drunkenness.[90]

Dr Littré was correct: cholera had indeed made 'cruel discoveries'. From sickness to incest, the labouring classes appeared inherently diseased and degenerate. Books such as Villermé's *Tableau* suggested that doctors and public authorities couldn't integrate industrial workers into French national life, thereby undermining the cherished aspirations associated with physical and moral hygiene inherited from the previous century. Lifestyle and habitat had become totally pathological; and cholera was only the most virulent symptom.[91] In this manner, sanitarians framed the 'social question' of early industrial France as a public health problem, but they weren't sure whether it could be cured by medical means. Whereas the Idéologue doctors of the French Revolution had wanted to use physical and moral hygiene to regenerate society – and create a new society – post-revolutionary doctors used moral hygiene to establish boundaries between social classes and keep the poor docile and disciplined. They feared that the labouring classes contaminated the entire urban environment and doctors and public authorities needed to quarantine them and clean them up.[92] Here, sanitarians stumbled upon another cruel discovery: this physical and moral degradation was potentially biologically inherited.

Inheritance and degeneration

If habitat predisposed the working classes to cholera, sanitarians reasoned, then perhaps other, more innate biological factors were also to blame. Consequently, heredity increasingly became an important element in discussions about disease aetiology. This hereditarian turn in medical discourse was not necessarily predetermined, but sociopolitical considerations certainly made it useful. Hereditarian ideas first emerged as a public health concern during the last third of the eighteenth century. At this time, a number of physicians and naturalists focused upon innate biological factors that potentially limited human faculties and aptitude. For these thinkers, inherited biological 'types' demonstrated that nature made social hierarchies independently of social and political factors. In other words, people had a natural-born identity – the self, the *moi* – that existed outside any environmental influences. Human nature just *was* and so it would remain. Of course, individuals could degenerate or improve themselves, but only within preordained biological confines. Georges Cuvier expressed a similar belief when he claimed that changing

---

90   Ibid., vol. 1, pp. 83. In a footnote, Villermé declared that two physicians and a police commissioner had verified that 'incest is oftentimes committed' in the working-class household (vol. 1, p. 83 n. 2).

91   On the moral causes of cholera, see J.-J. Virey, *Petit manuel d'hygiène prophylactique contre les épidémies, ou de leurs meilleurs préservatifs* (Paris, 1832); cf. the review by Leuret in *Annales d'hygiène publique et médecine légale* 9 (1833): 235–36.

92   Benoiston de Châteauneuf, *Rapport*, pp. 193–94.

biological 'conditions of existence' caused self-annihilation and species extinction, suggesting that environmental change and individual initiative could not overcome inborn biological realities.

Ironically, the French Revolution had abolished heredity. Between 1789 and 1793, as Jean Borie has argued, revolutionaries dismantled hereditary privilege 'in the name of a *natural* equality founded upon the biological universality of the notion of man'.[93] This belief appears in the constitution of 1793 (arguably the most radical legislative document of the Revolution). Article 28 of the *Déclaration des droits de l'homme et du citoyen* maintained, 'A people maintains the right to review, reform and change its constitution. A generation cannot subordinate future generations to its laws.'[94] The Revolution baptized all citizens and cleansed them of past sins and transgressions; afterwards, all newborn children – at least in a juridical sense – were born free and innocent. But some intellectuals wondered why inequality persisted in French society; others wanted to reinstate social distinctions based upon birth and privilege. In this general context, ideas about 'blood' and 'descent' began to permeate intellectual discussions about the social question in early industrial France.

Here again, cholera intensified beliefs because it forced physicians to ask more pointed questions about the relation between heredity and social difference. In this regard, doctors were motivated by powerful fears of crime, violence and madness in the urban areas.[95] The most concerned doctors were psychiatrists,[96] who framed the question over biological inequalities in terms of an inherited degeneration, something which they called *dégénérescence*.[97]

This idea had important pedigree. Eighteenth-century physicians had argued that degenerative diseases such as syphilis, scurvy, gout, phthisis and scrofula were hereditary and that treatment depended on careful attention to disease patterns within the family's genealogy. Doctors particularly worried about congenital disease and

---

93   Jean Borie, *Mythologies de l'hérédité au XIXe siècle* (Paris, 1981), pp. 11–19.

94   Ibid., pp. 11–12.

95   Cf. the comments in J.-E.-D. Esquirol, 'Mémoire lu dans le séance publique de l'Académie royale de médecine, le 23 juillet 1824: Existe-t-il de nos jours un plus grande nombre de fous qu'il n'en existait il y a quatre ans?' *Mémoires de l'Académie royale de médecine* 1 (1828): 32–50. Esquirol suggested that higher statistical rates of crime and madness, for example, were perhaps due to improved data-collection agencies, rather than merely reflecting a rising crime wave.

96   On the intellectual and social history of French psychiatry, see Robert Castel, *L'ordre psychiatrique: l'âge d'or de l'aliénisme* (Paris, 1976); and especially Jan Goldstein, *Console and Classify: The French Psychiatric Profession in the Nineteenth Century* (Cambridge and New York, 1987).

97   See the superb discussion in Daniel Pick, *Faces of Degeneration: A European Disorder, c. 1848–c. 1918* (Cambridge and New York, 1989); and Sander Gilman and J. Edwards Chamberlin, eds., *Degeneration: The Dark Side of Progress* (New York, 1985). For France, the work of Robert A. Nye remains of singular importance; see his *Crime, Madness, and Politics in Modern France: The Medical Concept of National Decline* (Princeton, 1984), and *Masculinity and Male Codes of Honor in Modern France* (Oxford and New York, 1993).

how patients acquired morbid traits in the process of reproduction and growth.[98] Most observers, such as C.-A. Vandermonde, remained optimistic in their prognosis, claiming that obstetric care and physical education could meliorate many inherited defects. In his lengthy book on nervous disease, Samuel Tissot expressed a generally held faith when he declared that moral hygiene could cure most hereditary vices.[99]

By the turn of the century, however, physicians defined inheritance in broader terms, especially when they discussed insanity and nervous disease.[100] For instance, Philippe Pinel, the venerable father of French psychiatry, suggested that heredity substantially shaped mental disease in his *Traité médico-philosophique sur l'aliénation mentale* (1809). His pupil J.-E.-D. Esquirol, however, expanded his arguments and claimed that inheritance predisposed certain patients to idiocy, alcoholism and mania.[101] These concerns permeated both clinical and private practice. For example, patient registers at the Salpêtrière and Bicêtre hospitals show that doctors asked, whenever possible, about family history, especially in cases of insanity and alcoholism.[102]

Crucially, both naturalists and pathologists had also used the idea of degeneration in their research. Georges-Louis Leclerc de Buffon first used the word to identify how groups or individuals of a specific type deviated from a pristine or primordial form, particularly in cases of domestication.[103] Following the publication of Xavier Bichat's pathbreaking *Recherches physiologiques sur la vie et la mort* (1800), pathologists isolated degenerative processes within specific tissues.[104] Bichat, in effect, put the exterior manifestations of degeneration in the interior spaces of the body. For naturalists, degeneration had caused morphological variation; but for

---

98   On eighteenth-century constructs of heredity, see Carlos López-Beltrán 'Forging Heredity: From Metaphor to Cause, a Reification Story', *Studies in the History and Philosophy of Science* 25 (1994): 211–35; and my 'Inheriting Vice, Acquiring Virtue: Hereditary Disease and Moral Hygiene in Eighteenth-Century France', *Bulletin of the History of Medicine* 80 (2006): 649–76.

99   Samuel Tissot, *Traité des nerfs et de leurs maladies* (5 vols, Paris, 1778), vol. 3, pp. 5–14, 20–25, vol. 4, pp. 459–60.

100   See Antoine Portal, *Considérations sur la nature et le traitement des maladies de famille et des maladies héréditaires, et sur les moyens les mieux éprouvés de les prévenir*, 3d edn (Paris, 1814); and A. Petit, *Essai sur les maladies héréditaires, considérées sous les rapports de leur nature, de leur origine ou formation* (Paris, 1817).

101   Philippe Pinel, *Traité médico-philosophique sur l'aliénation mentale*, 2d edn (Paris, 1809), pp. 13, 46; and J.-E.-D. Esquirol, *Des maladies mentales* (Paris, 1838), pp. 64, 341, 683.

102   See 6 R 21 Salpêtrière, Registres d'observations médicales, 5e division, 2e section (1815–51), nos. 299, 357, 358, 388, 451; 6 R 1 Salpêtrière, Registres d'observations médicales, 5e division, 1e section (1820–51), nos. 34, 43, 67, 293; 6 R 3 Salpêtrière, Registres d'observations médicales (1835–52), nos. 119, 155, 156, 159, 239, 263, 324, 340; 6 R 1 Bicêtre, Registres d'observations, 5e division, 2e section (1818–53), nos. 27, 81, 88, 98, 127, 152, 169, 175, 292, 303, 317, 352, 378. Diagnoses increased after the 1820s.

103   G.-L. Leclerc de Buffon, *Oeuvres complètes* (32 vols, Paris, 1825–28), vol. 19, pp. 1–114.

104   Xavier Bichat's work on degeneration had a racial tinge, as he said that blacks were internally and externally degenerated; see *Anatomie générale, appliquée à la physiologie et à la médecine* (4 vols, Paris, 1801), vol. 4, 657–59, 763–66.

Bichat, it caused internal anomalies and lesions and became a factor in disease. Following Bichat, doctors now examined the patient's body for pathological signs of hereditary degeneration. In fact, dating from the advent of vitalist physiology in France in the second half of the eighteenth century, medical researchers said that the nervous system – the 'centre of government in the individual body' – caused all these degenerative diseases.[105]

These developments influenced medical theories of hereditary degeneration in a number of ways. Foremost, early and mid-century hygienists and alienists hoped to realign public health and psychiatric studies with the dominant regularities of organic medicine. Under the leadership of Claude Bertrand and his experimental followers, physicians sought to discover material causes for pathological processes. Psychiatry, for example, was no exception to this trend. Psychiatrists thus wanted to find the causes of mental illness in the anatomical recesses of the body. For researchers well-versed in microscopy, the key to this organic validity lay in the morbid appearances of the nervous tissue.[106] This was an important change. Now, doctors saw the nerves as a palimpsest upon which an inherited identity inscribed itself. As one physician explained in 1843:

> [The nervous] system is acted upon by exterior objects and reacts. It proves itself the agent of a power that is intermediary to impression and reaction. It is simultaneously the seat of sensibility, material instrument of intelligence and will, and the source of movement. If [the nervous system] is very developed and if it predominates in the [animal] economy over other systems, it shall necessarily result that sensations will be more lively, delicate, profound and numerous; moral activity will be greater; and muscular mobility shall be more readily activated, more rapid, or more energetic.[107]

As a result, doctors insisted that reproductive strategies could meliorate immorality and sedition, since they feared that hereditary diseases were largely incurable and were thus beyond immediate therapeutic skills.[108] Procreation became the ultimate signifier of the biological individual's past and present health, an event which encapsulated their entire physical and moral existence leading up to that point. Given that everything was potentially at stake, in terms of the individual and future descent, patients should never leave reproductive health to chance: the essential elements became self-control and foresight. These demands were fine for members of the urban bourgeoisie, who could be largely trusted to manage lifestyle and sexuality in

---

105 J.-J. Virey, *De la physiologie dans ses rapports avec la philosophie* (Paris, 1844), p. 310. Prosper Lucas discussed this issue in his *Traité physiologique et philosophique de l'hérédité dans les états de santé et de maladie du système nerveux* (2 vols, Paris, 1848–50), vol. 2, pp. 670–02.

106 See Nye, *Masculinity*, pp. 74–75; and John E. Lesch, *Science and Medicine in France: The Emergence of Experimental Physiology, 1790–1855* (Cambridge, MA, 1984), pp. 197–224.

107 M. E. Guitrac, 'Mémoire sur l'influence de l'hérédité sur la production de l surexcitation nerveuse, sur les maladies qui en résultent, et des moyens de les guérir', *Mémoires de l'Académie royale de médecine* 11 (1845): 193–382 (at p. 212).

108 AM 259, Moreau de Tours, 'Mémoire sur les causes prédisposantes héréditaires de l'idiotie et de l'imbécillité', 4 Jan. 1853.

an appropriate matter. However, this was not necessarily the case with the labouring classes and the urban poor. For this reason, several physicians urged the government to aggressively promote sexual hygiene and family planning amongst the lower levels of French society. As Dr Brémont de Valuejols explained:

> If our resources are hardly efficacious against hereditary diseases which have already developed, it would be essential to prohibit their transmission; without doubt, the first, the most direct and the most powerful of our means would consist in suitably furnishing the nuptial couch, since one can at will (so to speak) degrade or perfect the organization of man, as one can degrade or perfect that of domestic animals. However, the doctor is almost never consulted when his advice would be so useful, since he could neutralize the evil by attacking at its source, when it would be so easy for him to indicate what the temperament, intelligence and constitution of the individual ought to be that when [he] is choosing [a partner], so to remove organic conditions, or even to counteract those which exist in the person carrying the sinister disposition of a hereditary malady.[109]

Within this highly charged intellectual context, Dr Prosper Lucas published his massive *Traité physiologique et philosophique de l'hérédité* between 1847 and 1850. This pivotal book established the mid-century medical position on heredity and sexual hygiene. Despite Lucas's apparent obscurity – he wrote his medical thesis on the question of moral contagion and later penned a short book on education – his *Traité de l'hérédité* was one of the most influential scientific treatises of the nineteenth century, inspiring Charles Darwin and literary figures ranging from Jules Michelet to Émile Zola.[110] Historians often credit Lucas with providing the psychiatric model of degeneration, although he scarcely used the term or provided a precise definition for it.[111] Rather, Lucas wanted to explore the relation between heredity disease and public health, and he hoped to establish a causal link between neurological disorder and morbid inheritance. Indeed, this particular problem consumed nearly a third of his 1,500-page work. On the one hand, Lucas sympathized with pathologists who said that nervous pathology caused all hereditary and congenital disorders. On the other hand, he disagreed with those psychiatrists who claimed that heredity caused all forms of insanity. Lucas thus alternated between the two schools of psychiatric treatment: the first which emphasized the moral causes of mental sickness and the intrinsic qualities of therapeutic treatment, and the second which looked for medicinal remedies and specific pathological processes in insanity.[112]

Beyond these therapeutic concerns, Lucas also had a social agenda. According to him, heredity dominated all debates over the 'physical and moral' nature of man, and

---

109 Brémont de Valuejols, *Essai sur les maladies héréditaires, considérées sous les rapports de leur nature et des théories dont elles ont été le sujet* (Paris, 1832), p. 16.

110 For Lucas's place in the health movement, see Erwin Ackerknecht, *Medicine at the Paris Hospital, 1794–1848* (Baltimore, 1967), p. 160; and on Lucas and the mid-century conception of heredity, see Frederick B. Churchill, 'From Heredity Theory to *Vererbung*: The Transmission Problem, 1850–1915', *Isis* 78 (1987): 337–64 (at pp. 342–43).

111 Note, however, that Lucas insisted degenerates were 'réjetées par leur nature, par leur origine, par leur cause, de la sphère du type spécifique, les maladies rentrent donc, sans exception, dans celle du type individuelle'; Lucas, *Traité*, vol. 2, p. 512.

112 Ibid., vol. 2, p. 755.

it shaped human nature and society itself. 'Physicians, philosophes or legislators', he declared, 'they have simply but largely grasped its influence on the being; they have placed the principle within the first source of physical nature and all states of health and disease.'[113] From the opening of his work, Lucas associated heredity and civil society and he evinced strong bourgeois sensibilities. For him, heredity offered a new set of natural laws to govern society, and he interpreted these laws in the broadest possible manner. Accordingly, doctors should consider heredity in its 'natural' and its 'institutional' bases. The first assured the 'physical and moral characters of our existence'; and the second concerned 'rights and goods', finding its origins 'in society and ... the laws of the State'.[114] As he explained:

> the generating principle of every convention that takes a character of universality and permanence is always nature; and from the instant where we recognize in the institution of *hérédité* this same character, we shall not limit ourselves to say there exists in this great phenomena a relation of descent [*origine*] between *nature* and the *institution*. In our profound faith, always, in these cases, *it is from the vital fact that the social fact proceeds*, we say, in our eyes, this relation is one of cause and effect. The cause is *nature*, the effect is the *institution*; the first is the principle, the second is only the expression, the application and the consequence; the *hérédité* of *nature* becomes in a word, for us, the primordial reason and the true source of the *hérédité* of the institution ... . In the institution, we want, like everything else these days, to trace its legitimacy from its source and scrutinize it to its base; one must trace [it] to nature, in which only virtue, substance and the life of the law resides.[115]

Note his usage: 'It is from the vital fact that the social fact proceeds.' Like other physicians, Lucas assumed that the same natural laws that governed the individual body also governed society; but in this case, he literally *congenitalized* the social body, putting laws, institutions and civil society itself under the long shadow of genealogy and descent. Lucas was not unique. In the years following the 1848 Revolutions, many prominent intellectuals sought the basis of social authority in the natural laws of heredity. The implications were not always comforting. At a meeting of the Academy of Moral and Political Sciences, Villermé and Benoiston de Châteauneuf presented a statistical study of noble genealogies (including the Bourbon heirs), suggesting that interclass marriages and ubiquitous transfer of aristocratic titles had debased the noble 'races' and bloodlines. The inference was clear. As noble bloodlines faded, traditional social hierarchies and values had also faded. Benoiston de Châteauneuf concluded:

> We see that noble families, and above all those whose origins can be traced back to removed times, have only continued to the present not on account of their line but because

---

113 Ibid., vol. 1, p. vii.
114 Ibid., vol. 1, pp. 3–4.
115 Ibid., vol. 1, pp. 4–5. I have retained usage of the French word *hérédité*, for, as it should be clear, the term held a precise signification and raised particular connotations in the mid-nineteenth century mind about status and solidity, and was central to Lucas's – and later B. A. Morel's – conceptions of inheritance.

of their name, which is older than the majority of their pedigree, and [is perpetuated] with the help of fictions of every species and by [mixing] with foreign families.[116]

Cholera had intensified upper-class anxieties, but everything changed after the 1848–52 Revolutions. After the intense violence and vicious class warfare, intellectuals revised their liberal faith in progress, doubting that society could ever progress to a higher stage, let alone to get along. One extreme example of this deepening pessimism is Arthur de Gobineau's *Essai sur l'inégalité des races humaines* (1853–55), a book which is arguably the founding text of modern racist ideology. In this sprawling text, Gobineau dramatically reconceptualized traditional society in the wake of Revolution and civil war. To be sure, Gobineau's belief that racial interbreeding and degeneracy had caused the demise of the Notables, mass democracy and proletarian revolution did not sit well with his compatriots.[117] Nevertheless, his work suggests that contemporary anxieties about the values attached to blood, descent and sexuality ran very deep. More often than not, intellectual elites again picked up the cry that this new physical and moral crisis contaminated that basic element of society: the family. Much like post-Thermidorean thinkers after the Reign of Terror, social conservatives again dreamed about regenerating family values in order to provide law-and-order solutions. As the Romantic historian Michelet explained it:

> In 1849, when our social tragedies had just broken our hearts, the air was filled with a terrible cold; it seemed that our blood had been drained from our veins. In presence of the phenomena which seemed to be the extinction of all life, I called upon that little heat that still remained; I invoked, with the help of laws, a renovation of morals, a purification of love and the family.[118]

Where Lucas's ideas differed from earlier thinkers such as C.-A. Vandermonde or Pierre Cabanis was that Lucas juxtaposed an older fear – sexual degeneracy – and a new panic – proletarian revolution – and thus telescoped bourgeois anxieties in an unprecedented way. When discussing heredity, Lucas implicitly raised the spectre of communism and working-class barricades. Hence, Lucas argued that heredity remained a central force (and therefore a legitimate object of social/scientific inquiry) in the transmission of property (the basis of social order), of sovereignty (the basis of political succession) and even civil society (art, literature, science and industry). Lest his readers miss the point, he emphasized that heredity 'is a *law*, a *force* and a *fact*, and this fact is one of the greatest marvels of existence; and this force, the force of organization and this law, the law that seems to govern, produce, propagate and multiply everything, is the law of creation, of the propagation of life'.[119]

For these reasons, Lucas insisted that the French government should take prophylactic steps to eliminate criminal lineages and discourage fertility in

---

116 Benoiston de Châteauneuf, 'Mémoire sur la durée des familles nobles de France', *Annales d'hygiène publique et médecine légale* 25 (1846): 27–58 (at p. 30).

117 On how the 1848 Revolutions influenced medical and cultural thought, see Pick, *Faces of Degeneration*.

118 Jules Michelet, *L'amour* (1858; Paris, 1923), pp. 24–25.

119 Lucas, *Traité*, vol. 1, p. 6.

congenitally ill families.[120] As for present morbidity and mortality amongst urban workers, Lucas conceded that doctors and public authorities could meliorate urban conditions through hygiene and welfare reform. Unfortunately, just as soon as physicians had introduced health and sanitary reforms, unfathomable pathogenic entities could arrive again, most likely from the Orient.[121]

To explain these beliefs, Lucas offered a broad theory of heredity. In his study of growth and reproduction, Lucas identified two opposite mechanisms: dissimilarity and resemblance. These mechanisms formed the two basic laws of reproduction: *innéité* and *hérédité*. For Lucas, *innéité* created all organic variation and governed how the embryo developed. *Innéité*, above all, showed that procreation was an unpredictable (if not fickle) force in nature. By contrast, *hérédité* constantly reproduced the specific type and it governed stasis and predictable form. Thus, *hérédité* reproduced of the totality of the body.[122] Whilst *innéité* appeared as a creative (and potentially destructive) force in nature, *hérédité* preserved the original fixity of species, races, families and individuals.

Lucas struggled to explain how people transmitted characteristics they had acquired under the variable forces of *innéité*. Early in his work, he had drawn upon Cuvier's work to articulate his own belief in independent creation and the fixity of all species. Nevertheless, Lucas conceded that individuals could inherit changes, anomalies and mutilations under specific circumstances, although he stressed that these acquired changes could not alter organic form beyond the original species imprint. Individuals inherited acquired characteristics, but under precise conditions. These involved the so-called essence of the modification, the genealogical precedent for the modification and the continued action of the 'original cause'. Moreover, a number of environmental factors – education, discipline, exercise, nutrition, milieu and climate – influenced how individuals reproduced acquired anomalies.[123] Lucas concluded:

> Under the duality of the primordial laws of generation, we rediscover the two greatest principles of natural history: that of the eternal fixity of species, that of the eternal mutability of individuals; they do not merely offer a seminal expression: they give the theory of the ways and means of the perpetuity of these two great principles, across the infinite succession of beings, across the infinite revolutions of centuries and places.[124]

These observations notwithstanding, Lucas claimed that both *innéité* and environmental 'conditions of existence' (more so than *hérédité* itself) could keep on making diseases and anomalies appear in a given population. In essence, organisms mutated less because they could inherit acquired characters than because they could uniformly adapt to powerful environmental forces. By stressing that organisms

---

120 Ibid., vol. 2, p. 446.

121 Lucas was thinking of the cholera epidemics (both in 1832 and 1849); ibid., vol. 2, pp. 867–68. On his views on *fécondité*, see especially vol. 1, pp. 480–531, and vol. 2, pp. 909–29.

122 Ibid., vol. 1, p. 238.

123 Ibid., vol. 1, pp. 66–67, vol. 2, pp. 436–37, 893–95.

124 Ibid., vol. 2, pp. 900–01.

reacted in dynamic ways to conditions of existence, Lucas thus suggested that a constant environment could make organisms change in consistent ways. This could manifest itself in either positive ways – progressive adaptation – or negative ways – degeneracy and decline. In this case, *innéité* obeyed the same regular laws as *hérédité*.[125]

Lucas changed how doctors thought about heredity, human nature and society. A decade later another publication cemented these associations. In 1857, almost two years before Charles Darwin changed the face of biology with his *On the Origin of Species*, a reticent French country physician and psychiatrist, Bénédict-Auguste Morel, also produced a work that engendered massive discussion and a proliferation of writings in European medical, anthropological and biological communities. Whereas critics attacked Darwin for what they believed was a brutal, mechanistic model of struggle and evolutionary change, many scientific authorities praised Morel's *Traité des dégénérescences* for explaining what seemed to be cultural rot and social unrest. Degeneration theory, often framed as a psychiatric model of mental illness, enveloped scientific, political and cultural communities alike, and dominated the debates over heredity, insanity and criminology in the broader European context.[126]

Though historians often discuss Morel in tandem with fin-de-siècle fears of decadence and degeneracy, what I want to stress here is how his work grew out of the long-standing discourse about physical and moral hygiene, and that his ideas about *dégénérescences* directly engaged the sweeping changes affecting socio-medical thought between 1832 and 1848. In this manner, Morel's complex book directly combined both Villermé's outrage over lower-class immorality with Lucas's perspective on hereditary predisposition. Like Lucas, too, Morel hoped to classify neurological diseases in a grand nosological sweep. Though Lucas had avoided a taxonomy of nervous afflictions based solely upon hereditary predisposition, Morel declared in the introduction to his work:

> I now believe that the insane enclosed in our asylums are only, in the majority of cases, representatives of certain unhealthy varieties in the species, modifiable in certain circumstances and unmodifiable in others. Whatever may remain of their original affliction, they are all more or less stricken by this degenerative state that presents them, under observation, with the majority of characteristics proper to diseases of long duration, and under which the indubitable influence of hereditary disposition dominates.[127]

In this manner, Morel pushed medical ideas about heredity and opened a new area of medical and psychiatric research. He defined degeneration as an elusive, all-

---

125 Ibid., vol. 2, pp. 437–44.

126 On Morel and degeneration, see Ruth Friedlander, 'Bénédict-Auguste Morel and the Development of the Theory of Dégénérescence (The Introduction of Anthropology into Psychiatry)' (PhD thesis, University of California at San Francisco, 1973); and on broader cultural receptions, see Ian Dowbiggin, *Inheriting Madness: Professionalization and Psychiatric Knowledge in Nineteenth-Century France* (Berkeley, 1991); Pick, *Faces of Degeneration*; and Nye, *Crime*.

127 B.-A. Morel, *Traité des dégénérescences physiques, intellectuelles et morales de l'espèce humaine, et des causes qui produisent ces variétés maladives* (Paris, 1857), p. vi.

encompassing biological force that exerted powerful and disruptive influence over all organisms, explaining the 'origins and formations' of 'the natural and the unhealthy varieties in the human species'.[128] For Morel, *dégénérescence* caused more than mental disease; rather, his target was 'that state of profound moral malaise' found in 'modern society'.[129] One fundamental part of this 'profound moral malaise' stemmed from the so-called dangerous classes, and they required a new form of moral and sexual hygiene to control its spread. As he described it:

> In midst of this so civilized society exist veritable varieties ... which possess neither the intelligence of duty, nor the sentiment of morality of action, and which their spirit is not susceptible of being enlightened nor consoled by any idea of religious order. Several of these varieties have been rightly designated under the name *dangerous classes*. Everything that we have said ... tends to demonstrate the importance of studying the causes that lead the individual to physical and moral degradation, constituting a state of permanent danger for society.[130]

In fact, hereditary degeneration caused the entire gauntlet of social woes wrought by industrialization, such as black lung, lead poisoning, tuberculosis, venereal disease and alcoholism.[131] This degraded environment subsequently contaminated the genital organs and reproduced itself across generations.[132] Morel returned to urban debauchery and concluded:

> The working classes are equally, in many cases, the involuntary victims of hard necessities that bring forth misery and the disorder in intellectual, moral and religious education. Their physical health, compromised as much by the nature of their work as by the excess to which they abandon themselves, is reflected in the constitution of their children and incessantly tends to perpetuate and transmit itself with the type a progressive physical and moral degradation.
>
> It is therefore under thousands and thousands of diverse forms, more or less scientific, and consequently more or less in relation with the results of pure medical observation, that the application of moral hygiene must be made.[133]

Therefore, the incidence of disease, insanity, immorality and social unrest ultimately proved how degenerative the environment of working-class France had become. As Daniel Pick has shown, Morel's treatise contained 'hidden' narratives of pathology, as he imagined that modern life was inundated with a flood of diseases, perversities, madness and deviance. As he put it, families could accumulate degenerative materials just like other families accumulated wealth and titles.[134] Morel gave a bleak prognosis. In some case studies, the first generation afflicted with *dégénérescence* became

---

128 Ibid., pp. ix, xiii.

129 Ibid., p. 461.

130 Ibid., p. 461 n. 1.

131 Ibid., pp. 57–58.

132 Ibid., p. 72.

133 Ibid., p. 688.

134 B.-A. Morel, *De l'hérédité morbide progressive ou des types dissemblables et disparates dans la famille* (Paris, 1867), pp. 4–5.

immoral, depraved and drunken. The second generation suffered from hereditary alcoholism, delusional mania and occasional paralysis. The third generation enjoyed some relief, appearing more sober; but they were often hypochondriacs, suffered from paranoia and displayed homicidal urges. The final generation of degenerates evidenced low intelligence, adolescent madness, stupidity, idiotism and sterility. In this spiralling decline, Morel discovered a natural mechanism that produced heritable, 'maladive' variations within the species – a degeneration that caused the race to become sterile and, finally, extinct.[135]

Morel's analysis, however, evinced strong biblicist assumptions. If *dégénérescence* was the 'unhealthy deviation of the normal type of humanity', he had trouble defining what precisely constituted the actual 'normal type'.[136] To deal with this problem, he speculated that degeneration was the inevitable result of the fall of man from his original Adamic stock and the moral and physical stigmata of original sin. Consequently, he defined the normal type by appealing to Thomist theology. He readily identified with Buffon's belief in the unity of all humankind and Cuvier's insistence on the fixity of species and individual types. Whereas Morel's *Traité* provided a totally naturalistic theory of degeneration, he still believed that the fall from Eden corrupted man's health and all subsequent endeavours.[137] Therefore, Morel's idea of *dégénérescence*, so critical to later biomedical thinking on inheritance and deviance, interpreted biological maladaptation through the lens of Christian theology.

But Morel wasn't out of the scientific mainstream. Quite the contrary. To explain this negative evolutionary force, he stated that physicians should broaden their scientific horizons and study the mechanisms of inheritance:

> Without a doubt, to understand the formation and the evolution of the degenerative principle and its relationship to heritable influences, it is just to give to the word *hérédité* [emphasis in original] a definition much larger than that we have ordinarily assigned to it.[138]

Morel further argued that, given a pathological environment, people could inherit variations acquired during growth and reproduction. He eschewed Lucas's more tenuous conclusions:

> We do not exclusively understand by *hérédité* the same malady that has been transmitted from parents to children in its development and with the identity of symptoms of the physical and moral order observed in the ascendants; we understand under the word *hérédité* the transmission of organic dispositions from parents to children. It is not necessary ... to demonstrate the existence of this transmission, that the diseases of parents might be *reproduced identically* in children: it suffices that the latter are endowed with

---

135 Morel, *Traité*, pp. 116–30, 386.

136 B.-A. Morel, *De la formation du type dans les variétés dégénérés ou nouveaux éléments d'anthropologie morbide* (Paris, 1864), pp. 2–3.

137 Morel, *Traité*, pp. 1–2, 2 n. 1. This point was not lost on contemporary critics, who were quick to point on the theological underpinning of Morel's work. See Dally and Robin, 'Dégénérescence', *Dictionnaire encyclopédique des sciences médicales*, ed. A. Deschambre et al. (100 vols, Paris, 1864–89), vol. 26, pp. 212–54 (at p. 213).

138 Morel, *Traité*, p. 565.

an unfortunate organic predisposition that becomes the departure point for pathological transformations that the connection and reciprocal dependence produce new unhealthy entities, whether in the physical order, whether in the moral order, and often in the two orders reunited.[139]

In Morel's schema, therefore, the pathological milieu and the force of *innéité* allowed individuals to acquire diseases and anomalies that were consistently reproduced under the forces of *hérédité*. As parents acquired degenerative habits and sicknesses, they predisposed their children to disease, and these malignancies then intensified in subsequent generations. He did not, however, precisely explain how these pathologies were transmitted, nor did he localize these degenerative properties in post-mortem studies.

In stark prose and resigned despair, Morel charted how the labouring and dangerous classes declined into squalor, degradation and ignominious extinction. In his eyes, *dégénérescence* spread beyond its original class specificity, contaminating all of society. Whereas Xavier Bichat had identified life as the sum of parts that resisted the anarchy of death, Morel believed that the social body resisted decay from within and without. With his bleak commentary, Morel reversed the positivistic thought and advanced social theory of writers such as Henri de Saint-Simon, Auguste Comte, Charles Fourier and Louis Blanc. Clearly, Morel epitomized a generation that had literally exhausted itself on ideas of progress.[140]

Between hygienists such as Villermé, Lucas and Morel, what do we have when we examine this mid-century perspective on identity and inheritance? In metaphysical terms, Morel exposed post-lapsarian man's descent into depravity and destruction. His *dégénérescence* inverted William Paley's natural theology; but for Morel, disease, not the marvels of nature, revealed the ultimate designs of the creator. Not surprisingly, both Lucas and Morel rejected Lamarckianism and accepted Cuvier's essentialistic notion of species. Like many mid-century physicians, however, Lucas and Morel conceded that that patients could inherit some acquired anomalies, particularly if the environment exerted a constant and measured force on individuals.

More importantly, hereditary degeneration forcefully crystallized post-cholera fears surrounding industrialization, urbanization and proletarianization. Morel gave doctors a new tool to explain the moral and physical degradation of the lower classes; Morel explained, in mechanistic terms, how immorality became contagious within the factory and the foyer. In a bizarre contradiction, degeneration still expressed an underlying assumption of the early nineteenth-century hygienists: whilst civilization may well create destitution and disease, it nevertheless gave doctors the tools to eliminate the origins of such distress. The frontispiece of *Traité de dégénérescences* advertised Morel's proposed sequel, a volume entitled *Hygiène physique et morale, traité théorique et pratique de toutes les indications curatives de l'ordre intellectuel, physique et moral, capable de prévenir et de combattre les causes des dégénérescences dans l'espèce humaine*. Morel died in 1875, never having completed his promised work on the new means of regeneration.

---

139 Ibid.
140 Pick, *Faces of Degeneration*, pp. 11–27; and Nye, *Masculinity*, p. 73.

Conclusion

By mid-century, then, physical and moral hygiene had fragmented under new ideological, socioeconomic and epidemiological pressures. In 1832, the cholera outbreak accelerated this shift, focusing medical attention upon perceived biological factors that caused disease, dearth and death. Doctors explored these new ideas when they discussed urban conditions of existence and congenital maladaptation; crucially, they now doubted the benefits of demographic growth, preferring to see society as characterized by a struggle for limited resources. But doctors did not simply respond to pathological conditions and social stratification within Parisian society, as Louis Chevalier argued in his famous study.[141] Rather, the preceding analysis has suggested that ideas about degeneracy and worker fertility were part of a continuing debate about physical and moral hygiene, one that originated back in the mid-Enlightenment. Here, doctors were revising established ideas about the social body, substituting a new vision of a society divided by innate biological qualities – themes that were explored, in different ways, by Prosper Lucas and B.-A Morel.

After the 1848 Revolutions, the bloody tragedies, political reaction and intellectual despair forced many doctors to reject their basic ideas about physical and moral hygiene. Of course, some doctors still hoped that social medicine could cure sociopolitical crises. But not all agreed they could regenerate the nation at large – or that they should want to do so. As these doctors warned, human nature could not be changed for the better and society was ridden with conflict. Reforming doctors had stumbled upon intractable problems: human heredity and hostile 'conditions of existence'.[142] Consequently, many health activists now believed that innate biological qualities determined human nature; the self, for them, was something fundamentally embodied and could not be changed in radical fashion. In so doing, doctors overturned the Revolutionary meanings of 'physical and moral hygiene' – both for self-perfection and social improvement – by saying that personal, physical and moral improvement was impossible for large segments of the social body. Social improvement was to be effected by careful surgical strikes – targeting key groups in circumspect ways – rather than broader social reform and regeneration.

---

141 Louis Chevalier *Classes laborieuses et classes dangereuses à Paris pendant la première moité du XIXe siècle* (1958; Paris, 1984).

142 Pick, *Faces of Degeneration*, p. 59; and Borie, *Mythologies*.

Conclusion: Degeneration and Regeneration after 1850

During the Age of Revolution, medicine acquired unprecedented political, social and cultural centrality in modern France, both at home and in its colonies. In this period, a quintessential middle-class occupation – medicine – came to represent the middle-class social order that emerged from the dual revolution in economics and politics. Doctors became the primary spokesmen for bourgeois values because they defined key ideas about human nature, sexuality and the social order in France. At the same time, medicine changed how contemporaries thought about themselves and their surrounding world; it allowed them to explain complex social phenomena in general and issues relating to the individual body, health and pathology in particular. Fearing degeneracy and demographic decline, elites used medicine to understand bewildering social and political changes and give themselves agency and control over these events. Concerns over the morbid social body, in turn, shaped law and policy in modern France, such as public health, public assistance, administrative agencies, population policy and the civil code itself.

This medical involvement in public and private life raises far-reaching questions about politics, socioeconomic change, and class and gender relations in modern France. Between 1750 and 1850, revolutionary forces overturned absolutist, feudal and theological systems and thereby provoked a crisis in established values. As a result, contemporaries sought new forms of cultural meaning and authority, especially those structuring class and sexual hierarchies. For intellectual elites, medicine offered an objective and disinterested system of knowledge that allowed them to mediate social change through domestic and government controls. As doctors taught them, human nature was shaped by a complex interplay of physical and moral determinants. Within biological limits, the self was open-ended, dynamic and malleable; both nature and nurture contributed to individual development and aptitude. Through these physiological insights, doctors abstracted an ideal social world that promoted health and harmony, one that was characterized by self-control, domesticity and social interdependence. Doctors called this model 'physical and moral hygiene'.

As we have seen, physical and moral hygiene comprised several interdependent levels. On the first level, physiological science gave doctors a working model of health and pathology from which they deduced the practices to treat the health of the nation. Paradoxically, doctors hoped this social hygiene would help contemporaries distinguish between social class and – simultaneously – inculcate a shared sense of national belonging and interdependence amongst all social classes. In this manner, medicine could shape collective attitudes, marking society with a kind of 'sameness', whilst also acknowledging differences in social status, sexuality and even race. Second, health activists identified what they considered to be the natural relations between men and women and the proper organization of domestic life. They claimed that no child should be left behind: they outlined a child's physical education and emphasized the mother as the conduit of child health and happiness. At the same time, these practitioners advised their patients on marital choices and prescribed guidelines for good sexual hygiene to maintain fertility and good breeding. Finally, they hoped to spread this health gospel through the general population with sage legislation, instruction and public assistance. Medicine, said health activists, promoted a new civism. Good health created moral virtue, patriotism and social cohesion.

As we have seen, the idea of physical and moral hygiene underwent three distinct phases. During the first period, which lasted between 1750 and 1789, doctors developed a new model of human nature and social amelioration, using it to attack the luxury and libertinism associated with upper-class society. According to doctors such as Antoine Le Camus, Brouzet de Béziers, C.-A. Vandermonde, Samuel Tissot and Pierre Roussel – to name only the most prominent – immorality and decadent behaviour had caused nervous disease, infant mortality and infertility. At the same time, medical reformers believed that the lower classes were mired in filth and destitution and desperately needed public assistance and instruction. Taken together, these trends had caused the French population to degenerate and decline. To repair this sorry state of affairs, in 1776, the royal government took the important step of creating the Royal Society of Medicine under Félix Vicq d'Azyr, a step that offered the most important policy response to these perceived threats.

During the second period, which lasted between 1789 and 1804, doctors participated in the political effort to regenerate the body politic during the French Revolution. For their part, doctors wanted to make a rejuvenated, sanitary utopia that could transform society through physical and moral hygiene, both in France and its colonies. But this radical vision did not last. After the Reign of Terror, physicians such as Pierre Cabanis and Xavier Bichat developed a more conservative view of human nature. Doubting human aptitude for change, their followers hoped that domestic hygiene and instruction could inculcate moderate republican values and reconstruct social authority along paternalist lines – views that came to fruition with the adoption of the Napoleonic Code in 1804.

During the final period, which lasted between 1804 and 1848, medical views on human nature and improvement fragmented under the pressures of industrialization, urbanization and continued political radicalism. Social medical thought divided between pragmatists such as Paul Mahon and F.-E. Fodéré, who espoused a law-and-order *médecine politique*; reformers such as J.-J. Virey and Philippe Buchez, who sought a Rousseauvian or social-Christian regeneration of society; and new sanitarians such as L.-F. Benoiston de Châteauneuf and L.-R. Villermé, who espoused Malthusian social policies and incorporated statistical methods into their health studies. The turning point was the 1832 cholera epidemic. Sanitarians now hoped to inculcate morality and fertility controls within the labouring classes, claiming that the poor were predisposed to disease and disorder. Following the 1848 Revolutions, doctors such as Prosper Lucas and B.-A. Morel advanced new theories of hereditary degeneration to explain social disease and dysfunction.

Throughout, a series of health panics about degeneracy and demographic patterns drove ideas about physical and moral hygiene. In many ways, the fears and anxieties remained the same, but the causes, targeted groups, and consequences changed over time. In general terms, scholars have often disagreed on what concrete factors spark deep-seated panics about degeneracy and demographic decline. For Michel Foucault, degeneration helped the bourgeoisie impose their ideas about the body upon the general population; by contrast, for Daniel Pick, it responded to deep-seated anxieties about socioeconomic and political change in post-1848 Europe.[1] According to other historians, however, degeneracy fears are less nebulous and often appear in concrete ways following wars, national disasters or failed reforms. In Britain, for example, J. R. Seale has argued that concerns about bodily inadequacy and national efficiency emerged after the Boer War, just when public authorities and intellectuals concluded that progressive social reforms hadn't improved lower-class conditions. In the United States, as Chris Shilling has shown, degeneracy fears appeared following the full-scale draft in World War I and subsequent revelations about sexually-transmitted diseases, IQ levels and other anthropomorphic data generated by standardized examinations.[2] Given all these complex variables, J. Edward Chamberlain and Sander Gilman have emphasized that degeneration was often polyvalent and contradictory in its meanings: 'Degeneration was one of the most uncertain of notions, and – like some viruses – the most difficult to isolate. The idea of degeneration could comfortably be caught up in the tapestry of ambivalence, to be sure, and whether it was conceived as warp or woof could be a matter of taste.'[3]

Yet, by mapping the broader contours of physical and moral hygiene, we can identify key correspondences between health activism, health panics and broader sociopolitical and cultural anxieties. In this sense, degeneration theories responded to powerful social changes, but these theories also promoted political activism, forcing public officials and moral crusaders to act and try to control the threatening situation. Health activists, in this case, set about finding the ways to regenerate the sick body politic and creating public and private initiatives to do so. In France, at least in the period covered here, health activism expressed itself in various ways: the concerns over libertinism, luxury and fashionable women and children after the War of Austrian Succession and the Seven Years War; concerns about country people and urban tradesmen in a period of reform and heightened sociopolitical expectations after the Turgot ministry; the desire to regenerate the body politic to make moderate and responsible citizens following war, violence and social upheaval during the French Revolution; and the desire to control lower-class behaviour following urbanization, industrialization and continued political radicalism in the post-revolutionary period.

Given these different examples, we might characterize health crusaders as 'social strata fighting on two fronts'. Sociologists use this term to describe how middling

1   Daniel Pick, *Faces of Degeneration: A European Disorder, c. 1848–c. 1918* (Cambridge and New York, 1989), p. 2.

2   J. R. Searle, *Eugenics and Politics in Britain, 1900–1914* (Leyden, 1976), pp. 9, 20; and Chris Shilling, *The Body and Social Theory* (London, 1993), p. 30.

3   J. Edward Chamberlain and Sander Gilman, *Degeneration: The Dark Side of Progress* (New York, 1985), p. xiii.

social groups who seek social power and cultural legitimacy can wage a cultural war against groups who are both above and below them on the social ladder. According to Norbert Elias, these groups often carry on this struggle outside the political realm, and frame their social concerns or grievances in explicit moral terms. Of course, as this struggle continues, the middle strata can become more direct and even antagonistic, explicitly confronting their opponents and stating their concrete agendas in no uncertain terms.[4] As Klaus Theweleit further notes, these groups often see themselves as the ultimate defenders of moral and cultural values, setting up an ascetic lifestyle to contrast the perceived decadence of the rich and privileged, on the one hand, and the deviant and disorderly ways of the lower classes, on the other. In this manner, middling orders turn themselves into the standard-bearers of a 'new morality' – a set of values and behaviour they expect the rest of society to follow and upon which they base their own claims to social power and authority.[5]

These theoretical models provide insight to explain what motivated doctors in their ideas about degeneration, regeneration and health politics in France between roughly 1750 and 1850. Health activists fought a health battle against both the elite and poor classes, but here framed moral concerns in biomedical ideas and language. In the old regime, under the stress of foreign war and internal political crises, health crusaders self-consciously picked up the mantle of patriotic and moral values and demanded that fashionable elites mend their decadent ways. According to them, luxury, libertinism and gender confusion had weakened the body and caused an epidemic of nervous disease – an epidemic that sapped national vitality and power. Faced by outside enemies and domestic crises, upper-class elites had to reform their lifestyle to assure national strength and unity – and if they failed to do so, the upper classes would lose their cultural and social authority, because they threatened the vitality of the nation itself. Here, moral critics rallied under the banner of national defence. At the same time, health crusaders worried about the health and hygiene of the poor and labouring classes in the towns and countryside. Believing that poverty and population decline also threatened France's great power status, they advocated health and welfare reforms to keep the nation rich, strong and healthy. Health activists thus made public health issues into – for lack of a better phrase – national security issues.

The French Revolution transformed this original crusade against degeneracy and depopulation. Since health crusaders had associated their particular values with the health and security of the nation-state, they now wanted to share them within broader community to regenerate the nation. This approach, for example, characterizes the more utopian health plans associated with F.-X. Lanthenas and J.-M. Audin-Rouvière. But this health radicalism did not survive the Reign of Terror. Now health crusaders introduced another idea: physical and moral hygiene could contain political radicalism associated with Jacobinism and the popular movement. From here, doctors used physical and moral hygiene to contain enemies within: not

---

4   Norbert Elias, *The Civilizing Process*, trans. Edmund Jephcott (Oxford, 1994), pp. 15, 23–24.

5   Klaus Theweleit, *Male Fantasies*, vol. 1, *Women, Floods, Bodies, History*, trans. trans. Eric Carter, Stephen Conway, and Chris Turner (Minneapolis, 1987), pp. 364–68.

for the national or collective interest, but to preserve the middle-class social order. In the late Revolutionary period, presumably, doctors believed that they had reasonably solved the social threats coming from above (associated with luxury, libertinism and gender transgression) and turned to regenerating health problems and deviance from below.

During the Restoration and the July monarchy, this trend accelerated. Though doctors represented diverse social, political, epistemological and professional interests, they apparently felt secure in their professional status and identified, by and large, with the status quo. But to respond to industrial change and working-class radicalism, middle-class doctors now made cause with the upper crust they had once lambasted (it perhaps helped that the aristocracy became a conservative and reactionary group after the Revolution) – so long as the upper crust remained committed to 'law and order' issues and paid sufficient lip service to the 'principles of 1789'. (These beliefs were savagely parodied in Gustave Flaubert's *Madame Bovary*: the pharmacist Homais, for example, extols middle-class values, technological change, social improvement and the firm political hand of Louis-Philippe's 'bourgeois monarchy' while all along advancing his own professional and familial interests.)

The significance of this change needs to be underscored. As industrial and urban change accelerated, doctors applied ideas about physical and moral hygiene to contain social threats from lower social strata. In this process, doctors abandoned the idea that social reform helped guarantee national security, and thus rejected their pre-Revolutionary and Revolutionary ancestors. At times, these new sanitarians could be remarkably frank, as when B.-A. Richerand and L.-R. Villermé declared that the poor did not deserve public services and it was better that they simply died out, obliterated by their self-made 'conditions of existence'. It is likely that this attitude stemmed, in a paradoxical fashion, from both self-confidence and fear: self-confidence, in that doctors sincerely believed in the social order and doubted that progressive social change would ever come or last; fear, in that doctors worried that radicals would try to impose their hopeless utopian dreams by force and thus cause violence and destruction. In all this, sanitarians did not see lower-class health as a pressing national risk, something that might jeopardize France's great power status. The attitude, rather, was to let the market run its course and take the risks of open class conflict.

In the post-revolutionary period, health activism might have declined because of the remarkable international stability. Between 1815 and 1848 – with the exception of Greek independence – the Concert of Europe largely maintained diplomatic consensus and averted full-scale conflicts. Lacking armed threats from neighbouring states, ruling elites then focused upon what they saw to be a more pressing danger: not foreign enemies, but the red republicans that lurked *within* their national borders. As long as the social order held the line on the international front, public officials and doctors could avoid sustained reforms – and, in some cases, they could dismember the reforms established during the revolutionary and Napoleonic period.

In this manner, the discourse on physical and moral hygiene casts a fascinating light on the dynamics of social reform. In stark terms, the French government considered health reforms when there were pressing issues – real or imagined – that threatened the nation on the international stage. The key, as always, was population growth. In these cases, ruling elites believed that national power and productivity were undermined by social inequalities and dismal living conditions. By contrast, when international threats disappeared or seemed less worrisome, ruling elites curtailed or abandoned health reforms in particular and progressive policies in general. In this sense, widespread dearth and deprivation failed to motivate policy-makers to promote sustained reform. Rather, the motivating factors were national security risks. This is not to suggest that all public authorities, intellectuals and doctors shared these views, or that they didn't change their attitudes as circumstances changed. Nor do I mean to dismiss the reformers and charity workers who laboured in post-revolutionary France on behalf of the needy and less fortunate. But the post-revolutionary reality, however, highlights their humanitarian dedication and values, which they preservered in the face of widespread apathy or hostility.

This thesis is strengthened by events that followed the 1848–52 Revolutions. In terms of health activism, the Second Empire, which lasted from 1852 to 1870, proved a transitory period. During this period, contemporaries now turned, more than ever, to the biomedical sciences to help explain bewildering sociopolitical changes and to try to imagine a better way of life – both in the private and public realms. The best example is the Romantic historian and naturalist Jules Michelet. After 1848, Michelet was horrified by political violence and class hatred and he feared that society itself would soon collapse. In response, he penned two novels to call his bourgeois readers to regenerate themselves and broader society: *L'amour* and *La femme*. Rejecting materialism and self-absorption – his target may have been Honoré de Balzac's scandalous *La physiologie du mariage* – Michelet called upon the middle classes to adopt new family values. Like the moral hygienists of the revolutionary period, he argued that women were the key to physical and moral regeneration, saying they were 'sick' and could not 'live alone'.[6] Therefore, readers could regenerate the family by reinforcing sentimental bonds between husband and wife, so long as both understood that a woman had innate deficiencies that kept her from living and working outside domestic realm. Apparently, however, he had little faith that his readers would change their lifestyle. 'This century', Michelet predicted, 'shall be called the century of uterine disease – otherwise stated, of women's destitution and despair'.[7]

Of course, these were not new ideas. Michelet belongs to a long history of biomedical sexism whose modern antecedents included, as we have seen, Pierre Roussel's *Système physique et moral de la femme*, J.-L. Moreau de la Sarthe's *Histoire naturelle de la femme* and J.-J. Virey's *De la femme*. The point here, however, is that these ideas about biological and sexual incommensurability momentarily coalesced around specific political moments, whether in the crisis of the old regime, the traumatic experiences of war and revolution, or the post-cholera imagination. In this case, Michelet's biomedical language mediated a threatened sense of self

6   Jules Michelet, *L'amour*, intro. by Jules Lemaître (Paris, 1923), p. 52, and *La femme* (Paris: Calmann-Lévy, n.d.), pp. 55–69.

7   Michelet, *L'amour*, p. 4.

and society, and this language shaped how the author and his readers perceived, experienced and interacted with the surrounding social world.

Michelet's *L'amour* and *La femme* were commercial successes but critical flops; the Parisian literary community skewered his overwrought sentimentalism and ideas about female subordination.[8] But his words proved prophetic. In the following decade, violent conflict again swept French society: the virulent strike waves of 1869, the disastrous Franco-Prussian War of 1870 and the traumatic bloodshed of the Paris Commune in 1871. These disasters transformed elite attitudes. Instead of bourgeois independence and autonomy, public authorities, intellectuals and doctors now preached from another gospel: that of social interdependence. As anthropologist Paul Rabinow notes, 'important segments of the conservative *classes éclairées* began to face up to the obvious fact that far-reaching changes were not only necessary but inevitable in almost every sphere of French life'.[9]

In many circles, intellectuals and authorities agreed that change had to come. For them, reformers such as the moral economists and the social Catholics seemed unable to deal with the sheer magnitude of the 'social question', as it was being now called. At this juncture, contemporaries now took the social problems originally diagnosed by doctors such as L.-F. Benoiston de Châteauneuf, Alexandre Parent-Duchâtelet and L.-R. Villermé and sought new ways to reform this behaviour to make the nation healthy and strong. In other words, the leaders of the newly constituted Third Republic, more cautiously (if not cynically) than the idealistic legislators of 1789, wanted to solve social problems and conflicts by using biomedical knowledge and skills.

Like the health activists of the French Revolution, post-1870 reformers used hygiene to enforce a political agenda, hoping to curtail radicalism by instilling moral restraint throughout the populace. They feared not Jacobinism, but new forms of political radicalism: socialism and worker activism. In blunt terms, sociologist Gaston Richard predicted, 'social science will play the biggest role in the struggle against socialism'.[10] These reformers wanted, quite literally, to pacify a hostile terrain, and saw this process in terms of colonial conquest and administration. Like revolutionary doctors in the 1790s, they used biomedicine and the related human sciences – especially the socio-statistical and socio-medical prerogatives developed by the 'new sanitarians' of the 1830s and 1840s – to control social change and improve power and productivity.

In all this, the new buzzword was 'social paternalism'. For many reformers and public officials, paternalism served as convenient shorthand to describe the embourgeoisement of the lower classes. According to them, the family was the basic social unit and normative type upon which legislators and trained experts must focus.

---

8   James Smith Allen, '"A Distant Echo": Reading Jules Michelet's *L'Amour* and *La Femme* in 1859–1860', *Nineteenth-Century French Studies* 16 (1986–87): 30–46.

9   Paul Rabinow, *French Modern: Norms and Forms of the Social Environment* (Cambridge, MA, 1989), p. 105.

10   Gaston Richard, *Socialisme et la science sociale* (Paris, 1897), p. 193, quoted in Sanford Elwitt, *The Third Republic Defended: Bourgeois Reform in France, 1880–1914* (Baton Rouge, 1986), p. 19.

These ideas were developed, most famously, by thinkers such as Frédéric Le Play, Hubert Lyautey and Émile Cheysson. As these men described it, social paternalism could contain class conflict by inculcating middle-class values in the working-class family. Consequently, they promoted many public projects and voluntary organizations, ranging from the Musée Sociale to the Alliance d'Hygiène Sociale, working-class housing, urban design, education and profit sharing.[11] In the 1890s, these ideas developed into a full-scale political movement called 'Solidarism', which was spearheaded by Léon Bourgeois and Léon Duguit. In different ways from Saint-Simonianism, Solidarism emphasized societal cooperation and interdependence: for its supporters, social reform was a prophylactic, because it neutralized the infectious causes of social unrest.[12]

Recent historians argue that Solidarism broke decisively with the older policy ideas associated with the social economists and moral economists. But when seen in the *longue durée* of medical activism, Solidarism seems less a break than a return to the values associated with earlier health crusaders. Like Solidarists, these earlier doctors wanted to restore national greatness by regenerating the whole of the body politic, and they looked to hygiene and public services to do so. Of course, not all post-revolutionary social commentators had rejected melioration. As we have seen, the Idéologue tradition continued in some medical circles, and social Catholics had also picked up the banner of reform in 1830s and 1840s.[13] But there is an important difference between pre-revolutionary, revolutionary and post-revolutionary medical activism. In post-revolutionary society, social reformers wanted to control degeneracy and fertility within specific groups of the poor and working classes. They did not equate the health of these peoples with the health and future vitality of the body politic. By contrast, in 1789–1803 and in 1871–1914, social thinkers wanted to use biomedical science to create a larger national community and promote population growth. As they saw it, they served the national interest, not a class-conscious agenda.

There were powerful reasons for them to change their mind. During the Third Republic, public officials, intellectuals and doctors found themselves again facing an old nemesis: depopulation.[14] But this time, depopulation was less a mirage than

---

11   Rabinow, *French Modern*, Ch. 4–6; Elwitt, *Third Republic Defended*, passim.

12   See especially Judith Stone, *The Search for Social Peace: Reform Legislation in France, 1890–1914* (Albany, 1985); these political considerations later appeared in Émile Durkheim's classic *Division of Labor in Society* (1896).

13   Katherine A. Lynch, *Family, Class, and Ideology in Early Industrial France: Social Policy and the Working-Class Family, 1825–1848* (Madison, 1988); see also the overview of these theorists in Rachel G. Fuchs, *Poor and Pregnant in Paris: Strategies for Survival in the Nineteenth Century* (New Brunswick, 1992), pp. 35–55.

14   See Robert A. Nye, *Crime, Madness, and Politics in Modern France: The Medical Concept of National Decline* (Princeton, 1984), and *Masculinity and Male Codes of Honor in Modern France* (Oxford and New York, 1993); Joseph Spenglar, *France Faces Depopulation* (Durham, NC, 1979); and Karen Offen, 'Depopulation, Nationalism, and Feminism in Fin-de-Siècle France', *American Historical Revue* 89 (1984): 452–84. Joshua H. Cole, *Power of Large Numbers: Population, Politics, and Gender in Nineteenth-Century France* (Ithaca, 2000) provides an excellent overview.

a biological possibility, and the changed international scene added to the intensity of the debate. As early as the 1830s, the French death rate rose faster than the rate of birth and, by the 1850s, fertility exceeded mortality just enough to increase the population by no less than 5 per cent. Now before 1870, during the July monarchy and the Second Empire, most social commentators had praised this phenomena, claiming that the low birth rate proved that France had been civilized by bourgeois self-restraint.

But everything changed after the Franco-Prussian War and the Paris Commune. In the intense soul-searching and agony that followed these disasters, moral critics blamed the defeat on depopulation and moral degeneracy. As they saw it, depopulation evidenced great power decline, a degenerate and moribund population and even future national disintegration. Like pre-revolutionary and revolutionary thinkers, then, post-1871 observers found that demographic decline (rather than worker fertility) proved physical and moral degeneracy. This contrasts with the social thinkers of the Restoration and July monarchies, who believed the exact opposite: namely, that *high* birth rates indicated moral and physical degeneracy. Whereas early nineteenth-century social thinkers wanted to limit fertility in particular groups of the poor and working classes, fin-de-siècle activists wanted to increase fertility across the board – and by any means possible. As historians such as Robert Nye, Rachel Fuchs and William Schneider have demonstrated, the fear about demographic decline and racial degeneration powerfully influenced Third Republican politics and social reform, causing policy-makers to expand welfare services, and even stimulated the French eugenics movement.[15] Here, politicians justified public services and social planning by saying they protected republican and national values. In some senses, then, when the depopulation panic emerged again in the 1880s, physical and moral hygiene had come full circle, as social reforms and health activists returned to an earlier tradition in social medical thought.

Seen in this light, the original health panics over degeneracy and depopulation between 1750 and 1850 left an ineffaceable legacy of health activism. On a basic level, these health activists invented the modern idea of social medicine and hoped to treat the health and well-being of large-scale populations. In so doing, they put medicine in the public arena – for the first time – and helped solidify the image of the doctor as a figure of social and cultural authority. More importantly, health activists promoted the belief that doctors could explain serious social and moral issues and propose private and public initiatives needed to cure these blights. In many ways, physical and moral hygiene provided an ideology designed to explain and change the social world of modernizing France. It was not special-interest pleading, vapid rhetoric designed to justify class and professional dominion; rather, these ideas about human nature and society rested upon concrete material conditions and encompassed a genuine, deeply held understanding of the social world.

In this manner, this study has moved beyond sociological explanations of medical power and the social constructionism associated with the new cultural

---

15   See also the collection of essays by Rachel Fuchs, Joshua Cole, Jean Elisabeth Pederson, Cheryl Koos, and Andrés Horacio Reggiani in the forum on 'Population and the State in the Third Republic', *French Historical Studies* 19 (1996): 633–754.

history. Doctors, as we have seen, did not promote straightforward social control agendas; nor did they simply construct or imagine class and gender relations through the medium of discourse. Rather, the doctor's views on self and society were significantly interwoven with his class status and material interests, but these views evolved in mutual dialogue with public authorities, intellectuals and patients. In this sense, the doctor's social vision was not entirely hegemonic in that it presented a unified ideological front. During the French Revolution, for example, medical interests lacked doctrinal coherence; at other times, during the Restoration and July Monarchy, medical politics were inimical and even antagonistic. As should be expected, doctors expressed a plurality of disciplinary, political and social interests. At crucial moments, however, health activism and sociopolitical concerns proved reinforcing, and thus helped to define the new world that came out of the Age of Revolution.

Bibliography of Printed Sources

Primary Sources

Alibert, J.-L., 'De l'influence des causes politiques sur les maladies et la constitution physique de l'homme', *Magasin encyclopédique, ou Journal des sciences, des lettres et des arts* 5 (1795): 298–305.
——, 'Du pouvoir de l'habitude dans l'état de santé et de maladie', *Mémoires de la Société médicale d'émulation* 1 (Year IV [1798]): 396–415.
Astruc, Jean, *Traité des maladies des femmes* (6 vols, Paris, 1761–65).
Audin-Rouvière, Joseph-Marie, *Essai sur la topographie physique et médicale de Paris* (Paris, Year II).
——, *La médecine sans médecin, ou moyens préservatifs et curatifs d'un grand nombre de maladies* (Paris, 1823).
Ballexserd, Jacques, *Dissertation sur l'éducation physique des enfans* (Paris, 1762).
——, *Dissertation sur cette question: quelles sont les causes principles de la mort d'un grand nombre d'enfans?* (Geneva, 1775).
Barrère, Pierre, *Dissertation sur la cause physique de la couluer des nègres, de la qualité de leurs cheveux, et de la dégénération de l'un et l'autre* (Paris, 1741).
——, *Nouvelle relation de la France équinoxiale* (Paris, 1743).
Barthez, P.-J., *Nouveaux élémens de la science de l'homme*, 2d edn (2 vols, Paris, 1806).
Beauchêne, E.-P.-C., *De l'influence des affections de l'âme dans les maladies nerveuses des femmes* (Montpellier and Paris, 1781).
Belloc, J.-J., *Cours de médecine légale, théorique et pratique*, 2d edn (Paris, 1811).
Benoiston de Châteauneuf, L.-F. et al., *Mémoire sur la mortalité des femmes de l'âge de quarante à cinquante ans* (Paris, 1834).
Benoiston de Châteauneuf, L.-F., et al., *Rapport sur la marche et les effets du choléra-morbus dans Paris et les communes rurales du département de la Seine* (Paris, 1834).
Berthelon, Pierre, *De la salubrité de l'air des villes et en particulier des moyens de la procurer* (Montpellier, 1786).
Bertin, Antoine, *Des moyens de conserver la santé des blancs et des nègres, aux Antilles ou climats chauds et humides de l'Amerique* (Paris, 1768).
Bichat, Xavier, *Anatomie générale, appliquée à la physiologie et à la médecine* (4 vols, Paris, 1801).
——, *Physiological Researches Upon Life and Death*, trans. Tobias Watkins (Philadelphia, 1809).
Brillat-Savarin, J.-A., *Physiologie du goût* (2 vols, Paris, 1826).
Boerhaave, Hermann, *Traité des maladies des enfans*, trans. M. Paul, rev. by Gerard van Swieten (Avignon and Paris, 1759).

Bonnemain, A.-J.-T., *Régénération des colonies, ou moyens de restituer graduellement aux hommes leur état politique, et d'assurer la prospérité des Nations* (Paris, 1792).

Bonnet, Charles, *Considérations sur les corps organisés* (2 vols, Neuchâtel, 1779).

Boyveau-Laffecteur, Pierre, *Traité des maladies physiques et morales des femmes*, 4th edn (1798; Paris, 1812).

Brémont de Valuejols, *Essai sur les maladies héréditaires, considérées sous les rapports de leur nature et des théories dont elles ont été le sujet* (Paris, 1832).

Broussais, F.-J.-V., *Le choléra-morbus épidémique, observé et traité selon la méthode physiologique* (Paris, 1832).

——, *A Treatise on Physiology Applied to Pathology*, 3d American edn, trans. John Bell and R. La Roche (Philadelphia, 1832).

Brouzet de Béziers, N., *Essai sur l'éducation médicinale des enfans et sur leurs maladies* (2 vols, Paris, 1754).

Bruhier d'Ablaincourt, J.-J., *Dissertation sur l'incertitude de la mort et l'abus des enterremens et embaumens précipités*, 2d edn (2 vols, Paris, 1749).

Buard d'Agen, G.-A.-L., *Du choléra-morbus épidémique* (Paris, 1832).

Buchan, William, *Domestic Medicine, or, a Treatise on the Prevention and Cure of Diseases by Regimen and Simple Medicines* (London, 1772).

Buchez, Philippe and Ulysse Trélat, *Précis élémentaire d'hygiène* (Paris, 1825).

Buffon, Georges-Louis Leclerc de, *Œuvres complètes*, ed. M.-A. Richard (34 vols, Paris, 1825–28).

Cabanis, P.-J.-G., 'Considérations générales sur l'étude de l'homme et sur les rapports de son organisation physique avec ses facultés intellectuelles et morales', *Mémoires de l'Institut national des sciences et arts*, 2e classe, *Sciences morales et politiques* 1 (Year VI): 37–97.

——, *Rapports du physique et du moral de l'homme* (2 vols, Paris, Year X [1802]).

Capuren, Joseph, *Traité des maladies des femmes, depuis la puberté jusqu'à l'âge critique inclusivement* (Paris, 1812).

Cerfvol, Chevalier de, *Mémoire sur la population* (London, 1768).

Chambon de Montaux, Nicolas, *Des maladies des femmes* (2 vols, Paris, 1784).

——, *Des maladies de la grossesse* (2 vols, Paris, 1785).

——, *Des maladies des filles* (2 vols, Paris, 1785).

——, *Des maladies des enfans* (2 vols, Paris, Year VII).

Chervin, Nicolas, *Pétition contre la formation des lazarets projetés depuis 1822 dans la vue de mettre la France à l'abri de la fièvre jaune* (Paris, 1828).

Chevalier, Jean-Damien, *Lettres à M. le Jean, docteur-regent de la Faculté de Medecine en l'université de Paris. I. Sur les maladies de St.-Domingue* (Paris, 1752).

Cheyne, George, *An Essay of Health and Long Life* (London, 1724).

Clisson, F. Fougnot de, *Dissertation sur le choléra-morbus épidémique* (Paris, 1832).

Condillac, Étienne de. *Oeuvres complètes* (32 vols, Geneva, 1970).

Cousin, Victor, *Introduction to the History of Philosophy*, trans. H. G. Linberg (Boston, 1832).

Cugoano, Ottobah, *Réflexion sur la traite et l'esclavage des nègres, traduites de l'anglais d'Ottobah Cugoano, afriquain, esclave à la Grenade et libre en Angleterre*, trans. Antoine Diannyère (London and Paris, 1788).

Dazille, J.-B., *Observations sur les maladies des nègres, leurs causes, leur traitements et les moyens de les prevenir* (Paris, 1776).

——, *Observations sur les maladies des climats chauds, leurs causes, leurs traitements et les moyens de les prévenir* (Paris, 1785).

——, *Observations sur le Tétanos, ses différences, ses symptômes, avec le traitement de cette maladie et les moyens de prevenir* (Paris, 1788).

Desbordeaux, P.-F.-F., *Nouvelle orthopédie, ou précis sur les difformités que l'on peut prévenir our corriger dans les enfans* (Paris, Year XIII [1805]).

Desessartz, J. C., *Traité de l'éducation corporelle des enfans en bas-âge*, 2d edn (Paris, Year VII).

Destutt de Tracy, A.-L.-C., *De l'amour*, ed. Gilbert Chinard (Paris, 1926).

Dictionnaire des sciences médicales, par une société de médecins et chirurgiens, ed. N. P. Adelon et al. (60 vols, Paris, 1812–22).

Dictionnaire encyclopédique des sciences médicales, ed. A. Deschambre et al. (100 vols, Paris, 1864–89).

Dictionnaire universel des sciences morales, économiques, politiques et diplomatiques, ou bibliothèque de l'homme d'état et du citoyen, ed. Jean-Baptiste Robinet (London, 1777–83).

Discours sur la nécessité d'établir à Paris une Société pour concourir, avec celle de Londres, à l'abolition de la traite et de l'esclavage des Nègres (Paris, 1788).

Du commerce des colonies, ses principes et ses lois: la paix est de temps de régler et d'agrandir le commerce (n.p., 1785).

Dumas, C.-L., *Principes de physiologie, ou introduction à la science experimentale, philsophique et médicale de l'homme vivant* (4 vols, Paris, 1800–03).

——, *Discours sur les progrès futurs de la science de l'homme, prononcé dans l'École de médecine de Montpellier, le 20 germinal an XII* (Montpellier, n.d.).

Encyclopédie méthodique ou par ordre des matières: économie politique et diplomatique, ed. J. N. Démeunier (4 vols, Paris, 1784–88).

Encyclopédie méthodique ou par ordre des matières: jurisprudence (10 vols, Paris, 1782–91).

Encyclopédie méthodique ou par ordre des matières: médecine, ed. Félix Vicq d'Azyr (13 vols, Paris, 1782–1832).

Encyclopédie, ou dictionnaire raisonné des sciences, des arts, et des métiers, eds Denis Diderot et al. (36 vols, Geneva, 1777–79).

L'Esclavage des Nègres aboli, ou moyens d'améliorer leur sort (Paris, 1789).

Esquirol, J.-E.-D., *Des maladies mentales* (Paris, 1838).

Faiguet de Villeneuve, Joachim, *Discours d'un bon citoyen sur les moyens de multiplier les forces de l'État et d'augmenter la population* (Brussels, 1760).

——, *L'econome politique: projet pour enricher et pour perfectionner l'espèce humaine* (London and Paris, 1763).

Fitzgerald, Gérard, *Traité des maladies des femmes* (Paris, 1758).

Fodéré, F.-E., *Les lois éclairées par les sciences physiques, ou Traité de médecine-légale et d'hygiène publique* (3 vols, Paris, Year VI).

——, *Les lois éclairées par les sciences physiques, ou Traité de médecine-légale et d'hygiène publique* (6 vols, Paris, 1813).

——, *Essai historique et moral sur la pauvreté des nations, la population, la mendicité, les hôpitaux et les enfans trouvés* (Paris, 1825).

——, *Recherches historiques sur la nature, les causes et le traitement du choléra-morbus* (Paris, 1831).

Fourcroy, Antoine (ed.), *La médecine éclairée par les sciences physiques* (4 vols, Paris, 1791–92).

Frégier, H.-A., *Des classes dangeureuses de la population dans les grandes villes, et des moyens de les rendre meilleures* (2 vols, Paris, 1840).

Frossmand, B.-J., *Observations sur l'abolition de la traite des nègres présentées à la Convention nationale* (Paris, 1793).

Ganne, Ambroise, *L'homme physique et moral, ou recherches sur les moyens de rendre l'homme plus sage* (Strasbourg and Paris, 1791).

Gendrin, A.-N., *Monographie du choléra-morbus épidémique de Paris* (Paris, 1832).

Gilbert, N.-P., *Quelques réflexions sur la médecine légale et son état actuel en France* (Paris, Year IX).

Gilibert, J.-E., *L'anarchie médicale, ou la médecine considérée comme nuisible à la société* (3 vols, Neuchâtel, 1772).

Goyon de La Plombaine, Henri le, *L'homme en société, ou nouvelles vues politiques et économiques pour porter la population au plus haut degré en France* (2 vols, Amsterdam, 1763).

Grégoire, Henri, *Essai sur la régénération physique, morale et politique des juifs* (Mezt, 1789).

——, *Mémoire en faveur des gens de couleur ou sang-mêlés de St.-Domingue, et des autres isles françoises de l'Amérique* (Paris, 1789).

——, *An Enquiry concerning the intellectual and moral facilities, and the literature of negroes*, trans. D. B. Warden (Brooklyn, 1810).

Hallé, J.-N., *Recherches sur la nature des effets du méphitisme des fosses d'aisance* (Paris, 1785).

Hellis, E., *Souvenirs du choléra en 1832* (Paris and Rouen, 1833).

Henrion de Pansey, Pierre-Paul-Nicolas, *Mémoire pour un nègre qui réclame sa liberté* (Paris, 1770).

Hippocratic Writings, ed. G. E. R. Lloyd, trans. J. Chadwick and W. N. Monn (Harmondsworth, 1978).

Histoire de la Société Royale de Médecine (10 vols, Paris, 1779–98).

d'Holbach, P.-H. Thiry, *Système social ou principes de la morale de la politique, avec un examen de l'influence du gouvernement sur les moeurs* (3 vols, London, 1773).

Il est encore des Aristocrates, ou Réponse à l'infâme auteur d'un écrit intitulé: Découverte d'une conspiration contre les intérêts de la France (Paris, 1790).

Jackson, Robert, *A Treatise on the Fevers of Jamaica, with some Observations on the Intermitting Fever of America* (London, 1791).

Jacquin, A.-P., *De la santé, ouvrage utile à tout le monde*, 2d edn (Paris, 1763).

Jaubert, Abbé Pierre, *Des causes de la dépopulation et des moyens d'y remédier* (Paris and London, 1767).

Jouard, Gabriel, *Nouvel essai sur la femme considérée comparativement à l'homme* (Paris, Year XII [1804]).

Labat, Jean-Baptiste, *Nouveau voyage aux isles de l'Amérique, contenant l'histoire naturelle de ces pays, l'origine, les moeurs, la religion et le gouvernement des habitans anciens et modernes* (8 vols, Paris, 1742).

Lacaze, Louis de, *Idée de l'homme physique et moral* (Paris, 1755).

Lachaise, Claude, *Topographie médicale de Paris* (Paris, 1820).

Laclos, Pierre Choderlos de, *Les liaisons dangereuses*, ed. René Pomeau (Paris, 1996).

Lafosse, J.-F., *Avis aux habitans des colonies, particulièrement à ceux de l'isle S. Domingue, sur les principales causes des maladies qu'on y éprouve le plus communément, et sur les moyens de les prévenir* (Paris, 1787).

Landais, *Dissertation sur les avantages de l'allaitement des enfans par leurs mères* (Geneva and Paris, 1781).

Lanthenas, F.-X., *De l'infuence de la liberté sur la santé, la morale et le bonheur* (Paris, 1792).

Lavolley, M.-J., *Manuel d'hygiène, ou l'art de prolonger la vie et de conserver la santé* (Paris, n.d.).

Laya, Jean-Louis, *La régénération des comédiens en France, ou leurs droits à l'état civil* (Paris, 1789).

Le Bègue de Presle, Achille, *Le conservateur de la santé* (Paris, 1763).

Lebrun, J.-C., *Essai de topographie médicale de la ville du Mans et de ses environs* (Mans, 1812).

Le Camus, Antoine, *Médecine de l'esprit* (2 vols, Paris, 1753).

Le Cat, C.-N., *Traité de la couleur de la peau humaine en générale, de celle des nègres en particulier et de la métamorphose d'une de ces couleurs en l'autre, soit de naissance, soit accidentellement* (Amersterdam, 1765).

Lecointe-Marsillac, *Le More-Lack, ou essai sur les moyens le plus doux et les plus équitables d'abolir la traite et l'esclavage des Nègres d'Afrique, en conservant aux Colonies tous les avantages d'une population agricole* (London and Paris, 1789).

Le Couer, J., *Précis sommaire sur le choléra-morbus épidémique, ses premiers symptoms, et les moyens les plus propres à les combattre* (Caen and Paris, 1832).

Lefebvre de Beauvray, Pierre, *Dictionnaire social et patriotique, ou précis raisonné des connoissances relatives à l'économie morale, civile et politique* (Amsterdam, 1770).

Lejumeau de Kergaradec, *Quelques mots sur le choléra-morbus épidémique et sur les moyens de s'en préserver* (Paris, 1832).

Lescallier, Daniel, *Réflexions sur le sort des noirs dans nos colonies* (Paris, 1789).

Lépecq de la Clôture, Louis, *Observations sur les maladies épidémiques* (Paris, 1776).

——, *Collection d'observations sur les maladies et constitutions épidémiques* (2 vols, Rouen, 1778).

Leroy, Alphonse, *Recherches sur les habillemens des femmes et des enfans* (Paris, 1772).

Lignac, Abbé de, *De l'homme et de la femme considérés physiquement dans l'état du mariage* (2 vols, Paris, 1772).

Littré, Émile, *Médecine et médecins*, 3d edn (Paris, 1875).

Lucas, Prosper, *Traité physiologique et philosophique de l'hérédité dans les états de santé et de maladie du système nerveux* (2 vols, Paris, 1848–50).

Macquart, L.-C.-H., *Dictionnaire de la conservation de l'homme, ou d'hygiène et d'éducation physique et morale* (2 vols, Paris, Year VII).

Mahon, P.-A.-O., *Médecine légale et police médicale*, ed. M. Fautrel (3 vols, Rouen, 1801).

Maine de Biran, F.-P., *Oeuvres*, ed. François Azouvi (13 vols, Paris, 1984–).

Mandar, Théophile, *Observations sur l'esclavage et le commerce des Nègres: Pour répondre aux questions insérées dans le Journal de Paris* (Paris, 1790).

Marat, J.-P., *De l'homme* (3 vols, Amsterdam and Paris, 1775–76).

Marie de Valognes, J.-P.-F., *Quelques propositions de médecine, et en particulier sur l'hygiène prophylactique du choléra épidémique* (Paris, 1832).

Maupertuis, P.-L. Moreau de, *Dissertation physique à l'occasion du nègre blanc* (Leyde, 1744).

Ménuret de Chambaud, J.-J. *Essais sur l'histoire médico-physique de Paris*, 2d edn (Paris, Year XIII).

Messance, Louis, *Recherches sur la population des généralités d'Auvergne, de Lyon, de Rouen et de quelques provinces et villes du royaume* (Paris, 1766).

——, *Nouvelles recherches sur la population de la France* (Lyon, 1788).

Michelet, Jules, *L'amour*, intro. by Jules Lemaître (Paris, 1923).

——, *La femme* (Paris, n.d.).

Millot, J.-A.,.*L'art de procéer les sexes à volonté, ou système complet de génération*, 4th edn (1800; Paris, n.d.).

——, *L'art d'améliorer et perfectionner les hommes au moral comme au physique* (2 vols, Paris, Year X [1801])

——, *Médecine perfective, ou code des bonnes mères* (2 vols, Paris, 1809).

Mirabeau, Victor de, *L'ami des hommes, ou traité de la population* (7 vols, The Hague, 1758).

Moheau, J.-B., *Recherches et considérations sur la population de la France* (1778; Paris, 1994).

Montesquieu, C.-L. de, *Lettres persanes* (1721; Paris, 1964).

Moreau de Jonnès, Alexandre, *Rapport au Conseil supérieur de santé sur le choléra-morbus pestilentiel* (Paris, 1831).

——, *Eléments de statistique, principes généraux de cette science, sa classification, sa méthode, ses opérations, ses divers degrés de certitude, ses erreurs et ses progrès*, 2d edn (Paris, 1856).

Moreau de la Sarthe, J.-L., *Histoire naturelle de la femme, suivie d'un traité d'hygiène appliquée à son régime physique et moral aux différentes époques de la vie* (2 vols, Paris, 1803).

——, *Esquisse d'un cours d'hygiène, ou de médecine appliquée à l'art d'user de la vie et de conserver la santé* (Paris, n.d.).

Moreau de Saint-Méry, M.-L.-E., *Description topographique, physique, civile, politique et historique de la partie française de l'isle Saint-Domingue*, ed. Blanche Maurel and Étienne Taillemite (3 vols, Paris, 1958).

Morel, B.-A., *Traité des dégénérescences physiques, intellectuelles et morales de l'espèce humaine, et des causes qui produisent ces variétés maladives* (Paris, 1857).

——, *De la formation du type dans les variétés dégénérés ou nouveaux éléments d'anthropologie morbide* (Paris, 1864).

——, *De l'hérédité morbide progressive ou des types dissemblables et disparates dans la famille* (Paris, 1867).

Morgagni, J. B., *The Seats and Causes of Diseases, Investigated by Anatomy*, trans. B. Alexander (3 vols, London, 1769).

Navier, P.-N., *Réflexions sur les dangers des exhumations précipitées, et sur l'abus des inhumations dans les églises* (Amsterdam and Paris, 1775).

Nicolas, P.-F., *Le cri de la nature en faveur des enfans nouveaux-nés* (Grenoble and Paris, 1775).

'Nouvelle division de la Terre, par les differentes Espèces ou Races qui l'habitent, envoyée par un fameux Voyageur ... à peu près en ces termes', *Journal des Sçavans* 12 (1684): 148–53.

Paillard, H., *Histoire statistique du choléra morbus qui a régné en France en 1832* (Paris, 1832).

Parent-Duchâtelet, Alexandre, *De la prostitution dans la ville de Paris* (2 vols, Paris, 1836).

Patissier, Philibert, *Traité des maladies des artisans et de celles qui résultent de diverses professions d'après Ramazzini* (Paris, 1822).

Pepin, *Adresse d'un patriote françois à l'Assemblée nationale sur la Traite des Noirs. Avril 1791* (Paris, 1791).

Pétion, Jérome, *Discours sur la traite des noirs* (April 1790).

Petit, A., *Essai sur les maladies héréditaires, considérées sous les rapports de leur nature, de leur origine ou formation* (Paris, 1817).

Pinel, Philippe, *A Treatise on Insanity*, trans. D. D. David, with an introduction by Paul F. Cranefield (1800; New York, 1962).

——, *Traité médico-philosophique sur l'aliénation mentale*, 2d edn (Paris, 1809).

Plane, J.-M., *Physiologie ou l'art de connaître les hommes sur leur physionomie* (2 vols, Meudon, 1797).

Poissonnier-Desperrières, Antoine, *Traité des fièvres de l'isle de St.-Domingue*, 2d edn (Paris, 1766).

Pomme, Pierre, *Traité des affections vaporeuses des deux sexes*, 2d edn (Lyon, 1765).

——, *Nouveau recueil de pièces relatives au traitement des vapeurs* (Paris, 1771).

Portal, Antoine, *Considérations sur la nature et le traitement des maladies de famille et des maladies héréditaires, et sur les moyens les mieux éprouvés de les prévenir*, 3d edn (Paris, 1814).

Portal, Antoine et al., 'Rapport de la commission chargée de rédiger un report d'instruction relativement aux épidémies', *Mémoires de l'Académie royale de médecine* 1 (1828): 245–79.

Pouppée-Desportes, J.-B., *Histoire des maladies de Saint-Domingue* (2 vols, Paris, 1770).

Projet d'instruction sur une maladie convulsive, fréquent dans les colonies d'Amérique, connue sous le nom de Tétanos (Paris, 1786).

Quetelet, Adolphe, *A Treatise on Man and the Development of his Faculties* (1842; New York, 1968).

Ramazzini, Bernadino, *De morbis artificum* (Multinae, 1700).

——, *Essai sur les maladies des artisans ...avec des notes et additions*, trans. and ed. A.-F. Fourcroy (Paris, 1777).

Raulin, Joseph, *Traité des affections vaporeuses du sexe* (Paris, 1758).

——, *De la conservation des enfans* (2 vols, Paris, 1768).

Réflexions sur l'abolition de la Traite et la liberté des Noirs (Orleans, 1789).

Riballier and Cosson, *De l'éducation physique et morale des femmes* (Paris and Brussels, 1779).

Richerand, B.-A., *Nouveaux élemens de physiologie*, 2d edn (2 vols, Paris, 1802).

——, *De la population dans ses rapports avec la nature des gouvernemens* (Paris, 1837).

Robert, L.-J.-M., *Essai sur la mégalanthropogénésie, ou l'art de faire des enfans d'esprit, qui deviennent de grands-hommes* (Paris, Year X [1801]).

Rousseau, J.-J., *The First and Second Discourses*, trans. Judith R. Masters (New York, 1964).

Roussel, Pierre, *Système physique et moral de la femme* (Paris, 1775).

——, *Médecine domestique, ou moeurs simples de conserver la santé* (3 vols, Paris, 1790–92).

Saint-Simon, C.-H. de, *Oeuvres*, ed. E. Dentu (6 vols, Geneva, 1977).

Sarrau de Montmahoux, E., *Considérations médicales sur les moyens employés pour conserver la beauté* (Paris, 1815).

Sèze, Victor de, *Recherches phisiologiques et philosophiques sur la sensibilité ou la vie animale* (Paris, 1786).

Sibire, Sébastien-André, *L'aristocracie nègrière, ou Refléxions philosophiques et historiques sur l'esclavage et l'affranchissement des Noirs* (Paris, 1789).

Sieyès, Emmanuel-Joseph, *What is the Third Estate?*, ed. S. E. Finer, trans. M. Blondel, with an introduction by Peter Campbell (New York, 1963).

Sue, Pierre, *Apperçu générale, appuyé de quelques faits, sur l'origine de la médecine légale* (Paris, Year VIII).

Tacheron, *Statistique médicale de la mortalité du choléra-morbus dans le XIe arrondissement de Paris pendant les mois d'avril, mai, juin, juillet et août 1832* (Paris, 1832).

Tissot, S.-A., *Avis au peuple sur sa santé* (Lausanne, 1761).

——, *Onanism, or A treatise upon the disorders produced by masturbation* (London, 1766).

——, *De la santé des gens de lettres* (Lausanne, 1768).

——, *Essai sur les maladies des gens du monde*, 2d edn (Lausanne, 1770).

——, *An Essay on the Disorders of People of Fashion*, trans. Francis Bacon Lee (London, 1771).

——, *Traité des nerfs et leurs maladies* (5 vols, Paris and Lausanne, 1778).

Tourtelle, Étienne, *Élémens d'hygiène*. 3d edn (2 vols, Paris, 1815).

Traité des Nègres: A Messieurs les Députés à l'Assemblée nationale (Paris, 1789).

Trapham, Thomas, *A Discourse on the State of Health in the Island of Jamaica, with a Provision therefore Calculated from the Air, the Place, and the Water* (London, 1679).

Vandermonde, C.-A., *Essai sur la manière de perfectioner l'espèce humaine* (2 vols, Paris, 1756).

Venel, Gabriel, *Essai sur la santé et sur l'éducation médicinale des filles destinées au mariage* (Yverdon, 1776).

Vicq d'Azyr, Félix, *Pièces concernant l'établissement fait par le Roi d'une commission ou société de médecine* (Paris, n.d.).

Vigarous, J.-M.-J., *Cours élémentaire de maladies des femmes, ou essai sur un nouvelle méthode pour étudier et pour classer les maladies de ce sexe* (2 vols, Paris, Year X [1801]).

Vigné, Jean-Baptiste, *De la médecine légale* (Rouen, 1805).

Villermé, L.-R., *Des prisons telles qu'elles sont et telles qu'elles devraient être, ouvrage dans lequel on les considère par rapport à l'hygiène, à la morale et à l'économie politique* (Paris, 1820).

——, *Tableau de l'état physique et moral des ouvriers employés dans les manufactures de coton, de lane et de soie* (2 vols, Paris, 1840).

Virey, J.-J., *Histoire naturelle du genre humain, ou recherches sur ses principaux fondemens physiques et moraux* (2 vols, Paris, Year IX).

——, *De l'éducation publique et privée des français* (Paris, Year X [1802]).

——, *L'art de perfectionner l'homme, ou de la médecine spirituelle et morale* (2 vols, Paris, 1808).

——, *De la puissance vitale, considérée dans ses fonctions physiologiques chez l'homme et tous les êtres organisés* (Paris, 1823).

——, *De la femme, sous ses rapports physiologique, moral et littéraire*, 2d edn (1824; Paris, 1825).

——, *Hygiène philosophique, ou de la santé dans le régime physique, moral et politique de la civilisation moderne* (2 vols, Paris, 1828).

——, *Petit manuel d'hygiène prophylactique contre les épidémies, ou de leurs meillieurs preservatifs* (Paris, 1832).

——, *De la physiologie dans ses rapports avec la philosophie* (Paris, 1844).

——, *Des métamorphoses physiologiqes de l'homme dans l'éducation* (Paris, n.d. [1845]).

Volney, C.-F., *Voyage en Syrie et en Égypte, pendants les années 1783, 1784, et 1785* (2 vols, Paris, 1787).

——, *La loi naturelle, ou catéchisme du citoyen français*, ed. Gaston-Martin (1793 [Year II]; Paris, 1934).

Wildenstein, Daniel and Guy Wildenstein (eds), *Documents complémentaires au catalogue de l'oeuvre de Louis David* (Paris, 1973).

Winslow, J.-B., *Exposition anatomique de la structure du corps humaine* (Paris, 1732).

Secondary Sources

Ackerknecht, Erwin H., 'Anticontagionism Between 1821 and 1867', *Bulletin of the History of Medicine* 22 (1948): 562–93.

——, 'Hygiene in France, 1815–1848', *Bulletin of the History of Medicine* 22 (1948): 117–53.

——, *Medicine at the Paris Hospital, 1794–1848* (Baltimore: Johns Hopkins University Press, 1967).

Adams, T. M., *Bureaucrats and Beggars: French Social Policy in the Age of Enlightenment* (New York: Oxford University Press, 1990).

Agamben, Giorgio, *Homo Sacer: Sovereign Power and Bare Life*, trans. Daniel Heller-Roazen (Stanford: Stanford University Press, 1998).

Allen, James Smith, '"A Distant Echo": Reading Jules Michelet's *L'Amour* and *La Femme* in 1859–1860', *Nineteenth-Century French Studies* 16 (1986–87): 30–46.

Anderson, Warwick, 'Climates of Opinion: Acclimatization in Nineteenth-Century France and England', *Victorian Studies*, 35 (1992): 135–57.

Ariès, Philippe, *Centuries of Childhood: A Social History of Family Life*, trans. Robert Baldick (New York: Vintage, 1962).

——, *The Hour of Our Death*, trans. Helen Weaver (New York: Vintage, 1981).

Arnaud, André-Jean, *Essai d'analyse structurale du code civil français: la règle du jeu dans la paix bourgeoise* (Paris: R. Pichon et R. Durand-Auzias, 1973).

Arnold, David, 'Disease, Medicine, and Empire', in Arnold (ed.), *Imperial Medicine and Indigenous Societies* (Manchester: Manchester University Press, 1988).

Azouvi, François, 'Woman as a Model of Pathology in the Eighteenth Century', trans. Michael Crawcour, *Diogenes*, no. 115 (1981): 22–36.

——, *Maine de Biran: la science de l'homme* (Paris: Vrin, 1995).

Baasner, Frank, *Der Begriff 'sensibilité' im 18. Jahrhundert: Aufstieg und Niedergang eines Ideals* (Heidelberg: Winter, 1988).

Baczko, Bronislaw, 'La Constitution de l'an III et la promotion culturelle du citoyen', in François Azouvi (ed.), *L'institution de la raison: la révolution culturelle des Idéologues* (Paris: Vrin, 1992).

——, *Ending the Terror: The French Revolution After Robespierre* (Cambridge and New York: Cambridge University Press, 1994).

Baecque, Antoine de, 'L'homme nouveau est arrivé: la "régénération" du français en 1789', *Dix-huitième siècle*, no. 20 (1988): 193–208.

——, *The Body Politic: Corporeal Metaphor in Revolutionary France, 1770–1800*, trans. Charlotte Mandell (Stanford: Stanford University Press, 1993).

Baker, Keith Michael, 'Scientism at the End of the Old Regime: Reflections on a Theme of Professor Charles Gillispie', *Minerva* 25 (1987): 21–34.

——, *Inventing the French Revolution: Essays on French Political Culture in the Eighteenth Century* (New York: Cambridge University Press, 1990).

Barker-Benfield, G. J., *The Culture of Sensibility: Sex and Society in Eighteenth-Century Britain* (Chicago: University of Chicago Press, 1992).

Ben-David, Joseph, *The Scientist's Role in Society: A Comparative Study* (Engelwood Cliffs: Prentice Hall, 1971).

Bénichou, Claude and Claude Blanckaert (eds), *Julien-Joseph Virey: naturaliste et anthropologue* (Paris: Vrin, 1988).

Bernardi, Walter, *Le metafisiche dell'embrione: scienze della vita e filosofia da Malpighi a Spallanzani (1672–1793)* (Florence: Olschki, 1986).

Bianchi, Serge, *La révolution culturelle de l'an II: élites et peuple (1789–1799)* (Paris: Aubier, 1982).

Bideau, Alain, Jacques Dupâquier, and Hector Gutierrez, 'La mort quantifiée', in Jacques Dupâquier (ed.), *Histoire de la population française*, vol. 2, *De la Renaissance à 1789* (Paris: Presses universitaires de France, 1995).

Biondi, Carminella, *Mon frère, tu es mon esclave! Teorie schiaviste e diabtti antropologico-razziali nel Settecento francese* (Pisa: Goliardica, 1973).

Blum, Carol, *Rousseu and the Republic of Virtue: The Language of Politics in the French Revolution* (Ithaca: Cornell University Press, 1986).

——, *Strength in Numbers: Population, Reproduction, and Power in Eighteenth-Century France* (Baltimore: Johns Hopkins University Press, 2002).

Boas, George, *French Philosophies of the Romantic Period* (New York: Russell & Russell, 1964).

Bodemer, Charles W., 'Regeneration and the Decline of Preformationism in Eighteenth Century Embryology', *Bulletin of the History of Medicine* 38 (1964): 20–31.

Borie, Jean, *Mythologies de l'hérédité au XIXe siècle* (Paris: Galilée, 1981).

Bosco, Domenico, *La decifrazione dell'ordine: morale e antropologia in Francia nella prima età moderna* (2 vols, Milan: Università cattolica del Sacro Cuore, 1988).

Boudriot, Pierre-Denis, 'Essai sur l'ordure en milieu urbain à l'époque pré-industrielle: boues, immondices et gadoue à Paris au XVIIIe siècle', *Histoire, économie et société* 5 (1986): 515–28.

Boulle, Pierre H., 'In Defense of Slavery: Eighteenth-Century Opposition to Abolition and the Origins of a Racist Ideology in France', in Frederick Krantz (ed.), *History from Below: Studies in Popular Protests and Popular Ideology in Honor of George Rudé* (Montreal: Concordia University, 1986).

Bourdelais, Patrice and Jean-Yves Raulot, *Une peur bleue: histoire du choléra en France, 1832–1854* (Paris: Payot, 1987).

Brau, Paul, *Trois siècles de médecine coloniale française* (Paris: Vigot Frères, 1931).

Briggs, Asa, 'Cholera and Society in the Nineteenth-Century', *Past and Present*, no. 19 (1961): 76–96.

Brockliss, Laurence and Colin Jones, *The Medical World of Early Modern France* (Oxford: Clarendon Press, 1997).

Burkhardt, R. W., Jr., *The Spirit of System: Lamarck and Evolutionary Biology* (1977; Cambridge: Harvard University Press, 1995).

Butler, Judith, *Gender Trouble: Feminism and the Subversion of Identity* (London: Routledge, 1990).

Canguilhem, Georges, *La connaissance de la vie*, 2d edn (Paris: Vrin, 1969).

Carlisle, Robert B., *The Proffered Crown: Saint-Simonianism and the Doctrine of Hope* (Baltimore: Johns Hopkins University Press, 1987).

Cassedy, J. H., 'Meteorology and Medicine in Colonial America: Beginnings of the Experimental Approach', *Journal of the History of Medicine and Allied Sciences* 24 (1969): 193–204.

Castel, Robert, *L'ordre psychiatrique: l'âge d'or de l'aliénisme* (Paris: Minuit, 1976).

Chamberlain, J. Edward and Sander Gilman, *Degeneration: The Dark Side of Progress* (New York: Columbia University Press, 1985).

Charlton, D. G., *New Images of the Natural in France: A Study in European Cultural History* (Cambridge and New York: Cambridge University Press, 1984).

Chartier, Roger, *The Cultural Origins of the French Revolution*, trans. Lydia G. Cochrane (Durham, NC: Duke University Press, 1991).

Chevalier, Louis, *Classes laborieuses et classes dangereuses à Paris pendant la première moité du XIXe siècle* (1958; Paris: Hachette, 1984).

Chisick, Harvey, *The Limits of Reform in the Enlightenment: Attitudes Toward the Education of the Lower Classes in Eighteenth-Century France* (Princeton: Princeton University Press, 1981).

Churchill, Frederick B., 'From Heredity Theory to *Vererbung*: The Transmission Problem, 1850–1915', *Isis* 78 (1987): 337–64.

Clarke, Edwin and L. S. Jacyna, *Nineteenth-Century Origins of Neuroscientific Concepts* (Berkeley: University of California Press, 1987).

Cobban, Alfred, *A History of Modern France* (2 vols, Harmondsworth: Penguin, 1963–65).

Cohen, William B., *The French Encounter with Africans: White Response to Blacks, 1530–1880* (Bloomington: Indiana University Press, 1980).

——, 'Malaria and French Imperialism', *Journal of African History* 24 (1983): 23–36.

Cole, Joshua, *Power of Large Numbers: Population, Politics, and Gender in Nineteenth-Century France* (Ithaca: Cornell University Press, 2000).

Coleman, William, *Georges Cuvier, Zoologist: A Study in the History of Evolution Theory* (Cambridge: Harvard University Press, 1964).

——, 'Health and Hygiene in the *Encyclopédie*: A Medical Doctrine for the Bourgeoisie', *Journal of the History of Medicine and Allied Sciences* 29 (1974): 399–421.

——, *Death is a Social Disease: Public Health and Political Economy in Early Industrial France* (Madison: University of Wisconsin Press, 1982).

——, *Yellow Fever of the North: The Methods of Early Epidemiology* (Madison: University of Wisconsin Press, 1987).

Conrad, Peter and Joseph W. Schneider, *Deviance and Medicalization: From Badness to Sickness*, 2d edn (Philadelphia: Temple University Press, 1992).

Cooter, Roger, 'Anticontagionism and History's Medical Record', in P. Wright and A. Treacher (eds), *The Problem of Medicial Knowledge* (Edinburgh: Edinburgh University Press, 1983).

Corbin, Alain, *Le miasme et la jonquille: l'odorat et l'imaginaire social, XVIIIe–XIXe siècles* (Paris: Flammarion, 1986).

Crawford, Catherine, 'Legalizing Medicine: Early Modern Legal Systems and the Growth of Medico-Legal Knowledge', in Michael Clark and Catherine Crawford (eds), *Legal Medicine in History* (New York: Cambridge University Press, 1994).

Cross, Stephen J., 'John Hunter, the Animal Oeconomy, and Late Eighteenth-Century Physiological Discourse', *Studies in the History of Biology* 5 (1981): 1–110.

Curran, Andrew, 'Monsters and the Self in the *Rêve de d'Alembert*', *Eighteenth-Century Life* 21 (1997): 48–69.

Curtin, Philip, '"The White Man's Grave": Image and Reality, 1780–1850', *Journal of British Studies* 1 (1961): 94–110.

——, *The Image of Africa: British Ideas and Action, 1780–1850* (Madison: University of Wisconsin Press, 1964).

——, *Death by Migration: Europe's Encounter with the Tropical World in the Nineteenth Century* (New York: Cambridge University Press, 1989).

Daget, Serge, 'Les mots esclave, nègre, noir et les jugements de valeur sur la traité négrière dans la littérature abolitionniste française de 1770 à 1845', *La Revue française d'histoire d'outre mer* 221 (1973): 511–48.

Darmon, Pierre, *Le mythe de la procréation à l'âge baroque* (Paris: Seuil, 1981).

Darnton, Robert, *The Great Cat Massacre and Other Episodes in French Cultural History* (New York: Basic Books, 1984).

——, *The Forbidden Best-Sellers of Pre-Revolutionary France* (New York: Norton, 1996).

Davis, Natalie Zemon, 'Women on Top', in *Society and Culture in Early Modern France* (Stanford: Stanford University Press, 1975).

Debien, Gabriel, *Les esclaves aux Antilles françaises (XVIIe–XVIIIe siècles)* (Basse-Terren et Forte-de-France: Société d'histoire de la Martinique, 1974).

De Certeau, Michel, *Heterologies: Discourse on the Other*, trans. Brian Massumi (Minneapolis: University of Minnesota Press, 1985).

Delaporte, François, *Disease and Civilization: The Cholera in Paris, 1832*, trans. Arthur Goldhammer (Cambridge: MIT Press, 1986).

Delasselle, Claude, 'Les enfants abondonnés à Paris au XVIIIe siècle', *Annales: E.S.C.* 30 (1975): 187–218.

Desan, Suzanne, 'Reconstituting the Social After the Terror: Family, Property, and the Law in Popular Politics', *Past and Present*, no. 164 (August 1999): 81–121.

——, 'What's After Political Culture? Recent French Revolutionary Historiography', *French Historical Studies* 23 (2000): 163–96.

Donzelot, Jacques, *The Policing of Families*, trans. Robert Hurley (New York: Pantheon, 1979).

Douthwaite, Julia V., *The Wild Girl, Natural Man, and the Monster: Dangerous Experiments in the Age of Enlightenment* (Chicago: University of Chicago Press, 2002).

Dowbiggin, Ian, *Inheriting Madness: Professionalization and Psychiatric Knowledge in Nineteenth-Century France* (Berkeley: University of California Press, 1991).

Drescher, Seymour, 'The Ending of the Slave Trade and the Evolution of European Scientific Racism', *Social Science History* 14 (1990): 415–50.

Duchet, Michèle, *Anthropologie et histoire au siècle des Lumières: Buffon, Voltaire, Rousseau, Helvétius, Diderot*, 2d edn (Paris: Albin Michel, 1995).

Duesterberg, Thomas J., 'Criminology and the Social Order in Nineteenth-Century France' (PhD thesis, Indiana University, 1979).

Dziembowski, Edmond, *Un nouveau patriotisme français, 1750–1770: la France face à la puissance anglaise à l'époque de la guerre de Sept Ans* (Oxford: Voltaire, 1998).

Efron, John M., 'Images of the Jewish Body: Three Medical Views from the Jewish Enlightenment', *Bulletin of the History of Medicine* 69 (1995): 349–66.

Egret, Jean, *La pré-Révolution française, 1787–1788* (Paris: Presses universitaires de France, 1962).

Elias, Norbert, *The Civilizing Process: The History of Manners and State Formation and Civilization*, trans. Edmund Jephcott (Oxford: Blackwell, 1994).

Elwitt, Sanford, *The Third Republic Defended: Bourgeois Reform in France, 1880–1914* (Baton Rouge: Louisiana State University Press, 1986).

Emch-Dériaz, Antoinette, *Tissot: Physician of the Enlightenment* (New York: Peter Lang, 1992).

Epstein, Steven, *Impure Science: AIDS, Activism, and the Politics of Knowledge* (Berkeley: University of California Press, 1996).

Etlin, Richard A., *The Architecture of Death: The Transformation of the Cemetery in Eighteenth-Century Paris* (Cambridge: MIT Press, 1984).

——, *Symbolic Space: French Enlightenment Archictecture and Its Legacy* (Chicago: University of Chicago Press, 1994).

Evans, Richard J., 'Epidemics and Revolutions: Cholera in Nineteenth-Century Europe', in Terence Ranger and Paul Slack (eds), *Epidemics and Ideas: Essays on the Historical Perception of Pestilence* (New York: Cambridge University Press, 1992).

Fanon, Frantz, 'Medicine and Colonialism', in John Ehrenreich (ed.), *Cultural Crisis of Modern Medicine* (New York: Monthly Review Press, 1978).

Farge, Arlette, 'Les artisans malades de leur travail', *Annales: E.S.C.* 32 (1977): 993–1006.

Farley, John, *Gametes and Spores: Ideas About Sexual Reproduction, 1750–1914* (Baltimore: Johns Hopkins University Press, 1982).

Farmer, Paul, *Pathologies of Power: Health, Human Rights, and the New War on the Poor* (Berkeley: University of California Press, 2003).

Faure, Olivier, 'La médicalisation vue par les historiens', in Pierre Aïach and Daniel Delanoë (eds), *L'ère de la médicalisation: Ecce homo sanitas* (Paris: Anthropos, 1999).

Favre, Robert, *La mort dans la littérature et la pensée françaises au siècle des Lumières* (Lyon: Presses universitaires de Lyon, 1978).

Febvre, Lucien, '*Civilisation*: Evolution of a Word and a Group of Ideas', in Peter Burke (ed.), *A New Kind of History and Other Essays*, trans. K. Folca (New York: Harper & Row, 1973).

Figlio, Karl, 'Sinister Medicine? A Critique of Left Approaches to Medicine', *Radical Science Journal* 9 (1979): 14–68.

Fissell, Mary E., 'Making a Masterpiece: The Aristotle Texts in Vernacular Medical Culture', in Charles E. Rosenberg (ed.), *Right Living: An Anglo-American Tradition of Self-Help Medicine and Hygiene* (Baltimore: Johns Hopkins University Press, 2003).

Flynn, Carol Houlihan, 'Running Out of Matter: The Body Exercised in Eighteenth-Century Fiction', in G. S. Rousseau (ed.), *The Languages of Psyche: Mind and Body in Enlightenment Thought* (Berkeley: University of California Press, 1990).

Foisil, Madeleine, 'Les attitudes devant la mort au XVIIIe siècle: sépultures et suppressions de sépultures dans le cimetière parisien des Saints-Innocens', *Revue historique*, no. 510 (1974): 303–30.

Foucault, Michel, *Histoire de la folie à l'âge classique* (Paris: Gallimard, 1972).

——, *Discipline and Punish: The Birth of the Prison*, trans. Alan Sheridan (New York: Vintage, 1977).

——, *Power/Knowledge: Selected Interviews and Other Writings, 1972–1977*, ed. Colin Gordon, trans. Colin Gordon, Leo Marshall, John Mepham, and Kate Soper (New York: Pantheon, 1980).

——, *The History of Sexuality: An Introduction*, trans. Robert Hurley (New York: Vintage, 1990 [1978]).

——, *Naissance de la clinique*, 4th edn (Paris: Presses universitaires de France, 1994).

——, *Power*, ed. James D. Faubion, vol. 3, *The Essential Works of Foucault 1954–1984*, ed. Paul Rabinow (New York: New Press, 2000).

Fraisse, Geneviève, *Reason's Muse: Sexual Difference and the Birth of Democracy*, trans. Jane Marie Todd (Chicago: University of Chicago Press, 1994).

Friedlander, Ruth, 'Bénédict-Auguste Morel and the Development of the Theory of Dégénérescence (The Introduction of Anthropology into Psychiatry)' (PhD thesis, University of California at San Francisco, 1973).

Frye, Northrop, 'Towards Defining an Age of Sensibility', *English Literary History* 23 (1956): 144–52.

Fuchs, Rachel G., *Abandoned Children: Foundlings and Child Welfare in Nineteenth-Century France* (Albany: State University of New York Press, 1984).

——, *Poor and Pregnant in Paris: Strategies for Survival in the Nineteenth Century* (New Brunswick: Rutgers University Press, 1992).

——, 'France in Comparative Perspective', in Elinor Accampo, Rachel Fuchs and Mary Lynn Stewart (eds), *Gender and the Politics of Social Reform in France, 1870–1914* (Baltimore: Johns Hopkins University Press, 1995).

Furet, François, *Interpreting the French Revolution*, trans. Elborg Forster (New York: Cambridge University Press, 1981).

Furet, François and Mona Ozouf (eds), *A Critical Dictionary of the French Revolution*, trans. Arthur Goldhammer (Cambridge: Harvard University Press, 1989).

Galzinga, Mario, 'L'organismo vivente e il suo ambiente: nascita di un rapporto', *Rivista critica di storia della filosofia* 34 (1979): 134–61.

Garaud, Marcel and Romuald Szramkiewicz, *La Révolution française et la famille: histoire générale du droit privé française (de 1789 à 1804)*, ed. Jean Carbonnier (Paris: Presses universitaires de France, 1978).

Garraway, Doris Lorraine, *The Libertine Colony: Creolization in the Early French Caribbean* (Durham, NC: Duke University Press, 2005).

Gasking, Elizabeth B., *Investigations Into Generation, 1651–1828* (Baltimore: Johns Hopkins University Press, 1967).

Gautier, Arlette, *Les soeurs de solitude: la condition féminine dans l'esclavage aux Antilles du XVIIe au XIX siècles* (Paris: Éditions Caribéennes, 1985).

Geertz, Clifford, *The Interpretation of Cultures: Selected Essays* (New York: Basic Books, 1973).

Geggus, David P., *Slavery, War and Revolution: The British Occupation of Saint Domingue 1793–1798* (Oxford: Clarendon, 1982).

——, 'Racial Equality, Slavery and Colonial Secession during the Constituent Assembly', *American Historical Review* (1989): 1290–308.

Gelbart, Nina Rattner, 'The French Revolution as Medical Event: The Journalistic Gaze', *History of European Ideas* 10 (1989): 417–27.

——, *The King's Midwife: A History and Mystery of Madame du Coudray* (Berkeley: University of California Press, 1998).

Gelfand, Toby, *Professionalizing, Modern Medicine: Paris Surgeons and Medical Science and Institutions in the Eighteenth Century* (Westport: Greenwood, 1980).

——, 'The Decline of the Ordinary Practitioner and the Rise of a Modern Medical Profession', in Martin S. Staum and Donald E. Larson (eds), *Doctors, Patients, and Society: Power and Authority in Medical Care* (Waterloo, Ont.: Wilfrid Laurier University Press, 1981).

Gillispie, Charles C., 'Science in the French Revolution', *Behavioral Science* 4 (1959): 67–73.

——, 'The *Encyclopédie* and the Jacobin Philosophy of Science: A Study in Ideas and Consequences', in M. Clagett (ed.), *Critical Problems in the History of Science* (Madison: University of Wisconsin Press, 1969).

——, *Science and Polity in France at the End of the Old Regime* (Princeton: Princeton University Press, 1980)

——, *Science and Polity in France: The Revolutionary and Napoleonic Years* (Princeton: Princeton University Press, 2004).

Gilman, Sander and J. Edwards Chamberlin (eds), *Degeneration: The Dark Side of Progress* (New York: Columbia University Press, 1985).

Godechot, Jacques, *La vie quotidienne en France sous le Directoire* (Paris: Hachette, 1977).

Goldstein, Jan, *Console and Classify: The French Psychiatric Profession in the Nineteenth Century* (New York: Cambridge University Press, 1987).

—— (ed.), *Foucault and the Writing of History* (Oxford: Blackwell, 1994).

——, 'Enthusiasm or Imagination? Eighteenth-Century Smear Words in Comparative National Context', in Lawrence E. Klein and Anthony J. La Vopa (eds), *Enthusiasm and Enlightenment in Europe, 1650–1850* (San Marino: Huntington Library, 1998).

——, *The Post-Revolutionary Self: Politics and Psyche in France, 1750–1850* (Cambridge: Harvard University Press, 2005).

Goode, Erich and Nachman Ben-Yehuda, *Moral Panics: The Social Construction of Deviance* (Oxford: Blackwell, 1994).

Goodman, Dena, *The Republic of Letters: A Cultural History of the French Enlightenment* (Ithaca: Cornell University Press, 1994).

Gordon, Daniel, *Citizens Without Sovereignty: Equality and Sociability in French Thought, 1670–1789* (Princeton: Princeton University Press, 1994).

Goubert, Jean-Pierre, 'The Extent of Medical Practice in France Around 1780', *Journal of Social History* 10 (1976–77): 410–27.

—— (ed.), *La médicalisation de la société française, 1770–1830* (Waterloo: Wilfrid Laurier University Press, 1982).

Goubert, Jean-Pierre and Lepetit, Bernard, 'Les niveaux de médicalisation des villes françaises à la fin de l'Ancien Régime', in Jean-Pierre Goubert (ed.) *La médicalisation de la société française, 1770–1830* (Waterloo: Wilfrid Laurier University Press, 1982),

Goulemot, J.-M., 'Toward a Definition of Libertine Fiction and Pornographic Novels', trans. A. Greenspan, *Yale French Studies*, no. 94 (1998): 133–45.

Gramain-Kibleur, Pascale, 'Le monde du médicament à l'aube de l'ère industrielle: les enjeux de la prescription médicamenteuse de la fin du XVIIIe et au début du XIXe siècle' (thèse du doctorat, Université de Paris–VII, 1999).

Gusdorf, Georges, *La révolution galiléenne* (2 vols, Paris: Payot, 1969).

——, *L'avènement des sciences humaines au siècle des Lumières* (Paris, 1972).

——, *Dieu, la nature, l'homme à la siècle des Lumières* (Paris, 1972).

Gutierrez, Hector and Jacques Houdaille, 'La mortalité maternelle en France aux XVIIIe siècle', *Population* 38 (1983): 975–83.

Gutwirth, Madelyn, *The Twilight of the Goddesses: Women and Representation in the French Revolutionary Era* (New Brunswick: Rutgers University Press, 1992).

Hacking, Ian, *The Taming of Chance* (New York: Cambridge University Press, 1990).

Hahn, Roger, *The Anatomy of a Scientific Institution: The Paris Academy of Sciences* (Berkeley: University of California Press, 1971).

Haigh, Elizabeth L., *Xavier Bichat and the Medical Theory of the Eighteenth Century* (London: Wellcome Institute, 1984).

Haines, Barbara, 'The Inter-Relations Between Social, Biological and Medical Thought, 1750–1850: Saint-Simon and Comte', *British Journal for the History of Science* 11 (1978): 19–35.

Halpérin, Jean-Louis, *L'impossible code civil* (Paris: Presses universitaires de France, 1992).

——, *Histoire du droit privé français depuis 1804* (Paris: Presses universitaires de France, 1996).

Hamlin, Christopher, 'Predisposing Causes and Public Health in Early Nineteenth-Century Medical Thought', *Social History of Medicine* 5 (1992): 43–70

Hannaway, Caroline, 'Medicine, Public Welfare, and the State in Eighteenth-Century France: The Société Royale de Médecine of Paris (1776–1793)' (PhD thesis, Johns Hopkins University, 1974).

Hannaway, Caroline and Anne La Berge (eds), *Constructing Paris Medicine* (Amsterdam and Atlanta: Rodopi, 1998).

Hannaway, Owen and Caroline Hannaway, 'La fermature du cimetière des Innocents', *Dix-huitième siècle*, no. 9 (1977): 181–92.

Harrison, Mark, '"The Tender Frame of Man": Disease, Climate, and Racial Difference in India and the West Indies, 1760–1860', *Bulletin of the History of Medicine* 70 (1996): 68–93.

Headrick, Daniel R., *The Tools of Empire: Technology and European Imperialism in the Nineteenth Century* (New York: Oxford University Press, 1981).

Hertzberg, Arthur, *The French Enlightenment and the Jews* (New York: Columbia University Press, 1968).

Hesse, Carla, *The Other Enlightenment: How French Women Became Modern* (Princeton: Princeton University Press, 2001).

Higonnet, Anne, *Pictures of Innocence: The History and Crisis of Ideal Childhood* (London: Thames and Hudson, 1998).

Hoffmann, Paul, *La femme dans la pensée des Lumières*, 2d edn (Geneva: Slatkine, 1995).

Hofrichter, Richard, 'The Politics of Health Inequities: Contested Terrain', in Hofrichter (ed.), *Health and Social Justice: Politics, Ideology, and Inequity in the Distribution of Disease* (San Francisco: Jossey-Bass, 2003).

Hould, Claudette, *Images of the French Revolution* (Quebec: Musée du Québec, 1989).

Hufton, Olwen, *The Poor in Eighteenth-Century France, 1750–1789* (Oxford: Clarendon Press, 1974).

Hulme, Peter, *Colonial Encounters: Europe and the Native Caribbean* (New York and Cambridge: Cambridge University Press, 1987).

Hunt, Lynn A., *Politics, Culture, and Class in the French Revolution* (Berkeley: University of California Press, 1984).

—— (ed.), *Eroticism and the Body Politic* (Baltimore: Johns Hopkins University Press, 1991).

——, *The Family Romance of the French Revolution* (Berkeley: University of California Press, 1992).

—— (ed.), *The Invention of Pornography: Obscenity and the Origins of Modernity, 1500–1800* (New York: Zone, 1993).

——, 'Forgetting and Remembering: The French Revolution Then and Now', *American Historical Review* 100 (1995): 1119–35.

——, 'The Origins of Human Rights in France', *Proceedings of the Western Society for French History* 24 (1997): 9–24.

Illich, Ivan, *Medical Nemesis: The Expropriation of Health* (New York: Pantheon, 1982).

Jacob, James R. 'The Political Economy of Science in Seventeenth-Century England', in Margaret C. Jacob (ed.), *The Politics of Western Science, 1640–1990* (Atlantic Highlands: Humanities Press, 1994).

——, 'The Heavenly City of the Natural Philosophers: Boyle, Wilkins, and Locke as Social Engineers, *c.* 1649–89', unpublished ms, City University of New York.

Jacob, James R. and Margaret C. Jacob, 'The Anglican Origins of Modern Science: The Metaphysical Foundations of the Whig Constitution', *Isis* 70 (1980): 251–67.

Jacob, Margaret C., *Scientific Culture and the Making of the Industrial West* (New York and Oxford: Oxford University Press, 1997).

Johnson, Dorothy, *Jacques-Louis David: Art in Metamorphis* (Princeton: Princeton University Press, 1993).

Jones, Colin, '"New Medical History in France": The View from Britain', *French Historian* 2 (1987): 3–14.

——, *The Charitable Imperative: Hospitals and Nursing in Ancien Régime and Revolutionary France* (London: Routledge, 1990).

——, 'Bourgeois Revolution Revivified: 1789 and Social Change', in Colin Lucas (ed.), *Rewriting the French Revolution* (Oxford: Clarendon, 1991).

——, 'The Great Chain of Buying: Medical Advertisement, the Bourgeois Public Sphere, and the Origins of the French Revolution', *American Historical Review* 101 (1996): 13–40.

——, 'Plague and Its Metaphors in Early Modern France', *Representations*, no. 53 (1996): 97–127.

——, 'Pulling Teeth in Eighteenth-Century Paris', *Past & Present* 166 (2000): 100–45.

Jordanova, L. J., 'Earth Science and Environmental Medicine: The Synthesis of the Late Enlightenment', in L. J. Jordanova and Roy S. Porter (eds), *Images of the Earth: Essays in the History of the Environmental Sciences* (Chalfont St Giles: BSHS, 1979).

——, 'Guarding the Body Politic: Volney's Catechism of 1793', in Francis Barker (ed.), *1789: Reading, Writing, Revolution* (Colchester: University of Essex Press, 1982).

——, 'Naturalizing the Family: Literature and the Bio-Medical Sciences in the Late Eighteenth Century', in Jordanova (ed.), *Languages of Nature: Critical Essays on Science and Literature* (London: Transaction, 1986).

——, 'The Popularisation of Medicine: Tissot on Onanism', *Textual Practice* 1 (1987): 68–79.

——, 'Medical Mediations: Mind, Body and the Guillotine', *History Workshop*, no. 28 (1989), 39–52.

——, 'The Art and Science of Seeing: Physiognomy, 1780–1830', in W. F. Bynum and Roy Porter (eds), *Medicine and the Five Senses* (New York: Cambridge University Press, 1993).

——, 'Has the Social History of Medicine Come of Age?', *Historical Journal* 36 (1993): 437–49.

——, *Nature Displayed: Gender, Science, and Medicine, 1760–1820* (London: Longman, 1999).

Kaplan, Steven, 'Réflexions sur la police du monde du travail, 1700–1815', *Revue historique* 256 (1979): 17–78.

Kates, Gary, 'Jews Into Frenchmen: Nationality and Representation in Revolutionary France', in Ferenc Fehér (ed.), *The French Revolution and the Birth of Modernity* (Berkeley: University of California Press, 1990).

Kennedy, Dane, 'The Perils of the Midday Sun: Climatic Anxieties in the Colonial Tropics', in John M. MacKenzie (ed.), *Imperialism and the Natural World* (Manchester: Manchester University Press, 1990).

King, Lester S., 'Boissier de Sauvages and Eighteenth-Century Nosology', *Bulletin of the History of Medicine* 40 (1966): 43–51.

Kiple, Kenneth F. (ed.), *The Cambridge World History of Human Disease* (New York: Cambridge University Press, 1993).

Kiple, Kenneth F. and King, Virginia H., *Another Dimension to the Black Diaspora: Diet, Disease and Racism* (New York: Cambridge University Press, 1981).

Knibiehler, Yvonne, 'Les médecins et la "nature féminine" au temps du code civil', *Annales: E.S.C.* 31 (1976): 824–45.

Knibiehler, Yvonne and Catherine Fouquet, *La femme et les médecins: analyse historique* (Paris: Hachette, 1983).

Kudlick, Catherine, *Cholera in Post-Revolutionary Paris: A Cultural History* (Berkeley: University of California Press, 1996).

Kupperman, Karen O., 'Fear of Hot Climates in the Anglo-American Colonial Experience', *William and Mary Quarterly* 41 (1984): 213–40.

La Berge, Anne, *Mission and Method: The Early Nineteenth-Century French Public Health Movement* (New York: Cambridge University Press, 1992).

Lajer-Burcharth, Ewa. *Necklines: The Art of Jacques-Louis David After the Terror* (New Haven: Yale University Press, 1999).

Landes, Joan, *Women and the Public Sphere in the Age of the French Revolution* (Ithaca: Cornell University Press, 1988).

Langlois, C., 'Le renouveau religieux au lendemain de la Révolution', in Jacques Le Goff and René Rémond (eds), *Histoire de la France religieuse*, vol. 3, *Du roi Très Chrétien à la laïcité républicaine (XVIIIe–XIXe siècle)* (Paris: Seuil, 1991).

Laqueur, Thomas, 'Orgasm, Generation, and the Politics of Reproductive Biology', in Catherine Gallagher and Thomas Laqueur (eds), *The Making of the Modern Body* (Berkeley: University of California Press, 1987).

——, 'Amor Veneris, vel Dulcedo Appeletur', in M. Feher (ed.), *Fragments for a History of the Human Body* (New York: Zone, 1989).

——, *Making Sex: Body and Gender from the Greeks to Freud* (Cambridge: Harvard University Press, 1990).

——, *Solitary Sex: A Cultural History of Masturbation* (New York: Zone, 2003).

Latour, Bruno, *Science in Action: How to Follow Scientists and Engineers through Society* (Cambridge: Harvard University Press, 1987).

Lawrence, Christopher, 'The Nervous System and Society in the Scottish Enlightenment', in Barry Barnes and Steven Shapin (eds), *Natural Order: Historical Studies of Scientific Culture* (Beverly Hills: Sage, 1979).

Lebrun, François, *Se soigner autrefois: médecins, saints et sorciers aux XVIIe et XVIIIe siècles* (Paris: Temps actuels, 1983).

Lecuir, Jean, 'La médicalisation de la société française dans la deuxième moitié du XVIIIIe siècle en France: aux origines des premiers traités de médecine légale', *Annales de Bretagne* 86 (1979): 231–50.

Lécuyer, Bernard P., 'Démographie, statistique et hygiène publique sous la monarchie censitaire', *Annales de démographie historique* (1977): 215–45.

——, 'L'hygiène en France avant Pasteur', in Claire Bayet-Salomon (ed.), *Pasteur et la Révolution Pastorienne* (Paris: Payot, 1986).

Leith, James A., *Media and Revolution: Moulding a New Citizenry in France During the Terror* (Toronto: Canadian Broadcasting Corp., 1968).

Léonard, Jacques, *Les médecins de l'ouest au XIXe siècle* (3 vols, Lille: Atelier de reproduction des thèses de Lille-III, 1978).

Lesch, John E., *Science and Medicine in France: The Emergence of Experimental Physiology, 1790–1855* (Cambridge: Harvard University Press, 1984).

Livingstone, David N., 'Human Acclimatization: Perspectives on a Contested Field of Inquiry in Science, Medicine, and Geography', *History of Science* 25 (1987): 359–94.

Longmate, Norman, *King Cholera: The Biography of a Disease* (London: Hamilton, 1966).

López-Beltrán, Carlos, 'Forging Heredity: From Metaphor to Cause, a Reification Story', *Studies in the History and Philosophy of Science* 25 (1994): 211–35.

Loux, F. and Morel, M.-F., 'L'enfance et les savoirs sur les corps: pratiques médicales et pratiques populaires dans la France traditionelle', *Ethnologie française* 6 (1976): 309–24.

Lupton, Deborah, *The Imperative of Health: Public Health and the Regulated Body* (London: Sage, 1995).

Lynch, Katherine A., *Family, Class, and Ideology in Early Industrial France: Social Policy and the Working-Class Family, 1825–1848* (Madison: University of Wisconsin Press, 1988).

Manchuelle, François, 'The "Regeneration of Africa": An Important and Ambiguous Concept in Eighteenth and Nineteenth-Century French Thinking about Africa', *Cahiers d'Études africaines*, no. 144 (1996): 559–88.

Manuel, Frank E., 'From Equality to Organicism', *Journal of the History of Ideas* 17 (1956): 54–69.

——, *The New World of Henri Saint-Simon* (Cambridge: Harvard University Press, 1956).

——, *The Prophets of Paris* (Cambridge: Harvard University Press, 1962).

Marcovich, Anne, 'French Colonial Medicine and Colonial Rule: Algeria and Indochina', trans. A. J. Grieco and S. F. Matthews, in Roy MacLeod and Milton Lewis (eds), *Disease, Medicine, and Empire: Perspectives on Western Medicine and the Experience of European Expansion* (London: Routledge, 1988).

Marcuse, Herbert, *One-Dimensional Man: Studies in the Ideology of Advanced Industrial Society*, 2d edn (Boston: Beacon, 1991).

Marx, Karl, 'The Eighteenth Brumaire of Louis Bonaparte' [1852], in *The Marx–Engels Reader*, ed. Robert C. Tucker (New York: Norton, 1972).

Maza, Sarah, 'The Diamond Necklace Affair Revisited (1785–1786): The Case of the Missing Queen', in Lynn Hunt (ed.), *Eroticism and the Body Politic* (Baltimore: Johns Hopkins University Press, 1991).

——, 'Luxury, Morality, and Social Change: Why There Was no Middle-Class Consciousness in Prerevolutionary France', *Journal of Modern History* 69 (1997): 199–229.

McLaren, Angus, *Sexuality and the Social Order: The Debate over the Fertility of Women and Workers in France, 1770–1920* (New York: Holmes & Meier, 1983).

McClellan, James E., III, *Colonialism and Science: Saint Domingue in the Old Regime* (Baltimore: Johns Hopkins University Press, 1992).

McNeill, William H., *Plagues and Peoples* (New York: Anchor, 1976).

Merton, Robert K., 'Science and the Social Order', in *The Sociology of Science: Theoretical and Empirical Investigations* (Chicago: University of Chicago Press, 1973).

Meyer, Jean, 'L'enquête de l'Académie de Médecine sur les épidémies, 1774–1794', in *Médecins, climat et épidémies à la fin du XVIIIe siècle*, by Jean-Paul Desaive, et al. (Paris: Mouton, 1972).

Michelet, Jules, *Histoire de la Révolution française* (2 vols, Paris: Gallimard, 1961–62).

Miller, David Philip, 'Joseph Banks, Empire, and "Centers of Calculation" in Late Hanoverian London', in David Philip Miller and Peter Hanns Reill (eds), *Visions of Empire: Voyages, Botany, and Representations of Nature* (New York: Cambridge University Press, 1996).

Mintz, Sidney, *Sweetness and Power: The Place of Sugar in Modern History* (New York: Viking, 1985).

Mitchell, Harvey, 'Rationality and Control in French Eighteenth-Century Medical Views of the Peasantry'. *Comparative Studies in Society and History* 21 (1979): 81–112.

——, 'The Political Economy of Health in France, 1770–1830: The Debate Over Hospital and Home Care and Images of the Working-Class Family', in Martin S. Staum and Donald E. Larson (eds), *Doctors, Patients, and Society: Power and Authority in Medical Care* (Waterloo, Ont.: Wilfrid Laurier University Press, 1981).

——, 'Politics in the Service of Knowledge: The Debate Over the Administration of Medicine and Welfare in Late Eighteenth-Century France', *Social History* 6 (1981): 185–207.

Mitchell, Harvey and Samuel S. Kottek, 'An Eighteenth-Century Medical View of the Diseases of the Jews in Northeastern France: Medical Anthropology and the Politics of Jewish Emancipation', *Bulletin of the History of Medicine* 67 (1993): 248–81.

Moore, F. C. T., *The Psychology of Maine de Biran* (Oxford: Clarendon, 1970).

Moravia, Sergio, *Il tramonto dell'illuminismo: filosofia e politica nella società francese (1770–1810)* (Bari: Laterza, 1968).

——, 'Philosophie et médecine en France à la fin du XVIIIe siècle', *Studies on Voltaire and the Eighteenth Century* 89 (1972): 1089–151.

——, 'Dall' "homme machine" all' "homme sensible": meccanicismo, animismo e vitalismo nel secolo XVIII', *Balfagor* 29 (1974): 633–48.

——, *Il pensiero degli Idéologues: scienza e filosofia in Francia (1780–1815)* (Florence: La Nuova Italia, 1974).

——, *La scienza dell'uomo nel settecento* (Bari: Laterza, 1978).

Morel, M.-F., 'Ville et compagne dans le discours médicale sur la petite enfance au XVIIIe siècle', *Annales: E.S.C.* 32 (1977): 1007–24.

Mukerji, Chandra, *Territorial Ambitions and the Gardens of Versailles* (New York: Cambridge University Press, 1997).

Mullan, John, *Sentiment and Sociability: The Language of Feeling in the Eighteenth Century* (Oxford: Clarendon, 1990).

Murphy, Terence D., 'Medical Knowledge and Statistical Methods in Early Nineteenth-Century France', *Medical History* 25 (1981): 301–19.

Niebyl, Peter, 'The Non-Naturals', *Bulletin of the History of Medicine* 45 (1971): 486–92.

Nye, Robert A., *Crime, Madness, and Politics in Modern France: The Medical Concept of National Decline* (Princeton: Princeton University Press, 1984).

——, *Masculinity and Male Codes of Honor in Modern France* (Oxford and New York: Oxford University Press, 1993).

——, 'Biology, Sexuality, and Morality in Eighteenth-Century France', *Eighteeth-Century Studies* 35 (2002): 235–38.

Offen, Karen, 'Depopulation, Nationalism, and Feminism in Fin-de-Siècle France', *American Historical Review* 89 (1984): 452–84.

O'Neal, John C., *The Authority of Experience: Sensationist Theory in the French Enlightenment* (University Park: Pennsylvania State University Press, 1996).

Outram, Dorinda, *Georges Cuvier: Vocation, Science, and Authority in Post-Revolutionary France* (Manchester: Manchester University Press, 1984).

——, *The Body and the French Revolution: Sex, Class, and Political Culture* (New Haven: Yale University Press, 1989).

Ozouf, Mona, 'Symboles et fonctions des âges dans les fêtes de l'époque révolutionnaire', *Annales historiques de la Révolution française* 202 (1970): 569–93.

——, 'La Révolution française et l'idée de l'homme nouveau', in Colin Lucas (ed.), *The Political Culture of the French Revolution*, vol. 2, *The French Revolution and the Creation of Modern Political Culture*, ed. Keith Michael Baker (Oxford: Pergamon, 1988).

Passmore, John, *The Perfectibility of Man* (New York: Scribner, 1970).

Paul, James E., 'Medicine and Imperialism', in John Ehrenreich (ed.), *The Cultural Crisis of Modern Medicine* (New York: Monthly Review Press, 1978).

Payne, Harry G., *The Philosophes and the People* (New Haven: Yale University Press, 1976).

Pearl, J. L., 'The Role of Personal Correspondence in the Exchange of Scientific Information in Early Modern France', *Renaissance and Reformation* 8 (1984): 106–13.

Pelling, Margaret, *Cholera, Fever and English Medicine, 1825–1865* (New York: Oxford University Press, 1978).

Peronnet, Michel, 'L'invention de l'Ancien Régime en France', *History of European Ideas* 14 (1992): 49–58.

Peter, Jean-Pierre, 'Médecine, épidémies et société en France à la fin du XVIIIe siècle d'après les archives de l'Académie de médecine', *Bulletin de la Société d'histoire moderne*, 14th series, no. 14 (1970): 2–9.

——, 'Le corps du délit', *Nouvelle revue de psychoanalyse*, no. 3 (1971): 71–108.

——, 'Les mots et les objets de la maladie: remarques sur les épidémies et la médecine dans la société française de la fin du XVIIIe siècle', *Revue historique*, no. 246 (July–September 1971): 13–38.

Peterson, Alan and Deborah Lupton, *The New Public Health: Health and Self in the Age of Risk* (London: Sage, 1996).

Pick, Daniel, *Faces of Degeneration: A European Disorder, c. 1848–c. 1918* (New York: Cambridge University Press, 1989).

Pickstone, John V., 'Bureaucracy, Liberalism and the Body in Post-Revolutionary France: Bichat's Physiology and the Paris School of Medicine', *History of Science* 19 (1981): 115–42.

——, 'Dearth, Dirt, and Fever Epidemics: Rewriting the History of British "Public Health", 1780–1850', in Terence Ranger and Paul Slack (eds), *Epidemics and Ideas: Essays on the Historical Perception of Pestilence* (New York: Cambridge University Press, 1992).

Pluchon, Pierre (ed.), *Histoire des médecins et pharmaciens de marine et des colonies* (Toulouse: Privat, 1985).

——, *Vaudou, sorciers, empoisonneurs de Saint-Domingue à Haiti* (Paris: Karthala, 1987).

Pollitzer, R., *Cholera* (Geneva: World Health Organization, 1959).

Popkin, Richard H., 'The Philosophical Basis of Eighteenth-Century Racism', in Harold E. Pagliaro (ed.), *Racism in the Eighteenth Century*, vol. 3, *Studies in Eighteenth-Century Culture* (Cleveland: Press of Case Western Reserve University, 1973).

——, 'Medicine, Racism, Anti-Semitism: A Dimension of Enlightenment Culture', in G. S. Rousseau (ed.), *The Languages of Psyche: Mind and Body in Enlightenment Thought* (Berkeley: University of California Press, 1990).

'Population and the State in the Third Republic' (forum), *French Historical Studies* 19 (1996): 633–754.

Porter, Dorothy, *Health, Civilization, and the State: A History of Public Health from Ancient to Modern Times* (London: Routledge, 1999).

Porter, Roy, '"The Secrets of Generation Display'd": Aristotle's Master-Piece in Eighteenth-Century England', in Robert Purks MacCubin (ed.), *'Tis Nature's Fault: Unauthorized Sexuality During the Enlightenment* (New York: Cambridge University Press, 1987).

Porter, Roy and Andrew Wear (eds), *Problems and Methods in the History of Medicine* (London: Croom, 1987).

Porter, Theodore M., *The Rise of Statistical Thinking, 1820–1900* (Princeton: Princeton University Press, 1988).

Potts, Alex, 'Beautiful Bodies and Dying Heroes: Images of Ideal Manhood in the French Revolution', *History Workshop*, no. 30 (Autumn, 1990): 1–20.

Pratt, Mary Louise, *Imperial Eyes: Travel Writing and Transculturation* (London: Routledge, 1992).

Puckrein, Gary, 'Climate, Health and Black Labor in the English Americas', *Journal of American Studies* 13 (1979): 179–93.

Py, Gilbert, *Rousseau et les éducateurs: Étude sur la fortune des idées pédagogiques de Jean-Jacques Rousseau en France et en Europe au XVIIIe siècle* (Oxford: Voltaire, 1997).

Quinlan, Sean M., 'Apparent Death in Eighteenth-Century France and England', *French History* 9 (1995): 27–47.

——, 'Sensibility and Human Science in the Enlightenment', *Eighteenth-Century Studies* 37 (2003–04): 296–301.

——, 'Inheriting Vice, Acquiring Virtue: Hereditary Disease and Moral Hygiene in Eighteenth-Century France', *Bulletin of the History of Medicine* 80 (2006): 649–76.

Rabinow, Paul, *French Modern: Norms and Forms of the Social Environment* (Cambridge: MIT Press, 1989).

Raeff, Marc, *The Well-Ordered Police State: Social and Institutional Change Through Law in the Germanies and Russia* (New Haven: Yale University Press, 1983).

Ramsey, Matthew, *Professional and Popular Medicine in France: The Social World of Medical Practice* (New York: Cambridge University Press, 1987).

——, 'Public Health in France', in Dorothy Porter (ed.), *The History of Public Health and the Modern State* (Amsterdam: Rodopi, 1994).

Reddy, William M., *The Rise of Market Culture: The Textile Trade and French Society, 1750–1900* (New York: Cambridge University Press, 1984).

——, 'Sentimentalism and Its Erasure: The Role of the Emotions in the Era of the French Revolution', *Journal of Modern History* 72 (2000): 109–52.

Rey, Roselyn, *Naissance et développement du vitalisme en France de la deuxième moitié du 18e siècle à la fin du Premier Empire* (Oxford: Voltaire, 2000).

Riley, James C., *Population Thought in the Age of Demographic Revolution* (Durham, NC: Carolina Academic Press, 1985).

——, *The Eighteenth-Century Campaign to Avoid Disease* (London: Macmillan, 1987).

Roberts, Warren, *Morality and Social Class in Eighteenth-Century French Literature and Painting* (Toronto: University of Toronto Press, 1974).

Roche, Daniel, *Les républicains des lettres: gens de culture et Lumières au XVIIIe siècle* (Paris: Fayard, 1988).

Roger, Jacques, *Les sciences de la vie dans la pensée française au XVIIIe siècle: la génération des animaux de Descartes à l'Encyclopédie*, 3d edn (Paris: Albin Michel, 1993).

Rosen, George, 'Cameralism and the Concept of Medical Police', *Bulletin of the History of Medicine* 27 (1953): 21–42.

——, *A History of Public Health* (New York: MD Publications, 1958).

——, 'Mercantilism and Health Policy in Eighteenth-Century French Thought', *Medical History* 3 (1959): 259–77.

Rosenberg, Charles E., *The Cholera Years: The United States in 1832, 1849, and 1866* (Chicago: University of Chicago Press, 1962).

Rosenblum, Robert, *Transformations in Late Eighteenth-Century Art* (Princeton: Princeton University Press, 1967).

Rosenwein, Barbara H., 'Worrying about Emotions in History', *American Historical Review* 107 (2002): 821–45.

Rousseau, G. S., 'Nerves, Spirits, and Fibres: Towards Defining the Origins of Sensibility', in R. F. Brissendon and J. C. Eade (eds), *Studies in the Eighteenth Century*, vol. 3 (Canberra: Australian National University Press, 1976).

Rupke, Nicolaas A. (ed.), *Medical Geography in Historical Perspective* (London: Wellcome, 2000).

Rustin, Jacques, *La vice à la mode: étude sur le roman français du XVIIIe siècle de Manon Lescaut à l'apparition de la Nouvelle Héloïse (1731–1761)* (Paris: Éditions Ophrys, 1979).

Saddy, Pierre, 'Le cycle des immondices', *Dix-huitième siècle*, no. 9 (1977): 203–14.

Said, Edward, *Culture and Imperialism* (New York: Vintage, 1993).

Salerno, Luigi, 'La pittura di paesaggio', *Storia dell'arte* 24/25 (1975): 111–24.

Schaffer, Simon, 'Regeneration: The Body of Natural Philosophers in Restoration England', in Christopher Lawrence and Steven Shapin (eds), *Science Incarnate: Historical Embodiments of Natural Knowledge* (Chicago: University of Chicago Press, 1998).

Schama, Simon, *Citizens: A Chronicle of the French Revolution* (New York: Vintage, 1989).

Schiebinger, Londa, 'Skeletons in the Closet: The First Illustrations of the Female Skeleton in Eighteenth-Century Anatomy', in Catherine Gallagher and Thomas Laqueur (eds), *The Making of the Modern Body: Sexuality and Society in the Nineteenth Century* (Berkeley: University of California Press, 1987).

——, *The Mind Has no Sex? Women in the Origins of Modern Science* (Cambridge: Harvard University Press, 1989).

——, *Nature's Body: Gender in the Making of Modern Science* (Boston: Beacon, 1993).

Schiller, Francis, *Paul Broca: Founder of French Anthropology, Explorer of the Brain* (Berkeley: University of California Press, 1979).

Schwartz, Robert, *Policing the Poor in Eighteenth-Century France* (Chapel Hill: University of North Carolina Press, 1988).

Scott, Joan W. *Gender and the Politics of History* (New York: Columbia University Press, 1988).

Searle, J. R., *Eugenics and Politics in Britain, 1900–1914* (Leyden: Noordhoof, 1976).

Secord, Anne, 'Corresponding Interests: Artisans and Gentlemen in Nineteenth-Century Natural History', *British Journal for the History of Science* 27 (1994): 383–408.

Seeber, Edward D., *Anti-Slavery Opinion in France during the Second Half of the Eighteenth Century* (1937; New York: Greenwood Press, 1969).

Senior, Nancy, 'Aspects of Infant Feeding in Eighteenth-Century France', *Eighteenth-Century Studies* 16 (1983): 367–88.

Sewell, William H., Jr., *Work and Revolution in France: The Language of Labor from the Old Regime to 1848* (New York: Cambridge University Press, 1980).

——, '*Le citoyen/la citoyenne*: Activity, Passivity, and the Revolutionary Concept of Citizenship', in Colin Lucas (ed.), *The French Revolution and the Creation of Modern Political Culture*, vol. 2, *The Political Culture of the French Revolution* (Oxford: Pergamon, 1988).

Shapin, Steven, 'Social Uses of Science, 1660–1800', in Roy S. Porter and G. S. Rousseau (eds), *The Ferment of Knowledge* (New York: Cambridge University Press, 1980).

Shilling, Chris, *The Body and Social Theory* (London, 1993).

Shinn, Terry, 'Science, Tocqueville, and the State: The Organization of Knowledge in Modern France', in Margaret C. Jacob (ed.), *The Politics of Western Science, 1640–1990* (Atlantic Highlands: Humanities Press, 1994).

Sigerist, Henry, *Medicine and Human Welfare* (New Haven: Yale University Press, 1941).

Sonenscher, Michael, *Work and Wages: Natural Law, Politics, and the Eighteenth-Century French Trades* (New York: Cambridge University Press, 1989).

Sontag, Susan, *Illness as a Metaphor* (Harmondsworth: Penguin, 1983).

Spary, Emma C., *Utopia's Garden: French Natural History from Old Regime to Revolution* (Chicago: University of Chicago Press, 2000).

Spengler, Joseph J., *French Predecessors to Malthus: A Study in Eighteenth-Century Wage and Population Theory* (Durham, NC: Duke University Press 1942).

——, *France Faces Depopulation* (Durham, NC: Duke University Press, 1979).

Stafford, Barbara Maria, *Voyage Into Substance: Art, Science, Nature, and the Illustrated Travel Account, 1760–1840* (Cambridge: MIT Press, 1984).

Starr, Paul, *The Social Transformation of American Medicine: The Rise of Sovereign Profession and the Making of a Vast Industry* (New York: Basic, 1984).

Staum, Martin S., *Cabanis: Enlightenment and Medical Philosophy in the French Revolution* (Princeton: Princeton University Press, 1980).

——, *Minerva's Message: Stabilizing the French Revolution* (Montreal: McGill-Queen's University Press, 1996).

Stengers, Jean and Anne Van Neck, *Histoire d'une grande peur: la masturbation* (Brussels: Éditions de l'université de Bruxelles, 1984).

Stepan, Nancy, *The Idea of Race in Science: Great Britain 1800–1960* (London: Macmillan, 1982).

Stolberg, Michael, 'An Unmanly Vice: Self-Pollution, Anxiety, and the Body in the Eighteenth Century', *Social History of Medicine* 13 (2000): 1–22.

Stone, Judith, *The Search for Social Peace: Reform Legislation in France, 1890–1914* (Albany: State University of New York Press, 1985).

Sussman, George, 'From Yellow Fever to Cholera: A Study of French Government Policy, Medical Professionalism, and Popular Movements in the Epidemic Crises of the Restoration and the July Monarchy' (PhD thesis, Yale University, 1971).

——, *Selling Mother's Milk: The Wet-Nursing Business in France, 1715–1914* (Urbana: University of Illinois Press, 1982).

Sutton, Geoffrey, 'The Physical and Chemical Path to Vitalism: Xavier Bichat's *Physiological Researches on Life and Death*', *Bulletin of the History of Medicine* 58 (1984): 53–71.

Temkin, Oswei. *Galenism: Rise and Decline of a Medical Philosophy* (Ithaca: Cornell University Press, 1973).

Terrall, Mary, *The Man Who Flattened the Earth: Maupertuis and the Sciences in the Enlightenment* (Chicago: University of Chicago Press, 2002).

Thésée, F., 'Autour de la Société des Amis des Noirs', *Présence africaine* 125 (1983): 3–82.

Theweleit, Klaus, *Male Fantasies*, trans. Eric Carter, Stephen Conway, and Chris Turner (2 vols, Minneapolis: University of Minnesota Press, 1987–89).

Thompson, Kenneth, *Moral Panics* (London: Routledge, 1998).

Thomson, Ann, *Materialism and Society in the Mid-Eighteenth Century: La Mettrie's Discours préliminaire* (Geneva: Droz, 1981).

——, *Barbary and Enlightenment: European Attitudes towards the Maghreb in the Eighteenth Century* (New York: E. J. Brill, 1987).

Todd, Janet, *Sensibility: An Introduction* (London: Methuen, 1986).

Tognotti, Eugenia, *Il mostro asiatico: storia del colera in Italia* (Rome: Laterza, 2000).

Tomaselli, Sylvana, 'The Enlightenment Debate on Women', *History Workshop*, no. 20 (1985): 101–24.

Tomes, Nancy, 'The Making of a Germ Panic, Then and Now', *American Journal of Public Health* 90 (2000): 191–98.

Traer, James, *Marriage and the Family in Eighteenth-Century France* (Ithaca: Cornell University Press, 1980).

Tribe, Keith, *Governing Economy: The Reformation of German Economic Discourse, 1750–1840* (New York: Cambridge University Press, 1988).

Turner, James G., 'The Properties of Libertinism', in Robert Purks MacCubin (ed.), *'Tis Nature's Fault: Unauthorized Sexuality During the Enlightenment* (New York: Cambridge University Press, 1987).

Vartanian, Aram, 'Trembley's Polyp, La Mettrie, and Eighteenth-Century French Materialism', *Journal of the History of Ideas* 11 (1950): 259–86.

Vaughan, Megan, *Creating the Creole Island: Slavery in Eighteenth-Century Mauritius* (Durham, NC: Duke University Press, 2005).

Vedrenne-Villeneuve, Edmonde, 'L'inégalité sociale devant la mort dans la première moitié du XIXe siècle', *Population* 16 (1961): 665–99.

Veith, Ilza, *Hysteria: The History of a Disease* (Chicago: University of Chicago Press, 1965).

Vess, David M., *Medical Revolution in France, 1789–1796* (Gainesville: University Presses of Florida, 1975).

Vigarello, Georges, *Le propre et le sale: l'hygiène du corps depuis le moyen âge.* (Paris: Seuil, 1985).

——, *Le sain et le malsain: santé et mieux-être depuis le Moyen Âge* (Paris: Seuil, 1993).

Vila, Anne C., 'Sex and Sensibility: Pierre Roussel's *Système physique et morale de la femme*', *Representations*, no. 52 (1995): 76–93.

——, *Enlightenment and Pathology: Sensibility in the Literature and Medicine of Eighteenth-Century France* (Baltimore: Johns Hopkins University Press, 1998).

Wahrman, Dror, '*Percy*'s Prologue: From Gender Play to Gender Panic in Eighteenth-Century England', *Past and Present*, no. 159 (1998): 113–60.

Watts, Sheldon, *Epidemics and History: Disease, Power and Imperialism* (New Haven: Yale University Press, 1997).

Weiner, Dora B., *The Citizen-Patient in Revolutionary and Imperial Paris* (Baltimore: Johns Hopkins University Press, 1993).

Weisz, George, *The Medical Mandarins: The French Academy of Medicine in the Nineteenth and Early Twentieth Centuries* (New York: Oxford University Press, 1995).

Wellman, Kathleen, *La Mettrie: Medicine, Philosophy, and Enlightenment* (Durham, NC: Duke University Press, 1992).

——, 'Physicians and Philosophes: Physiology and Sexual Morality in the French Enlightenment', *Eighteenth-Century Studies* 35 (2002): 267–77.

Williams, Elizabeth A., *The Physical and the Moral: Anthroplogy, Physiology, and Philosophical Medicine in France, 1750–1850* (New York: Cambridge University Press, 1994).

——, *A Cultural History of Medical Vitalism in Enlightenment Montpellier* (Aldershot: Ashgate, 2003).

Wilson, Lindsay, *Women and Medicine in the French Enlightenment: The Debate Over 'Maladies Des Femmes'* (Baltimore: Johns Hopkins University Press, 1993).

Wokler, Robert, 'Rousseau's Perfectibilian Liberalism', in Alan Ryan (ed.), *The Idea of Freedom* (New York: Oxford University Press, 1979).

Worboys, Michael, 'The Emergence of Tropical Medicine: A Study in the Establishment of a Scientific Speciality', in Gerard Lemaine, Roy MacLeod, Michael Mulkay, and Peter Weingart (eds), *Perspectives on the Emergence of Scientific Disciplines* (The Hague: Mouton, 1976).

Young, Robert, *Mind, Brain, and Adaptation in the Nineteenth Century* (Oxford: Clarendon, 1970).

Index